T0094214

VARIATIONS IN SEX DEVELOPMENT

LIH-MEI LIAO is a licensed psychologist, independent scholar and trainer/supervisor for health professionals in the UK.

A compassionate, insightful, and necessary book from a foremost psychologist on intersex. A long-time advocate for improving care, Dr. Liao expertly guides readers through one of the most contested areas of medicine. With lucidity, urgency, and a unique blend of science and storytelling, *Variations in Sex Development* nimbly navigates complex debates that deepen our appreciation of what constitutes good care.

> – Katrina Karkazis, Professor of Sexuality, Women's, and Gender Studies, and author, Fixing Sex: Intersex, Medical Authority and Lived Experience.

This book will revolutionise psychological practice in the field. No other psychologist in the history of Intersex/differences in sex development (DSD) has forged and maintained such fruitful working relationships across the terrain of international professional and peer experts. EVERY psychologist in this field of practice should own this book and use it as a primer, guide and backbone for their clinical practice and professional development.

> – Julie Alderson, Consultant Clinical Psychologist, and Chair, Paediatric Psychology Network DSD Special Interest Group, UK.

"Dr. Liao's extensive experience in working with, alongside, and on behalf of people with variations in sex development makes her especially equipped to write this text. The inclusion of practice vignettes will enhance readers' skills in taking an intersectional, anti-oppressive approach to therapeutic work. This book promises to be the first to explain to mental health providers how to compassionately and ethically work with intersex people and their loved ones."

> – Lourdes Dolores Follins, psychotherapist, author, and co-editor, Black LGBT Health in The United States: The Intersection of Race, Gender, and Sexual Orientation.

This subject matter of this book should always make us think with an open mind. I thoroughly enjoyed reading this wonderful and thought-provoking book. You may agree or disagree with the author at times, but you will benefit from engaging with the challenges that the book poses.

> – Dan Wood, Professor of Urology, and senior editor, Journal of Pediatric Urology.

Dr Liao has distilled decades of knowledge and experience in a MUST READ for every care provider in differences in sex development (DSD). Away from dogmatic interpretations, the book portraits the evolution of DSD management and spells out what open-minded and holistic care may actually look like, so that it can be a compass for the future.

> – Lina Michala, Assistant Professor in Paediatric and Adolescent Gynaecology, University of Athens.

An insightful, compassionate and nuanced analysis of care needs, controversies and advocacy, with a long awaited focus on psychosocial concerns of individuals and families. A distillation of decades of expertise, this book is indispensable reading for peer workers and health, social care and education professionals.

> – Morgan Carpenter, Executive Director of Intersex Human Rights Australia.

VARIATIONS IN SEX DEVELOPMENT

Medicine, Culture and Psychological Practice

LIH-MEI LIAO

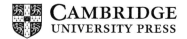

CAMBRIDGE
UNIVERSITY PRESS

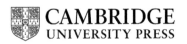

CAMBRIDGE
UNIVERSITY PRESS

Shaftesbury Road, Cambridge CB2 8EA, United Kingdom

One Liberty Plaza, 20th Floor, New York, NY 10006, USA

477 Williamstown Road, Port Melbourne, VIC 3207, Australia

314–321, 3rd Floor, Plot 3, Splendor Forum, Jasola District Centre, New Delhi – 110025, India

103 Penang Road, #05–06/07, Visioncrest Commercial, Singapore 238467

Cambridge University Press is part of Cambridge University Press & Assessment, a department of the University of Cambridge.

We share the University's mission to contribute to society through the pursuit of education, learning and research at the highest international levels of excellence.

www.cambridge.org
Information on this title: www.cambridge.org/9781316518373

DOI: 10.1017/9781009000345

First published 2023

Printed in the United Kingdom by TJ Books Limited, Padstow Cornwall

A catalogue record for this publication is available from the British Library.

Library of Congress Cataloging-in-Publication Data
NAMES: Liao, Lih-Mei, author.
TITLE: Variations in sex development : medicine, culture and
psychological practice / Lih-Mei Liao.
DESCRIPTION: Cambridge, United Kingdom ; New York, NY :
Cambridge University Press, 2022. | Includes bibliographical references and index.
IDENTIFIERS: LCCN 2022016865 (print) | LCCN 2022016866 (ebook) |
ISBN 9781316518373 (hardback) | ISBN 9781009000345 (epub)
SUBJECTS: LCSH: Intersexuality. | Intersex people–Medical care. |
Intersex people–Mental health services. | Intersex people–Identity.
CLASSIFICATION: LCC RC883 .L53 2022 (print) | LCC RC883 (ebook) |
DDC 616.6/94–dc23/eng/20220613
LC record available at https://lccn.loc.gov/2022016865
LC ebook record available at https://lccn.loc.gov/2022016866

ISBN 978-1-316-51837-3 Hardback

. . . .

For SheHan, memories of SangMin, Antonia, Jordana

Contents

Colour Plates section to be found between pp. 92 and 93

Preface

This book is about psychological practice for people and families impacted by a wide range of developmental presentations whereby the sex chromosomes, reproductive anatomy and urogenital characteristics – in combination – do not map clearly onto the social categories of female or male. The book goes some way to explain why this is a contested healthcare field and to visualize ethical psychological practices.

Irreconcilable Differences in Language

In the past, medical doctors and scientists referred to atypical biological sex as *intersex*. Today, the presentations are grouped under the collective term *differences in sex development* (DSD). Meanwhile, the term *variations in sex characteristics* (VSC) has been introduced as a less stigmatizing term than intersex and DSD. The irreconcilable debate on terminology is understandable. It is a contest about who gets to name whom. Therefore, it is unlikely that any one term will receive broad acceptance by those whom it describes.

Under the collective term(s) are highly variable bodily presentations. In medicine, diagnostic workup is triggered either by visible genital variations in an infant or by atypical or absent pubertal development in an adolescent. People who are born with the said physical variations are as different from one another as people without variations in terms of identity, sexuality and all human attributes. While many people with lived experience have reclaimed intersex as a personal/political identity, many more consider themselves as gender-normative with a bodily variation that does not define them.

The evolving terms and changing criteria make it important to emphasize that this book is about psychological practice in the field of intersex/ DSD/VSC, by which I mean nonsexually dimorphic combinations of genetic, reproductive and urogenital characteristics, as described in Chapter 2. As this is a healthcare book, it has to be in dialogue with the clinical literature. This means engaging with medical terminology when referencing medical publications. For example, I refer to *intersex medicine* when discussing past medical practices and to *DSD services* when discussing current medical practices. Otherwise, I use vocabularies such as variations in sex development, genital variations or just variations – descriptively. Furthermore, in this book, psychological service users are not just "patients" with variations but also caretakers, families and partners who are impacted by sex variations.

Why This Book?

This book is an attempt to bring social science research and critical analyses into interpersonal work with service users. Like many psychological care providers (PCPs), I inhabit both coalface and ivory tower with limited resource to digest the voluminous publications on the topic across disciplinary corridors. This book condenses several literatures to provide a background to enhance PCPs' understanding of the current debates, as a preparation for rigorous and ethical interpersonal work with service users.

Many physicians and nurses tell me that they wish to be more psychologically informed in order to engage more confidently with service users about uncertainty, stigma, loss, identity, marginalization, relationships and sex. Furthermore, medical providers who work in other regions of the world tell me that, without access to formally trained PCPs, they often double up as counselors for patients and families. Despite its Western focus, I hope that some of the content of this book is useful to them.

This book discusses healthcare for intersex/DSD/VSC as a lifelong concern. Lifelong care requires contributions from communities where people work, play, learn, worship, socialize, fall in love, grow up and grow old. Community-based providers such as family doctors, nursery nurses, teachers, sex educators and spiritual care providers have much to offer individuals and families. The problem is that people impacted by variations are often misunderstood outside specialist services. This book is a resource to orientate the nonspecialist to the field so that their capacity for care contributions can be realized.

Finally, the book is also for researchers new to sex development or new to critical psychology. My critical interpretation of psychosocial research in the field reflects my personal journey that criss-crossed paradigms. By paradigm I mean a philosophical framework that guides me to examine my values, assumptions, methods and interpretations. Experimental psychology was my strong point at the beginning of that journey, and I am grateful for the immersion. It has helped me to answer some questions but also opened my eyes to the arbitrariness of probabilistic computations. The formulaic nature of positivist research is reassuring but, in the interpersonal space that I occupy as a therapist, the way that feelings and intentions unfold is much more aptly captured by qualitative research. The privileging of intersubjective influences of language, values and power relationships in discursive research, which positions all researchers as already politically engaged, speaks most directly to my clinical practice, where talk is by nature dynamic and elusive yet context-bound. I hope that this book will stimulate debate about the future of psychosocial research, which can materially affect lives and carries social responsibilities.

How is the Book Structured?

Biogenetics is the dominant discourse of variations in sex characteristics. In a book that uniquely privileges psychosocial practice, it feels more appropriate to begin with stories of people, places, relationships, feelings and choices rather than body compounds like genes and enzymes. Therefore, in Chapter 1, I literally tell a story. Entitled "Circles and Squares," the story enables me to introduce salient psychological themes, which are addressed in different parts of the book. Thereafter, the book is split into three sections.

Psychological practice broadly involves the steps of familiarizing oneself with the service context, identifying the problem to be addressed, using explicit frameworks to contextualize the problems and working with clients towards agreed goals. The structure of this book approximates these steps. The introductory notes at the beginning of each section are there to orientate readers to the focus of the section.

The section "Medicalization and Resistance" is a portrayal of an evolving service context. It addresses medical understandings past and present and gives context to the call to demedicalize intersex. Demedicalization does not mean denying the materiality of genes, hormones and anatomy or negating the benefits of new technology. Rather, it halts the framing of psychosocial concerns as medical problems and argues for a social model of understanding lived experience and interpreting care needs.

The section "Psychological Theories and Applications" is, as the title suggests, a conversation about knowledge frameworks in healthcare psychology and their strengths and weaknesses in informing remedial interpersonal work. This section lays the ground for working with the clinical themes in subsequent chapters.

The final section, "Working Psychologically," is the practice area of the book. It comprises Chapters 9–14, which address six overlapping themes. In a researcher-practitioner spirit, each chapter begins with a narrative summary of relevant research and ends with a practice vignette. The vignettes are not recipes to follow. Quite the opposite; they are constructed to show that interpersonal work is by nature contingent and open to challenge. I hope that in future, more PCPs render their interpersonal work transparent in the interests of peer learning and practice improvement.

Whom to Thank?

Sarah Creighton and Gerry Conway have been the most important people on the journey that led me to this book. When we first gathered at University College London Hospitals (UCLH) in the UK in the mid-1990s, we did not anticipate the long and organic growth of our project. It began when we met Margaret Simmonds in 1995 at a Royal Society of Medicine symposium, *Management of Intersex into Adult Life*, at which she and another member of the Androgen Insensitivity Syndrome Support Group (AISSG) UK had been invited to speak. The 1990s was a time when the UK was without a service strategy for adults with sex variations. The idea of a multidisciplinary service for adults emerged in 1997 in conversations with Margaret and other AISSG UK members. Out of these early discussions grew the world's first known adult clinic that combined expertise in endocrinology, gynecology and clinical psychology and enabled service users to see specialists in any or all of these disciplines in the course of a single clinic visit.

Between the late 1990s and mid-2000s, our service quickly grew from once a month to three times a week. A person whose dedication was pivotal to coordinate this growth before she retired was a nurse specialist called Maligaye Bikoo. We were also supported by exceptional colleagues in urology, imaging and genetics and were so fortunate as to attract a continuous stream of outstanding trainees and fellows in medicine, nursing and psychology to keep us inspired. I had much to learn from colleagues not very far away from UCLH, at the pediatric DSD service at Great Ormond Street Hospital for Children. The geographical closeness meant that early on, service users had the chance to access the kind of lifespan care that is so talked about today.

The postmodern therapist has been likened to an *accidental ethnographer* who comes into the system from a position of not fixing. With neither lived experience nor professional guidance for working in the field, the analogy worked for me, if up to a point. While I knew neither what nor how to fix, I was already a feminist and critical psychologist and made sense of my experiences in a particular way. But it is true that for some years, my existence in intersex medicine was something akin to that of an ethnographer, though I did not know it at the time. Such a venture would not have been possible without the generosity and kindness of people who are too numerous to thank individually.

Among clinical experts, I need to thank the many medical and psychological professionals who invited me to meet with their teams in France, Italy, Sweden, Germany, the UK and the USA. My gratitude also goes to the many academic hosts who involved me in teaching and learning. I could not but be impressed by the progress made in the field in a very short time and humbled by the dedication and passion to improve care.

A person who offered me new dialogue in the early days was Iain Morland. When we met in 2002, I had no idea how much I was to profit from his unrivalled intellect and humor. Among other people who have also raised my game are Katrina Roen and Peter Hegarty, with whom I have enjoyed numerous projects. Franco D'Alberton's clinical acumen and camaraderie made me realize the importance of peer support for myself. I salute the dozens of contributors to the former European Network for Psychosocial Studies in Intersex (EuroPSI). The network was relaunched as Psychosocial Studies in Intersex International (PSI-I) in 2021. The enthusiasm to champion the fledgling efforts of this evolving network speaks volumes of the value that psychosocial researchers and practitioners place on mutual learning and support.

Working with peer advocacy groups has been inspirational. As well as the AISSG UK, it has been my deepest honor to connect with the following people and organizations: Magda Rakita, Anick Soni and Interconnected UK, Ellie Magritte and dsdfamilies, Arlene Smyth and the Turner Syndrome Support Society UK, Alison Bridges, Paul Dutton and the Klinefelter Syndrome Association UK, AISIA in Italy and grApSIA in Spain. Further afield, I thank pioneering intersex advocates Bo Laurent, Arlene Baratz and their colleagues in the USA for their friendship and collaboration.

Many people have provided me with helpful conversations and feedback regarding specific aspects of the book. Among those not already named are Julie Alderson, Mary Boyle, Morgan Carpenter and Dan Wood, whose expert advice has been indispensable. Jackie Doyle and Jackie Hughes' unconditional support for the book was an intellectual and spiritual well that kept me going.

My gratitude goes, of course, also to the hundreds of service users who shared their stories with me and to the dedicated supervisees, trainees, students and interns not just in DSD but across specialties – from perinatal to palliative care – for the time spent in thinking together about intrapersonal and interpersonal human concerns and the relevance and limitations of psychological approaches.

Writing is selfish and excluding and a risk to relationships. My family and friends have remained loving without the quality attention due to them.

Thank you all.

Abbreviations

5αR2D-5	alpha reductase 2 deficiency
17βHSD3D-17	beta hydroxysteroid dehydrogenase 3 deficiency
AIS	androgen insensitivity syndrome
ART	assisted reproductive technology
BPSM	biopsychosocial model
CAH	congenital adrenal hyperplasia
DSD	differences in sex development
ISNA	Intersex Society of North America
KS	Klinefelter syndrome
MDT	multidisciplinary team
MRKHS	Mayer-Rokitansky-Küster-Hauser syndrome
PCC	patient-centered care
PCP	psychological care provider
PTMF	Power Threat Meaning Framework
TS	Turner syndrome
UN	United Nations
VSC	variations in sex characteristics
WHO	World Health Organization

Ordinary Lives

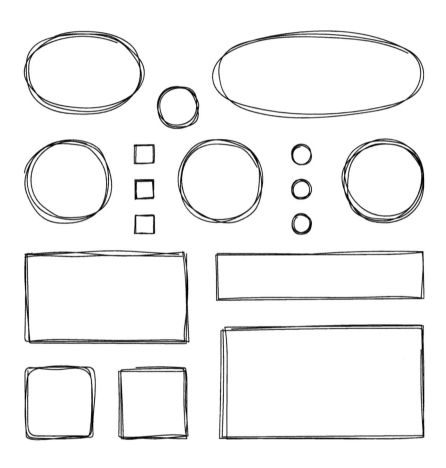

CHAPTER I

Circles and Squares

Jude can't sleep. It's been an overwhelming day. Eyes fixated on the red dot on the black screen, she tries to reorganize her memory of the afternoon. She'd been curious about the meeting for a while. It's a meeting that she'd signed up for and withdrawn from. But this time – this time – she's gone for it!

She goes over the afternoon's medical talk again and feels her headache coming back. The young doctor seemed kind, genuine, enthusiastic, but unreachable. Jude repeated her question three times, and the answers kept missing the mark. According to Dr. Vergoth's diagram of circles and squares, Jude is a son to her parents. But she is a daughter to her parents. Dr. Vergoth smiled in agreement, and then proceeded to talk about the diagram of circles and squares, just as before!

As sleep continues to evade Jude, she frets again – has she offended that poor doctor? Is she branded an argumentative newbie? At least two persons in the room had put their hand up to speak to the doctor but never got the chance. So-o-o embarrassing. There's still tomorrow to get through. . .

I will say nothing tomorrow.
In fact I don't have to turn up at all.
Am I giving up too soon?
I can take a walk in the morning and rejoin after lunch?

Jude is disappointed with herself. Her "self-soothing" techniques are trumped by the intensity of her "ruminations" – a peculiar psychology word from Lennox pops into mind. Starched sheets and fluffy pillows in hotel rooms are her favorites, yet sleep does not come.

She makes a plan for tomorrow: *I'll sit next to Dillon.* She resets the alarm to give herself extra time to arrive early and choose her seat: *I must park myself at the back of the room. That's the plan.* With a bit of luck, she'll catch Dillon walking in and get him to sit next to her.

Back at the beginning of the day, not long after she had gotten her badge from the organizers, Dillon was among the first to introduce himself to Jude. *"Hi, I'm Dillon,"* he shrugged his shoulders with a half-smile, *"I have hypospadias. This is my third meeting."* Jude's frozen expression revealed that she didn't know anything about hypospadias. Dillon continued, *"All the doctors told my parents to get me fixed before my first birthday. My mom didn't like their bedside manners. So she pushed back."*

Jude had struggled throughout the day to piece together all the things people at the meeting were saying about their surgeries and about being fixed. Too soon, too late, too many... She wanted to figure out whether Dillon was angry or happy with his doctors. She wanted to react correctly.

It would seem that Dillon's mother didn't manage to "push back" for very long. Apparently, a growing Dillon said one day, *"How come you sit down to pee and Dad doesn't? Does Grandma sit down too? How does Grandpa pee? I'm a boy, but I sit down like you and not Dad."* These might have been half-distracted musings of a little boy being his usual quizzical self. But they matched the language of Dillon's doctors too well. Dillon's mom berated herself for delaying her son's surgery. Five months later, Dillon had his first hypospadias surgery.

As she listened attentively to Dillon, Jude felt sure that the people behind her were also talking about surgery. She has only ever had one surgery in her life – a planned Caesarean section five years ago to deliver Sam. She did not want to talk about surgery. But there was no getting away.

Dillon picked up after a short pause:

> *I remember all my surgeries, I think seven in total? And I might go back one last time, just a small procedure, not sure if I should. I try not to think about all the anesthesia I've had. But my doctor's nice, treats me like a grown-up, doesn't rush me through my appointment. He's ok, Dr Da Silva, tells me to date, have relationships, don't get too hung up about anatomy he says, everyone's different.*

Dillon has on occasions lied to Dr. Da Silva about dating, that "sex" (with his dates) was working out just fine, even though he had yet to experience it.

Dillon regrets how he dealt with his first date. He was in his early twenties then. Having delayed sex with Shauna for some time, when it finally happened, he had not told her that his body might look and work differently. They were already undressed when he suddenly told her that he had never "had sex" before. This prompted many reassuring and loving expressions from Shauna. Their gentle exchanges somehow morphed into mutual apologies, and big hugs, when they abandoned the game. The young people agreed to have a conversation later. But neither of them got in touch.

Almost three years later, having read a few stories on the Internet and spoken to a few men with hypospadias, Dillon approached his next date differently. He met Clare at a bike hire shop in Vietnam. They got on so well that they decided to backpack together for a few days. They were blown away – literally, by a monsoon, on their last day.

Late into that evening, all was calm again. The sea had turned itself back to a lake. The sky withdrew its shimmering distractions and gave nothing away. Who knows what Clare might have done next. But what followed was not likely to have been on her radar. Under the obligatory straw parasol, with a fifth bottle of Saigon in hand, Dillon decided to spill out his entire medical history.

He spoke at a relaxed pace, with some degree of irreverence for chronology. Clare listened with interest. She asked questions. They were skillfully phrased. She wanted to know how Dillon felt about yet another operation, and whether the hospital had arranged some counseling for him.

To return Dillon's trust, Clare confided in him something she had told no one other than ex-girlfriend Simone. On the day before Clare's sixth birthday, her father left home unannounced. Clare had planned to make Singapore her last stop on this backpacking trip. It's where her father now lives, with his new family. It was to be their first meeting in eight years. But Clare had changed her mind. She was to travel home the next day – Simone was coming out of rehab and her family had asked Clare for help. Clare was happy to go home, really. The reunion thing didn't feel like such a good idea anymore.

Dillon and Clare exchanged sticky embraces without saying anything about keeping in touch. They left the hostel at dawn, separately. Dillon didn't need any promises. Feeling a huge weight lifted, he did a big star jump before crawling into a tuk tuk. He felt ridiculously happy. A few weeks later, he received a call from Clare.

They began a loving relationship. They traveled as much as they could afford to. They introduced their friendship groups to each other. They became passionately involved in climate activism. He showed her how to cook and take better photos. Sex was not such a big part of the relationship. It happened when it happened. And when it happened, it was pleasurable for both.

Clare encouraged Dillon to go back and finish his education. It struck her that Dillon would make a great teacher. Dillon however didn't have a good word to say about school. There were the hospital appointments and admissions of his youth that could not be timed to his vacations – despite his mom's best effort. At one point, he had missed so much school that he had to repeat a whole year. That brought on peer problems, which the school handled really badly – again, despite his mom's best effort. Dillon was severely bullied by younger kids for a time and had to change school in the end.

With Clare's help and support, Dillon was to pass his Math and English exams and became eligible for college. A year ago however, Clare broke up with Dillon. He had gone back on antidepressants, but this made no difference to the outcome of the relationship. Dillon would explain to friends and family that Clare could not cope with his moodiness. Privately, he thought their sex life was to blame. His mind went automatically to his hypospadias and all the surgeries, forgetting that Clare had her own sexuality journey to charter, not to mention attachment issues – legacy from times past.

Jude wonders that Dillon does not see a therapist. She and Yuri had couple therapy. Okay, it didn't save their marriage, but it did help them with co-parenting. Childcare between them just works. Yuri is happily taking care of Sam this weekend and the whole of the coming week.

Despite a bad night, Jude feels better today – perhaps because there are fewer people at the meeting. Everyone is walking around with dark circles round the eyes looking absolutely pooped. All those empty seats – *did they all have a bad night too?*

Behind Jude sits a young family. Father and child move away at break. Karla, the mother, leans forward to speak to Jude. Jude is taken aback: *Is Karla really asking if I'm "an XY"?* Jude feels under pressure to talk about herself. But, again, there is no need. Karla is quite happy to chat about her little girl. Lulu goes to a famous pediatric clinic – a *"one-stop DSD clinic"* that seems to be all the rage.

Karla is worried that Lulu's surgery is not yet scheduled. The resurfacing of surgery doesn't surprise Jude. She is getting used to recantations of vagina, scarring, glans, clitoris, dilators, scrotal resection, curvature and fistula. She discerns no sensations on hearing words like intersex and differences in sex development. They don't apply to her. *Or do they?* She attends to Karla's chatter with interest, glad for the support that Karla is getting from an online group for *"CAH [congenital adrenal hyperplasia] parents."* But Karla's experience sounds kind of complicated.

Shortly after birth, Lulu had been offered surgery to make her more *"girl-like, down at the front."* Karla and her husband had chosen to delay this move. They wanted more time to enjoy Lulu first. Having done their research and taken the time to get to know Lulu, they now feel confident to move forward with her surgery before school.

The surgery will make Lulu's clitoris smaller. The doctors might do other small stuff, but the net effect is that the little girl will look more normal. Lulu can't wait to go back to the hospital. She's been promised swimming lessons *"when the doctors have made everything ok."* Lulu would be able to use the same changing rooms and toilets as other girls. There would be no need for her new school to take special steps. In a classroom of 30 youngsters, it's unreasonable to expect overstretched teachers to protect Lulu from being seen and then teased by other children. After the surgery, well, there would be no need to tell the school anything at all. Lulu would not have to be "special."

Karla has been outraged by some of the comments on the Internet about surgery. Someone even calls it "female genital mutilation." Karla can't get over why people, including clever clogs like college professors, could be so cruel to parents doing the best they can: *Have they ever brought up a girl with a. . .?* Karla does not waver. It is her job to do the best for Lulu; other people are welcome to come to their own conclusions.

Karla confides in no one about Lulu's condition except three other CAH parents. These parents live in Sweden, Belgium and Australia. She has never met any of them in person, but they have compared detailed notes about steroid treatments, and they have shared their hopes and fears about their daughters' future. They are like a little peer group within a peer group.

These mutually supportive parents reassure each other that it's fine if their daughter turns out to be a little tomboy. That would be kind of cute, in a way. Of course it would be better if the child were to play with girls too, not just boys. Sometimes the topic of sexuality would come up. They only want their daughter to be happy. So what if the girl turns out to be gay? But, of course, it would be so much easier if they were to turn out straight.

Almost four years ago, Baby Lulu's debut caused mayhem in the labor ward of the local maternity hospital. The doctors eventually diagnosed CAH and reassured the parents that they had a little girl – "*absolutely.*" The parents were given excellent written information and upbeat videos on CAH. Between them, the couple have managed Lulu's steroids beautifully. She is a happy, healthy little girl. As a family, they go to as many support group meetings as possible. They don't want to miss out on anything. Somewhere along the line, they have even gotten comfortable with Lulu's somewhat wrinkly and protruding genitals – something once thought unimaginable.

When it comes to surgery, Karla and her husband have gone over the pros and cons and uncertainties for months. It has been exhausting. They have even gone as far as to find before and after photos in medical journals. It's clear to them that those after photos look really good. They have been warned that in the future Lulu may disagree with their decision. But, you know, parents get the flak no matter what they do. The couple are fully prepared to shoulder any parent-blaming in the years to come.

A good while back, Karla was given the option to see the hospital psychologist. It was hard for her to find the time. Besides, they were quite catered for in terms of support. When the surgery was agreed, however, Lulu's doctor raised the subject again. He said that pediatric psychology was the only gap missing in Lulu's care plan, and that the child psychologist could prepare Lulu for the surgery and Karla for talking to Lulu about it later.

Karla thinks to herself: "*I don't get this. Isn't talking to Lulu something for me to figure out? How many more times do I have to go over the grounds about surgery?*" Nevertheless, the doctor insisted that psychology was part of "*the team approach.*"

That sounded like a tick box exercise to Karla. She was unimpressed. She accepted an appointment to humor the doctor but had no intention of keeping it. Privately, much as she was grateful to the clinic, she was not prepared to travel for two hours to have Lulu's surgery rubber stamped by a psychologist: *I am not depressed; I am perfectly capable of deciding for my child.* Karla has a great relationship with her daughter and has no doubt that she can talk to Lulu when the time comes: *There really isn't anything else to discuss.*

There are moments, however, when Karla is dazed. These moments can come randomly – in the middle of cutting up carrots or waiting for the coffee to brew, in the car at the traffic lights, in the middle of the night. . . Memories, questions, fears, hopes and dreams would pile on:

Did that really happen to us?
What would Lulu be like now, if she didn't have the CAH?
She won't wear her new dress, is she a tomboy?
Does she know she's a girl – absolutely?
Will she get a moustache in her teens?
Why am I still sad? Can she see through me? Will this affect her?
They say "acceptance," am I "acceptance" enough?

Karla's husband is very quiet. He never says his name at support group meetings. Today he looks lethargic and disinterested. It's hard to tell whether he is troubled by the same thoughts as his wife or just bored. He only repeats that he wants what's best for Lulu: "*For her to grow up happy, meet someone who loves her and takes care of her, for her to have kids.*"

With a headful of tumbling locks, Lulu's eyes are permanently fixed on the tray of chocolate brownies at the back of the room. Jude muses over those things that every parent in the room says they want for their kid. She has done them all. She has been in love. She has been married. And she has a kid. Born with a womb but no ovaries, a fertility clinic implanted in Jude "high quality embryos" created with sperms from Yuri and eggs donated by someone far away. Sounds simple enough. It took almost four years before she conceived Sam. Another story.

Jude was only 15 years old when doctors told her that she had "Swyer syndrome." From memory, the process is best described as firefighting. At one point, someone in the hospital room pulled out a medical journal, and the team of experts argued with each other in front of the family. The letters SRY were blurted out several times. The family had no idea what that meant. Jude's mother broke down and sobbed uncontrollably. Her father fell silent.

Jude thinks back on that weird time. She sees herself watching the event unfold in her mind's eye, a bit like a film clip. She was only interested in the estrogen, because she wanted breasts. What did she care about the biology! Frankly, as a horny teenager, unless the doctors could have gotten her a love life, she couldn't wait to be shot of them.

The hormone did change her body. But her breasts are still quite small. She once mentioned this to a doctor. He immediately suggested a referral to a breast surgeon. *How doctors like to give presents!* Jude rather enjoys her lanky looks – "*very Charlotte Rampling*," an ardent admirer once remarked.

At this very moment, in the middle of her first "support group" weekend, something flashes through her mind. Her first operation was not the C-section! It was the keyhole surgery to remove her "gonads." She can't remember much and hasn't thought about it at all.

Since that weird animated debate between overexcited doctors by her bedside, Jude's father has not set foot in the hospital again. He was to retreat from any discussion about Swyer syndrome. Perhaps it was to make up for his neglect that he decided to teach his daughter to sail. Father and daughter were to sail across the Atlantic in due course. And now, daughter has even more seafaring qualifications and trophies than father.

It is not the diagnosis of Swyer syndrome but the horror of Jude's fertility journey that still makes her hold her breath. She shudders to recall how she might have survived those blighted years of being controlled like a ragdoll. The actual procedures were disgusting. But it was more than that. She and Yuri had to stay in their hated jobs – for the money. There was neither the time nor energy to sail, even if they could afford to hold on to the boat. Her one passion in life was up in smoke. In fact, everything that meant anything to her at all had to be suspended. She simply acquiesced. Her relationship with Yuri was never the same again. Sam will be five soon. The question of how to tell him about his conception is closing in: *The clinic didn't say anything about that!*

Doing female things hasn't made Jude feel more female – a thought best kept to herself today. In the natural world, females are circles and men are squares. She has a Y chromosome. In the young doctor's diagram, she is a square. Every time she clicks "female" on a form, she feels just that little bit disingenuous. It's as if she doesn't have. . . "*legitimacy.*" That's the weighty word that she once blurted out to Lennox. Maybe that weird SRY argument between the doctors did seed some weird ideas in her.

Jude feels some envy toward the nonbinary youths on the front row this morning. Their crazy hair, funky clothes and big laughs. "*How liberating,*" she thinks, "*to be free from herd mentality.*" Jude has seen them talking to the meeting organizers and other youngsters in the room. She wonders if all of the young people have gotten from the meeting what they had come for. She regrets not making her way to the front of the room to introduce herself before they left. But then it's been so full on!

Trains don't run well on Sunday. Jude's journey home is another classic. Physically and emotionally drained after the most intense two days of her life, Jude finds herself running full pelt with her heavy bag for the train. She collapses onto a seat and feels sick. She switches on the playlist compiled by Yuri but passes out and has very little idea of the rest of the journey home.

The alarm says she's slept round the clock. She is ravenous and remembers having eaten next to nothing over the weekend. She swallows something vaguely edible as she listens to the news, leaning over the sink to avoid dribbling on her silk blouse.

Back at Desk 48, she sips a thick coffee. She has never felt happier looking at the mess on her desk. Her work demands total concentration. Her job title is Assistant Director of Workforce, a destination she did not foresee when she chose to major in French Studies at college.

This is a big week for Jude. She is childfree. And she has tickets! She feels the urge to light a cigarette, but makes do with a few long exhalations. *I love my job.* She never thinks these words without gratitude – but especially this morning. Her new friend Dillon ain't so lucky. He lost his job as a chef last year. Postpandemic, who knows what the future holds for his industry: *Will he train as a teacher now? Shall I call to find out – is it a done thing? Will he be at the meeting next year?*

A colleague asks about the weekend. Jude collects herself and mutters something about a big party at a hotel. She longs to debrief with Lennox. She rehearses her conversation with him. She places her hand over her mouth to suppress an unfamiliar sensation. It feels something like – yes, she dares – triumph. Yes. Yes.

Medicalization and Resistance

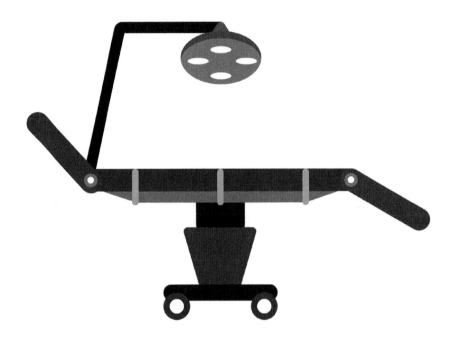

Introductory Notes

This section of the book provides some basic information on how biological sex characteristics develop in human beings and how the characteristics can vary. It portrays how medical understanding has evolved. It summarizes how people with lived experience are resisting medical authority and how medicine has responded to the dissenting voices of care users.

Chapter 2 begins with a brief summary of typical embryonic development of the urogenital and reproductive systems. Where the sex chromosomes, reproductive organs and genitalia in combination do not fit the social categories of female and male, doctors and scientists used to call these physical outcomes hermaphroditism and intersex. They debated for a long time on the "true sex" of the individuals but could not agree on which of the biological sex characteristics should count as their true sex – should it be the sex chromosomes, the gonads or the genitals? For more than a hundred years, many doctors and scientists settled on a gonadal definition of sex. This means that people who have testes are male, people who have ovaries are female and only those with both testicular and ovarian tissue are considered *true* hermaphrodites, regardless of their sex chromosomes and their genital structures. The rest of the people with physical sex variations were considered *pseudo*hermaphrodites. In the age of genetics, much more is known about how the atypical features have developed. At the same time, however, people who are impacted by sex variations are increasingly disputing the medical framing of their differences. The twenty-first century was to seed a new and ongoing debate between the new medical term, differences in sex development, and intersex, with the latter being reclaimed by an increasing number of impacted adults.

Not all sex variations are apparent at birth. Sometimes they are internal and therefore not visible on the outside, that is, the child is born looking like a typical boy or girl. The child may be brought to medical attention much later, for example when puberty does not follow the expected path. Many of these care users were not told the truth about their biological variation because health professionals and sometimes parents believed that the information would harm the person. At the same time, the growing child and adult "patient" noticed that they were fascinating to health professionals, who may have examined them in droves. Some care users did not discover the truth about their diagnosis and the treatment until they accessed their medical records in mid-life. This discussion forms the first part of Chapter 3.

For children whose external genitalia look different at birth, when surgical safety and techniques improved, it became routine to align the urogenital anatomy of newborns and young children to the assigned gender. The gender–genitalia alignment was believed to be important psychologically for child and family. Because surgeons found it easier to *feminize* than *masculinize* the genitalia, most babies with genital variations were assigned female. From the 1990s, some of the adults who had been so treated in their childhood have been speaking out about their negative experiences. They talk of having had too many operations, being too often examined by too many people and not understanding what was happening to them. These experiences are summarized in the latter half of Chapter 3.

In a gendered world, doctors and caretakers took it for granted that making atypical bodies more typical was a humane way out of a difficult situation for child and family. Had the health professionals carried out proper research, they would have learned from their young patients that the approach was physically and psychologically risky. But research on the long-term effects was not carried out, certainly not from the patients' perspective. There was also no comparison group made up of people growing up with unaltered genital variations, because surgery was so widespread. Since the 1990s, a number of outcome studies with adults have identified many problems of childhood surgery, such as multiple operations, scarring, shrinkage, sensitivity loss, unusual genital appearance and sexual difficulties. Research with adults is the topic of Chapter 4.

Some former patients mounted street protests in front of medical conferences to draw attention to their trauma in the 1990s. They reclaimed intersex as a personal identity and campaigned for healthcare reform. These developments are the focus of Chapter 5. Intersex is coming out of the medical closet more and more, through being a topic in television documentaries, novels, films and other art forms. Intersex activists challenge medical authority to change practice. Furthermore, they are not waiting for doctors and scientists to come to their viewpoints. They have successfully lobbied human rights agencies to position childhood genital surgery as a violation of their human rights. They demand that surgery is delayed until the child can give informed consent or is at least old enough to participate in the discussion and offer their agreement.

Chapter 6 summarizes the changes to medical care in recent years. There is now a greater recognition that the projected social and psychological challenges of genital variations cannot be fixed by surgery. The first international consensus statement on intersex was published in 2006. The statement makes a number of recommendations to improve care. Controversially however, a new term *disorders of sex development* (and, later, differences in sex development, or DSD) was introduced to refer to biological sex variations. Biotechnological developments have been advancing rapidly since then. More has been learned about "normal" and "abnormal" sex development. However, parents still struggle to talk to children about their bodily variations, young people still worry about getting into relationships, psychological expertise is still a low priority even in specialist multidisciplinary services and the full potential of peer support is not yet realized. Because there is not enough commitment to develop a wider range of solutions, too many doctors and parents still see childhood genital surgery as the only way out of stigmatization for child and family.

In summary, this section describes how doctors and scientists have been making sense of nondimorphic sex development. It draws attention to the human costs of controversial medical practices in the past. It highlights a thriving intersex movement in the present. It outlines aspirations of the new era of medical practice but also exposes the gap between aspiration and practice.

CHAPTER 2

Evolving Terms and Definitions

Chromosomal, reproductive and urogenital sex characteristics do not always map clearly onto the social categories of female or male. Social responses to the diverse developmental outcomes have been highly variable, depending on time and place. Had the variations been common knowledge, they might have been considered rather unremarkable. However, they have been shrouded in secrecy and, in modern societies, are considered the domain of specialist medical doctors and scientists.

Where the external genitalia appear to be somewhere along the female-typical or male-typical spectrum, as opposed to at either pole, medical investigations are often triggered in early childhood. Where the external genitalia look female or male typical, the internal variation may become apparent much later, for example when pubertal development is absent or is unexpected in some way. Sometimes the diagnosis is made even later, such as when a heterosexual couple present at fertility clinics because they cannot conceive, and tests reveal a genetic variation in one of the couple.

This chapter starts with a brief summary of dimorphic sex development. It outlines how medical understandings of nondimorphic development have evolved and how these understandings are still being disputed. My summary here is intended to provide basic information for nonmedical specialists and a context for subsequent chapters.

2.1 Dimorphic Sex Development

Most human beings have 23 pairs of chromosomes (bundles of genes). The 23rd pair is known as the sex chromosomes, because they largely (but not exclusively) determine sex characteristics, that is, hormones, reproductive organs and genitalia. The pair typically comes as either two X chromosomes (46,XX) or one X and one Y chromosome (46,XY). Regardless of chromosomal complement, human embryos have two tube-like structures called the Müllerian duct and the Wolffian duct.

Usually, one structure proliferates and the other regresses, resulting in what we recognize as an either female or male form.

With a 46,XY chromosomal complement, male-typical development is triggered in the embryo by the SRY gene located on the short arm of the Y chromosome that, in conjunction with genes elsewhere, induces the gonads to differentiate into testes. Anti-Müllerian hormone secreted by the testes regresses the Müllerian duct. Testosterone produced by the testes stimulates the Wolffian duct to develop into the spermatic ducts. Testosterone is converted to dihydrotestosterone (DHT) in the skin of the external genitalia by an enzyme called 5α-reductase type 2. Stimulated by DHT, the labio-scrotal swelling fuses to become the scrotum and the proto-phallus develops into the penis. The urethra migrates distally to be finally sited at the tip of the penis. Testicular production of testosterone at puberty contributes to further sex differentiation.

There has been a long-held view that "internal and external prenatal sex development is constitutively female" (Hughes, 2002, p. 769). With a 46, XX chromosomal complement, that is, without the SRY and other genes to trigger testicular development, the Wolffian duct regresses by default. The Müllerian duct becomes the uterus, fallopian tubes, cervix and vagina. The bipotential gonads develop into ovaries and, because ovaries do not produce testosterone, the proto-phallus becomes a clitoris, the labioscrotal folds become the labia and the urethra and vagina open separately onto the perineum. At puberty, the ovaries produce estrogen and other hormones that contribute to further sex differentiation. Recent research suggests that ovarian development and elimination of the Wolffian duct do not happen by default. Rather, complex molecular events interact to inhibit male-typical development and maintain the female-typical trajectory.

In summary, the urogenital and reproductive systems are outcomes of a sequential pattern of molecular activations and suppressions occurring at specific moments. Any deviation from the path may result in an atypical combination of chromosomes, reproductive anatomy and urogenital con-figurations along the gestational axis. Many of the atypical presentations have been named (see Section 2.4). For the remainder of this chapter, I briefly summarize how medical doctors and scientists have sought to understand atypical sex development over the centuries.

2.2 "Hermaphroditism"

In one version of ancient Greek mythology, Hermaphrodite is the son of Hermes and Aphrodite, 2 of the 12 gods that rule the world from Mount

Olympus. So desirable is Hermaphrodite to the water nymph Salmacis that, after a seduction debacle on her part, she appeals to the gods to be permanently intertwined with him as a single individual. The wish is granted. The unwitting Hermaphrodite is now doubly sexed – a godly configuration, but a human impossibility, at least not after the first six weeks of conception. Nevertheless, people with nondimorphic physical sex characteristics have been so named since ancient times.

Prior to the advent of modern medicine, it is not certain whether people with atypical sex traits knew their anatomy to be different or considered it to be inherently negative. Even today, the number of people with sex development variations known to health services and communities falls well short of population estimates (Ahmed et al., 2014). It is possible that many people today are either unaware of their variation or do not experience it as a problem. Post-Napoleonic Europe saw an end to the privacy of many hermaphrodites who, if discovered, were increasingly researched and exhibited in ways that would have been considered barbaric even then.

As the nineteenth century progressed, public recognition of disciplinary authority on societal ills and moral laxity was gradually transferred from the clergy to medicine in the West. Built on scientific knowledge rather than unproven faith, medicine was increasingly looked upon for expert guidance on social deviance. Doctors and scientists were poised to scrutinize people who broke the cultural codes of the time, and the status of abnormality was conferred on a wide range of physical and behavioral presentations that did not fall in line with social expectations. From the 1830s, learned men began to publish anatomical and histological findings of animals and humans to build a scientific understanding of hermaphroditism (Dreger, 1998).

Classification turned out to be a complicated business, which went through layers of revision throughout the nineteenth century, with contemporary experts disputing and reinterpreting observations of their predecessors. With today's advanced knowledge, it is easy to see why. A newborn with external genital variations may have any of the following current medically classified conditions: congenital adrenal hyperplasia, partial androgen insensitivity syndrome, 5α-reductase 2 deficiency, to name a few. The external genital variations may look the same, but the internal structures, underlying causes and healthcare needs are different. These variations are so complex that scientists continue to take account of new discoveries to redefine and regroup them.

Whereas early experts saw their task as mapping out different forms of hermaphroditism, their successors from about the mid-nineteenth century, according to scholars of intersex studies, began to interest themselves in separating the real hermaphrodites from the arbitrary ones. This task must have been mindboggling (see Karkazis, 2008). Scientists could not agree on which physical marker should be the separator of the two sexes. As knowledge of the gonads improved, some scientists began to accept the gonad-based classification developed by German pathologist Theodor Albrecht Edwin Klebs (see Dreger, 1998). In Klebs' version of the truth about sex, a person must possess ovarian and testicular material to qualify as a true hermaphrodite. The rest are of the *pseudo* varieties. Based on Klebs' definitions, five sex anatomies were later described:

1.   Females – defined by standard female sex anatomy and XX karyotype
2.   Males – defined by standard male sex anatomy and XY karyotype
3.   Female pseudohermaphrodites – defined by the presence of ovaries and absence of testes and XX karyotype
4.   Male pseudohermaphrodites – defined by the presence of testes in the abdomen or inguinal canal and absence of ovaries and XY karyotype
5.   True hermaphrodites – defined by the presence of ovarian and testicular tissues in one or both of the gonads regardless of genital anatomy and reproductive tracts; the majority of this group have XX karyotype but not exclusively

Gonad-based definition of true sex was not without its critics and, prior to the age of consensus and national and international guidances, medical practice was likely to have been idiosyncratic (Reis, 2009). In time, the gonads came to be understood not just as merely egg or sperm factories but glands that secrete chemicals that affect overall bodily functioning. Nevertheless, in the absence of a better offer, the Klebs taxonomy served as a conceptual platform for medical observations for the ensuing decades. One major consequence of the gonadal definitions was the drastic reduction of the number of hermaphrodites. Historians suggest that the scheme was driven by a need to maintain the sex divide, which would have been made more awkward by the presence of too many nonbinary bodies (Dreger, 1998). However, there was still the question of what gender should true hermaphrodites be. Since they had both types of gonads, should they be allowed to have a gender other than female or male (Karkazis, 2008)? There was much unfinished business.

2.3   "Intersex"

The term hermaphroditism remained in use in medicine until the beginning of the twenty-first century. Meanwhile, in 1917, Richard Goldschmidt, another German scientist, introduced the term intersex to the English language. The zoologist summarized the "vast amount of information" already collated on sex development via methods in "cytology, genetics, teratology, physiology, serology, endocrinology, etc." in his review (Goldschmidt, 1917, p. 433). Although his review was at the invitation of the editor of the journal *Endocrinology*, Goldschmidt drew attention to the limitations of endocrinology as a discipline and advocated for an open mind that draws from diverse knowledge bases.

Goldschmidt and his colleagues did not set out to overturn Klebs' taxonomy. Rather, they tried to synthesize multidisciplinary data sources based on studies of vertebrates. The term intersex became extended to humans before long and, throughout much of the twentieth century, hermaphroditism and intersexuality were interchangeable terms in medical publications.

Uncovering the true sex of intersexuals was not straightforward. There was no question of having to assign everyone to one or the other sex. However, what should it be based on, when biology was revealing more and more "conflicting and contradictory signifiers of sex" (Karkazis, 2008, p. 43)? Failure to find the true sex could have huge legal and social ramifications. Assigning the wrong sex to someone could result in that person having sexual desires for people of the same sex. It could also mean a person wrongfully inheriting an estate.

As knowledge of anesthesia and asepsis improved, the role of surgery was to change from confirming a gonad-based diagnosis to reducing genital atypicality (Karkazis, 2008, p. 43), that is, to give less dichotomized bodies a boost. US surgeon Hugh Hampton Young, regarded as a major force in urology during the first half of the twentieth century (Meldrum et al., 2001), is credited as the first to describe removal of both of the adrenal glands to suppress bodily masculinization in girls and women with congenital adrenal hyperplasia (CAH), or a form of female pseudohermaphroditism, according to the terminology of the day. With emergent new knowledge of gonads, hormones and genetics and the mainstreaming of investigative and surgical techniques from the 1930s, it became ever more compelling to find a way to be more systematic about researching and managing intersex that takes account of psychology (e.g., gender identity, sexual attraction) as a contending marker of true sex.

It is important to consider the broader social, economic and cultural backdrop for these developments. The postwar decades saw the unprecedented growth of biomedicine into one of the largest industries in

Anglophone and Western European nations. The development and regulation of health services at state and national levels began to grow into the
complex infrastructures that we take for granted today. To give a sense of
the scale of this development, in the USA, the healthcare industry currently employs one in nine working people, without taking account of the
breathtaking scale of the pharmaceutical industry (see Stam et al., 2018).
Integral to these developments is the creation and propagation of medical
research as a government-sponsored enterprise and the mushrooming in
numbers of academic physicians. Medicine was becoming synonymous
with biology and technology, and the importance of the family physician, a
person much more closely connected to patient, family and community,
began to shrink in parallel. The development of new modes of communication made it ever more possible for biomedical specialists to share
expertise and standardize approaches across regions for particular diseases
or disease groups. I mention these macro, generic developments here,
because they are integral to contemporary intersex medicine and highly
relevant for understanding the state of play.

By the end of the twentieth century, medical and affiliated specialists
were blessed with many more tools to scrutinize in increasing detail
nondimorphic sex characteristics. The gonadal classification scheme had
long been failing as a conceptual platform for biomedical advances. There
was a lot of catching up with the age of genetics. However, just as
laboratory research on sex variations was gaining credibility in the world
of molecular science, not least for its potential to map out "normal" sex
development, the credibility of clinical management of intersex was
increasingly publicly challenged. From the 1990s, adults who had been
silent and seemingly without agency started to publish gut-wrenching first-
person accounts that exposed and shamed the medical profession. They
claimed intersex as their personal and political identity, mounted public
protests at medical venues and made specific demands to change medical
practice. These developments are briefly summarized in Chapter 5.

2.4   "'Disorders of Sex Development"

The year 2005 is often considered by many to be a watershed moment in
intersex medicine. The age of genetics had entered into its golden period.
Advances in biotechnology had enabled isolation of an increasing number
of genetic variants in sex development. That year, an invitation-only
group of 50 experts met in Chicago to review medical research and revise
the nomenclature. The product was a seminal publication in multiple

venues – *Consensus Statement on Management of Intersex Disorders* (Lee et al., 2006), hereafter the Chicago consensus. The authors of the Chicago consensus explained, "[a] modern lexicon is needed to integrate progress in molecular genetic aspects of sex development" (Lee et al., 2006, p. e488). It was thought that the ideal nomenclature should be flexible enough to make sense of research to date and to accommodate advances on the horizon. The impact of the new nomenclature on service users is examined in more detail in Chapter 6 – from a psychosocial perspective.

Significantly, the terms hermaphroditism and intersex were dropped in favor of disorders of sex development, to denote atypical combinations of sex chromosomes, reproductive anatomy and genital morphology (Lee et al., 2006). The term has since been substituted by *differences in sex development*, hereafter DSD, in many medical publications. The main subcategories of DSD are 46,XX DSD, 46,XY DSD, ovotesticular DSD and sex chromosome DSD. Each of these subcategories has its own set of discrete diagnoses that are increasingly split into subtypes as a result of finer-grained analyses.

Currently the DSD designation includes at least 50 variations in urogenital and reproductive differentiation and every one of them is a spectrum condition (Hiort et al., 2014). This means that the physical manifestations are rarely identical between two persons with the same diagnosis, let alone lived experience and personal identities. A genetic diagnosis is now possible for the majority of 46,XX DSDs, but the same level of specificity is not yet available for the majority of 46,XY DSDs. The genotype-phenotypic (genetic-anatomy) relationship is less predictable than anticipated. Uncertainty continues to haunt care providers and users.

Psychological practitioners are required to have a level of biological knowledge of DSD, not least because today's service users are expected to process complex information about their diagnosis. For the purpose of educating individuals and caretakers about the biology of variations in sex development, a UK-based peer advocacy group (dsdfamilies, 2019) published a booklet called *The Story of Sex Development*. The lesson starts from "The First 8 Weeks" (of gestation) as in Figure 2.1a. It ends with "Bringing It Together," as some of the best-known conditions are listed along the gestational axis as diagrammatically represented in Figure 2.1b. Some of the conditions most often encountered by psychological practitioners working in the field and discussed in this book are seen in Figure 2.1b. They are briefly described below, albeit impacted people may not identify with the descriptions.

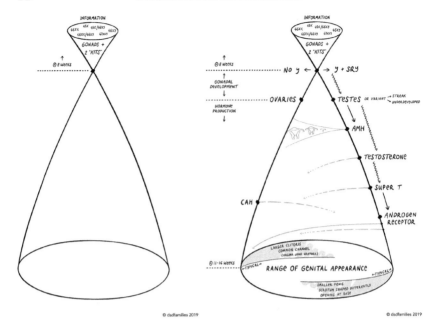

Figure 2.1a   *The Story of Sex Development* (p. 5), reproduced with permission from dsdfamilies.org

Figure 2.1b   *The Story of Sex Development* (p. 21), reproduced with permission from dsdfamilies.org

2.4.1   46,XX DSD

2.4.1.1   *Mayer-Rokitansky-Küster-Hauser Syndrome (MRKHS)*

The reported incidence of MRKHS is 1:5 000 live births. The syndrome is associated with female-typical external genitalia and secondary sex characteristics. Internally, individuals with MRKHS have healthy ovaries and a smaller vagina that does not lead to a cervix. Without a womb and cervix, they ovulate but do not menstruate and cannot carry a pregnancy. A diagnosis is usually triggered in adolescence when menstruation does not occur as expected.

2.4.1.2   *Congenital Adrenal Hyperplasia (CAH)*

CAH is a family of conditions that affect approximately 1:10 000 to 1:15 000 people; about two-thirds have XX (female-typical) chromosomes. In embryonic development, cholesterol is typically converted to cortisol by several enzymes in the adrenal gland. The majority of people with CAH have a deficiency of the enzyme 21 hydroxylase. The deficiency impairs cortisol biosynthesis, resulting in increased adrenocorticotropic hormone concentrations and chronic adrenal stimulation causing hyperplasia. A baby with CAH does not have enough cortisol and often also aldosterone, which results in salt loss. The metabolic effects are usually evident in the first few days of life (Speiser et al., 2010), and treatment involves daily replacement of cortisol and mineralocorticoid. Both XX and XY children may undergo puberty earlier than average and be under average in final height.

Because of the high levels of androgens, internally, an XX fetus with CAH typically has ovaries and a uterus, but the vagina and urethra are joined together as a single opening to the perineum. The external genitalia may appear to be somewhere along the female- to male-typical spectrum, that is, the clitoris is usually enlarged and the labia are often fused, wrinkled and ridged giving a more scrotal appearance.

2.4.2   46,XY DSD

2.4.2.1   Androgen Insensitivity Syndrome (AIS)

In complete AIS, the fetus has testes that produce androgens as per typical in the presence of XY chromosomes. However, the fetus does not have receptors to respond to androgens, so that the usual male-typical development does not take place. The newborn presents female-typical external genitalia but with a smaller vaginal canal that does not lead to a cervix or womb. Complete AIS may remain unrecognized until adolescence, when a typical girl does not menstruate. In partial AIS, there is some response to androgens. Therefore, the external genital appearance may be somewhere along the female- to male-typical spectrum.

2.4.2.2   5α-Reductase 2 Deficiency (5αR2D)

5αR2D is the primary enzyme that converts testosterone into DHT in early male-typical development. With reduced or absent enzymatic activity, the external genital morphology falls somewhere along the female- to male-typical spectrum. At puberty, there are other pathways through which the body can make DHT and stimulate the external genitalia and the rest of the body to develop in the male-typical direction. If left unaltered, individuals with a diagnosis of 5αR2D may appear to be more female-typical at birth and spontaneously transition to a more male-typical form at puberty.

2.4.2.3   17β-Hydroxysteroid Dehydrogenase-3 Deficiency (17βHSD3D)

17β-hydroxysteroid dehydrogenase-3 is one of several enzymes that regulate the activity of steroid hormones at the prereceptor level. Deficiency of this enzyme affects how testosterone is processed and actioned. The testes do not produce enough testosterone and tend to stay in the abdomen. At birth, the anatomical outcome is female-typical or along the female- to male-typical spectrum. At puberty, the testes may become more active. With more testosterone being released, male-typical secondary sex characteristics usually develop.

2.4.2.4   XY Complete Gonadal Dysgenesis (Swyer Syndrome)

The condition is defined by an absence of testicular and ovarian tissue and hormonal production and intact Müllerian structures, that is, womb, fallopian tubes and upper vagina and female-typical external genitalia. As for complete AIS, the newborn presents female-typical external genitalia and the condition usually becomes apparent in a typical adolescent girl for whom pubertal changes do not happen. Unlike complete AIS, however, early hormone replacement is necessary to induce the development of secondary sex characteristics and achieve peak bone mass. Furthermore, there is a significant risk of germ cell tumor in the gonads for which bilateral gonadectomy is currently recommended. With the womb present, pregnancy is possible via egg donation (Michala et al., 2008).

2.4.3   Ovotesticular DSD

The majority of people with ovotesticular DSD have a 46,XX karyotype. The diagnosis is defined by the presence of both ovarian and testicular tissue in the same person. The external genitalia are likely to be somewhere along the spectrum. In XX individuals the uterus is usually present and pregnancy is possible with assisted reproductive technology and gamete donation.

2.4.4   Sex Chromosome DSD

The sex chromosome conditions can affect multiple body systems and the two best-known conditions are mentioned below.

2.4.4.1   Turner Syndrome (TS)

The reported incidence of TS is 1 in 2 500 live female births. It is usually associated with partial or total deletion of the second X chromosome (45, XO). A significant number of individuals may not be diagnosed. For example, it has been estimated that active medical records exist for fewer than one in five of the predicted 15 000 women in the UK (Conway, 2022). People with TS have a female-typical external sex anatomy. Diagnosis at birth is often triggered by low birth weight, shorter neck and swelling of hands and feet. TS is associated with increased risks of thyroid disease, celiac disease, hearing loss, hypertension and diabetes. TS expressions are highly variable and may also include cardiac and renal anomalies, shorter stature and delayed puberty. Women with TS can carry a pregnancy but usually via egg donation because of depletion of egg reserve before puberty.

2.4.4.2 Klinefelter Syndrome (KS)

KS is associated with an extra X in the chromosomal complement (47, XXY). The reported incidence is 1 in 500–1 000 live births. As for TS, a significant number of individuals may not have been diagnosed and are without symptoms, and some individuals may not consider themselves as having a medical condition even if diagnosed (Conway, 2022). Individuals with KS do not produce the usual level of testosterone. They may have a male-typical external sex anatomy and smaller testes, delayed puberty, some breast development, infertility and taller stature. KS is thought to be associated with elevated risks of cognitive and behavioral concerns for some individuals, but these variations are harder to ascertain and quantify.

2.4.5 Other Genital Variations

The DSD nosology excludes certain genital variations such as those described below. Yet in some publications, the below variations are discussed in the same light as other DSD diagnoses.

2.4.5.1 Hypospadias

Hypospadias is, most commonly, an isolated congenital anomaly affecting the penis. It is defined by the proximal location of the urethral meatus on the ventral surface of the penis, dorsal chordee and an incomplete or "hooded" foreskin (Wood & Wilcox, 2022). It has been suggested that the incidence of hypospadias may be variously increasing or decreasing over time. Although there is uncertainty, it is generally accepted that there are regional differences in prevalence, with the number lowest in Asia (0.6–69/10 000) and highest in North America (34.2/10 000).

Fitchner et al. (1995) investigated the meatal location, curvature of the penis, voiding position and reports of erection and coitus in 500 healthy men. They found that only 55% of their sample had the meatus located at the tip of the penis and 32% located in the mid third of the glans. With a small handful of exceptions, the men were unaware of any cosmetic or functional concern. Thus while some patients with hypospadias could have long-term voiding problems and difficulty with sexual penetration (e.g., due to curvature) and, for heterosexual couples, conception difficulties, many will have no long-term problems (Wood & Wilcox, 2022).

2.4.5.2 Cloacal Anomalies

The cloaca is the embryonic structure that divides to form the rectum, bladder and genitalia. Cloacal variations are not covered in the DSD family but some are considered iatrogenic DSDs. Where the rectum, vagina and urethra merge as one exit out of the body instead of three separate outlets in 46,XX individuals, the condition is sometimes called a persistent cloaca or cloacal anomaly. The ovaries and fallopian tubes are typically unaffected.

2.4.5.3 Bladder Exstrophy-Epispadias Complex (BEEC)

Epispadias is the least severe form of BEEC. It refers to the urethra not forming fully during fetal development. Because it is open where it should be closed, urine can leak from wherever the opening occurs. Epispadias can affect XX and XY infants.

Children with bladder exstrophy also have epispadias. Bladder exstrophy is defined by the bladder developing outside the fetus and is visible when the baby is born. The exposed bladder does not store urine and, because the bladder is exposed, urine constantly trickles onto the skin causing a range of problems. The condition can affect the structure and function of the bladder, intestines, pelvic bones, reproductive organs and genitalia.

Cloacal exstrophy is the most serious form of BEEC. The rectum, bladder and genitals may not fully form and do not fully separate. The gastrointestinal tract and bladder are not sealed in the abdominal wall and are visible outside the abdomen. The anus may not be open. In XX babies, the clitoris may be split, and there may be two vaginal openings. In XY babies, the penis may be absent or shorter and split in two, the testes are undescended and the epispadias is severe. The condition is typically associated with abnormal kidney and spinal development. The kidneys, pelvic bones, backbone and spinal cord may be affected. Most children with cloacal exstrophy have spinal abnormalities, including spina bifida. Life expectancy is improving with modern life-saving surgical techniques.

2.5 Dispute over Naming

The main text of the Chicago consensus begins with: "Terms such as 'intersex,' 'pseudohermaphroditism,' 'hermaphroditism,' 'sex reversal' and gender-based diagnostic labels are particularly controversial. These terms are perceived as potentially pejorative by patients and can be confusing to practitioners and parents alike" (Lee et al., 2006, p. e488). The opening statement is so promising that the next sentence comes as something of a surprise: "We propose the term disorders of sex development." The term has turned out to be the most controversial of all. Its widespread adoption in the medical community means that people whom it describes are left to engage with it and to deal with the "tremendous amount of new tension in the intersex community" over their differences in how to relate to the term (Davis, 2015, p. 88).

Articles defending the new nomenclature appeared almost immediately. One of the arguments in favor of the word disorder is that it labels the condition rather than the person. Furthermore, by equalizing the syndromes with other medical conditions, evidence-based healthcare is expected. The argument against the word intersex is that it describes the person and implies a gender identity or a certain political stance. Among intersex activists and advocates, the concern is that in naming benign atypical physical features as disordered, their bodies are pathologized and people are more compelled to (have their children) undergo elective medical interventions that can be invasive and high risk.

Descriptive terms such as variations of reproductive development have been proposed (e.g., Simmonds, 2007). In some psychosocial and humanities publications, the word disorder is substituted by "divergence" and "diverse," to preserve the acronym DSD so that the works are in dialogue with the medical literature (Liao & Roen, 2014).

The proponents for the term DSD might have been quick to claim their victory based on its widespread adoption (Hughes, 2010, p. 161); however, the dissent is refusing to quieten down, so much so that reactions to the disorder vocabulary have prompted its own line of investigation. A number of reports of variable quality are now available, based on research with people to whom the term is applied.

A group of pediatric experts in the UK constructed their own questionnaire for a convenient sample of 19 parents of children attending a DSD clinic and 15 health professionals (Davies et al., 2011). The group added an opportunistic sample of 25 parents of children without DSD. The authors claimed to have obtained broad support for the disorder terminology. They interpreted their results with uncritical optimism relating to the term and offered no further thought about the myriad factors that might have affected their results. The optimism, however, is not supported in a subsequent study in the USA, whereby medical specialists surveyed the views of actual people to whom the term applies. The study involved 128 women with CAH and 408 parents or other family members via email. Only 1% of the cohort expressed a favorable opinion of the term disorder. As many as 71% of respondents responded to the term with "dislike" or "strongly dislike" and the rest mainly ticked "neutral" or "don't mind" (Lin-Su et al., 2015).

An international European cohort recruited by medical professionals from their services in six countries were asked to rate their attitudes to disorders of sex development on a Likert scale (Bennecke et al., 2021). The authors noted that 31% of the sample did not consider the term relevant to them. They also noted that fewer people with XY conditions objected to DSD compared to people diagnosed with KS, TS and CAH. No favorable alternative label was found. A sizable minority, 179/941 participants, reported a preference for intersex. The authors concluded that a large majority (69%) reported that the term disorders of sex development applied to them *or* that they felt neutral about it (Bennecke et al., 2021). This conclusion seems rather uncritical, when close to one-third of the sample disagreed or strongly disagreed with the term DSD, despite being part of a medical cohort that had self-selected to participate in a study called DSD-Life.

Mixed and complex reactions were reported in a qualitative study with 37 affected adults and caretakers of affected children recruited from peer groups (Davis, 2015). All of the interviewees were familiar with the term DSD, indicating how unavoidable it had become. The author observed that participants who opposed the term often described more positive conceptualizations of the self but spoke of troubled relationships with family members and medical professionals. Participants who were more open to the term generally described positive relationships with families and medical professionals, but it was not uncommon for them to express feeling abnormal. Some individuals expressed a degree of exasperation at the terminology dispute. To these individuals, the priority is better health-care for children and families. As far as the term intersex was concerned, some of the research participants felt that the term was too political or had connotations of a third sex or a limbo state.

A recent quantitative study on the topic in the USA was carried out in collaboration with the largest US care advocacy group. The researchers surveyed the group membership, that is, outside the clinical environment (Johnson et al., 2017). The authors were honest about the low participation rate of 35%, though this was no lower than the aforementioned European study. The 202 participants comprised affected adults with a range of gender identities as well as caregivers of affected children with variations. The participants expressed negative emotional experiences of the use of the DSD term in clinics. Most of these individuals reported having changed their care as a result. About half of the participants expressed a preference for "intersex," "variation in sex development" and "difference of sex development," with "disorder" being preferred by the lowest number of people. Importantly, about a third of the sample expressed that they would not attend a service named as a disorder of sex development clinic. Most of the participants (81%) answered the open questions in the survey. The most frequent expression derived from the verbatim responses was the importance of flexible terminology by service users (Johnson et al., 2017).

Thus far, there is broad agreement that diagnoses of specific syndromes (e.g., TS, KS) are least objected to (Bennecke et al., 2021; Guntram, 2013; Lundberg et al., 2018). In general, care users appear to prefer to use direct descriptors, such as the adrenal gland not working, not having periods or not being able to have biological children.

As the Chicago consensus was approaching its tenth anniversary, several leading pediatric endocrinologists called for an ambitious global update to assess progress along multiple dimensions. Diverse stakeholders worked in separate virtual groups on key themes. The naming group involved medical specialists, psychologists, intersex advocates and humanities scholars. Described as long and complex, the process lasted many months. The working group, which appeared to have shrunk significantly in size presumably due to withdrawal and disengagement, had had their work made needlessly more difficult by an unclear agenda and oscillating remit. Despite the many challenges, those who remained in the group carried out a painstaking analysis of email exchanges of 80 000 words alluding to 300 points, comments and queries. The product was a nuanced account by Delimata et al. (2018) of passionate feelings about terminology and the complex reasons for the strong feelings, which vindicate Davis' (2015) comment that the renaming of intersex as DSD has not been a "victimless victory" for service users (Davis, 2015, p. 46). Debate over terminology is a contest between people from irreconcilable epistemological standpoints. The impressive contribution by Delimata et al. (2018) to the literature is an indispensable starting point for any future debate on terminology.

2.6 Disputes over Inclusion and Prevalence

Although prevalence is a most frequently asked question about DSD, it is not very meaningful, because DSD is not a fixed and stable entity but a collective concept still being debated. Just as the scientists in the nine-teenth century disputed their predecessors' classification, so contemporary scientists are doing exactly the same. For example, some experts have argued for CAH to be removed from the DSD taxonomy. The argument is that gender assignment and gender identity is unproblematic for the majority of chromosomal females and males with CAH who do not present problems of the reproductive development tract (González & Ludwikowski, 2018). This concurs with a pre-Chicago observation that CAH (and the other rare causes of masculinized sex anatomy in XX babies) is "not strictly disorders of sex determination and sex differentiation" (Hughes, 2002, p. 771). A clinical guidance for CAH does not reference intersex or DSD at all (Speiser et al., 2010) and described "early single-stage genital repair (a new term for one-stage childhood feminizing geni-toplasty) for severely virilized (defined as Prader staging 3 or above) girls" (p. 4143). Moving certain diagnoses out of the DSD nomenclature could mean evasion from potential restrictions of cosmetic genital surgery on children with DSD in future.

The term *variations in sex characteristics* (VSC) has been introduced to refer to the same phenomena as those under the DSD banner. In using the term VSC, Roen and Lundberg (2020) does not limit it to specific medical diagnoses, genital variations or medical interventions but highlight expe-riences of living with bodily difference coded as relating to *sex development*. The problem is, research findings based on a range of definitions are often discussed together as if they relate meaningfully to each other when cross-comparisons are being made across heterogenous populations. This may not matter for some research questions but can be hugely problematic for others.

Using a rather broad definition that includes any "individual who deviates from the Platonic ideal of physical dimorphism at the chromo-somal, genital, gonadal or hormone levels" (Blackless et al., 2000, p. 161), prevalence of atypical sex traits is estimated to be in the region of 1.7% of the population. This definition is said to be too broad (Sax, 2002), though one might ask too broad or too narrow for what purpose and in whose interests.

Prevalence of conditions associated with atypical external genitalia is estimated to be in the range of 1:2 000–1:4 500 live births (Hughes et al., 2007). In terms of overall prevalence as defined by the Chicago nosology, prevalence is estimated to be 0.1%–0.5% of live births (Ahmed et al., 2014). The Chicago consensus notes that if all congenital genital anoma-lies are included, including crytorchidism and hypospadias, then the rate may be as high as 1:200 or 1:300. Prevalence is likely to be variable in different regions of the world, with some being more common in regions where consanguinity is practised, for example parts of the Middle East, north and sub-Saharan Africa and west, central and south Asia. In more privileged nations where prenatal diagnosis of DSD is becoming more common and continuation with a pregnancy is a choice, prevalence of a range of variations (not just DSD) can be expected to reduce.

2.7 Implications for Psychological Practice

The goalpost of the biomedical odyssey that began in the nineteenth century has moved from separation of real and pseudo hermaphrodites, to finding the true sex of all patients, to giving every patient a genetic diagnosis. The new classification scheme drawn up in 2006 has facilitated biomedical advances, but the terminology remains vehemently debated. It is doubtful that substitution of the word disorder with differences, divergence or diversity of/in sex development would enhance acceptance or reduce stigma. Intersex is also a negative term for the majority of people impacted by sex variations. Specialist psychological practitioners are required to be fluent in the language of medicine in order to participate in DSD services. The language of medicine is, however, just the starting point. The end point is its deconstruction and the construction of preferred meanings. How to do this work in an intensely biomedical space is an ongoing question for psychological care providers. Reflections with care users on the dilemma of how to talk and think about bodily differences are not a means to an end but the very substance of a rich, moving and mutually transformative dialogue.

CHAPTER 3

Medical and Psychological Controversies

For a very long time, information about sex variations was concealed from care users, especially (but not exclusively) women with XY chromosomes whose variations were internal and who were diagnosed in adolescence or adulthood. This practice held the individuals back from understanding about their bodies and having a say in what was being done to them. Not surprisingly, many people later said that despite not being told the truth, they were aware that they were somehow different, not least because their bodies seemed to arouse such intense professional interests.

In terms of children whose variations were visible at birth, gender assignment used to revolve around the size of the phallus and surgical expedience. Children whose phallus was considered too small for them to live as male were assigned female. Once assigned female, the phallus, which was now considered too large as a clitoris, would be surgically reduced in size to achieve a more "feminine" appearance. This practice was meant to protect children from anticipated stigmatization in the social sphere. Genital "normalization" was taken for granted to the extent that there appeared to have been no need to methodically research the long-term effects. For several decades, the widespread practice of "normalizing" surgery was conveniently justified by contemporary psychological theories about gender development.

Voices of adult survivors of prevailing medical practices have become increasingly audible since the early 1990s. Many adults have spoken of their experiences of *medical trauma* and demanded healthcare reforms. Their voices have evolved and diversified to articulate a buoyant, energetic and influential worldwide advocacy movement with many creative strands. These developments are the subject of Chapter 5. The current chapter is a succinct narrative of controversial medical and psychological practices spanning the latter half of the twentieth century.

3.1   Concealment

In 2020, a publication in the *British Journal of General Practice* (Williams, 2020) reads:

> Although I was diagnosed with androgen insensitivity syndrome (AIS) shortly after I was born, it took over 23 years until I was finally told the truth about my diagnosis. (p. 598)

The author, now a medical doctor herself, tells about the time when she had her testes removed:

> When I was 14, my childhood doctor gave me a devastating and fictional story of how my ovaries were pre-cancerous and needed to be removed – and wrapped this up in a cloak of secrecy and the advice that I never needed to tell anyone. I was offered no psychological support and was sent home with a prescription for HRT and a deep feeling of shame about my body. (p. 598)

Gender-normative women with XY chromosomes used to be the most likely group to have been lied to, although the first ever such stories told to me were actually by men who had found photographs of themselves as children in medical textbooks. Indeed the incidents triggered the referral to me by their then treating physician. Dissatisfied by evasive answers, the men had taken upon themselves to search for information in medical libraries. Imagine their surprise.

In 2002, two women with complete AIS gave permission to a group of UK clinicians to publish their experiences of seeing their childhood clinical photographs in medical journals (Creighton et al., 2002). XY conditions were considered so shocking that it was in the women's interests that "no information regarding the precise nature of their abnormality should be made available to these patients" (Perez-Palacios & Jaffe, 1972, p. 665). But many XY women recounted how medical curiosity about their body and evasive answers by adults had raised suspicion early on that they were "different" to other girls.

The practice of total and partial concealment of information was far from unique to intersex/differences in sex development (DSD) medicine. Rather, it reflected broader medical paternalism in time and place. Furthermore, professional assumptions of the risks of full diagnostic and prognostic information were not entirely unfounded. Eugen Bleuler, a German psychiatrist in the nineteenth century, is reported to have invented the term "iatrogenic illness" to describe a patient's psychological distress caused by a physician's communication of a poor medical prognosis (see Prigerson et al., 2016). Studies have demonstrated that mishaps and injuries are higher in the weeks before and after a cancer diagnosis (Prigerson et al., 2016). Of course, this is not an acceptable reason for lying to patients. Research with care providers in other clinical settings has demonstrated that concealment of diagnosis is often motivated by the care providers' own need to protect themselves and stay in control. In fight-flight mode, they often choose to manage their own anxiety of imaginary reactions from patients by not telling them the whole story (Panagopoulou et al., 2008).

Between the mid-1990s and 2000s, stories about haphazard, incidental discovery of sex variations were a regular feature in my practice as a clinical psychologist. Some women told me that they did not have full disclosure of their diagnosis and treatment history until midlife (Liao, 2003). Their explanations for not having pressed harder for information included a fear of upsetting family members, whose responses to being questioned included bursting into tears, walking out of the room or saying they had "been through hell" (p. 231). Care users also feared recrimination from doctors as they thought perhaps they had a life-threatening illness. Their confusion was at times exacerbated by outlandish remarks by health professionals, for example to the effect that they would "never have sex" or that they would never get pregnant so why not "lie back and enjoy it" (p. 231).

Care users described muddling through the years and at times stumbling upon information, such as seeing someone on a television program who described similar characteristics or experiences, or listening to a lecture on sex development at college. The information fragments from multiple sources often confused rather than clarified, as in an example of a woman with complete AIS who told me that she had learned about having testes and XY chromosomes at age 16 years but, 9 years on, at age 25, she still thought that she was having a hysterectomy when her testes were being removed (Liao, 2003). In line with medical recommendations, "genetic males" who "act, behave, and think of themselves as women" should be persuaded to have their testes removed due to the risk of cancer and for the testes to be "referred to as ovaries in discussion with the patient" (Perez-Palacios & Jaffe, 1972, p. 664). In the 1990s, when peer support and intersex activism groups were formed, many people self-diagnosed by comparing themselves to narratives in newsletters and websites.

Similar stories of concealment were identifiable across several countries (Alderson et al., 2004; D'Alberton, 2010; Davis & Feder, 2015; Dreger, 1999), suggesting that the practice was widespread. Across available accounts was a consistent observation that secrecy had had care users fearing the worst (e.g., that they might have cancer), and that this practice had caused far more suffering than the diagnosis might have done. However, concealment of information had other serious implications, not least an ethical and legal breach of self-determination relating to receiving treatment and to being researched. As expressed by pediatric psychologist Franco D'Alberton (2010), without full disclosure, a person receives medical interventions under a false pretext and that to be deceived in this way is to be pulled along the path of rage, sorrow and regret. Concealment also meant that care users had no way of reaching out to each other for mutual support. The arrival of the Internet in the home was a catalyst that enabled many individuals to find each other and come out of total isolation. Feelings of anger and betrayal were expressed in a proliferation of care user publications in the 1990s and 2000s (see also Chapter 5).

3.2 The Gaze

Assessment of genital morphology is integral to diagnosing sex variations in infancy and adolescence, but conversations about ethically and psychologically informed protocols did not make their way into intersex medicine for quite some time. Intersex services are highly specialized and generally located in teaching hospitals, where learners and observers congregate. Even today, it is not uncommon for an infant to be examined by a large team of senior physicians and trainees – hands on. Health professionals may consider it acceptable because the infant or child purportedly does not know what is happening. From a psychological perspective, however, such acts devalue the child and demean the caretakers who have to witness them. Caretakers have expressed feeling troubled by these encounters, which made them feel as if their baby was a "show-horse" (Crissman et al., 2011, p. 7). After discharge, the child usually attends clinics as an outpatient. Further evaluation takes place at each visit, by the same specialists, often joined by additional colleagues and learners passing through. The genitals may be photographed time and again. The absence of flat refusals by patients may have been mistaken as unproblematic acceptance. Feder (2006), for example, told the story of her informant "Mary," who had consented to her young daughter "Jessica" to be examined by "scores of male residents" (p. 199) because Mary believed that being observed in that way was a nonnegotiable trade-off for receiving care in teaching hospitals. Jessica was only able to speak of the devastating sense of violation as an adult.

References to the potential for children to experience genital examinations and photography as sexually abusive were mooted early on (Money & Lamacz, 1987). Memories of degrading and shaming childhood experiences were an important finding of the first known large-scale qualitative study by sociologist Sharon Preves (1998). Psychological therapists have drawn attention to adults' overwhelming distress as they recount experiences of pediatric management (Williams, 2002). More recent research echoes the finding that adult survivors report childhood genital examinations as stigmatizing (Meyer-Bahlburg et al., 2017). Care users have spoken to me of being "paraded" in front of large numbers of clinicians without knowing for what purpose (Liao, 2003, p. 231).

Children on genital surgery paths are particularly vulnerable, because clinicians need to examine the anatomy of the growing child in order to evaluate their intervention and to take photographs for teaching and learning purposes. Genital assessment practices may vary between services but, in the absence of a binding protocol that centralizes patient welfare, it is left to individual practitioners and clinics to interpret what is appropriate and what counts as a sensitive approach.

The psychological impact of such potentially toxic exposure begs investigation, but methodical research dedicated to this specific topic is sparse (Tishelman et al., 2017). A groundswell of first-person accounts of traumatic medical encounters has emerged in the grey literature. On reviewing the 18 care user narratives in a special issue edited by Davis and Feder (2015), I ponder over the extent of parental compliance with what appeared to be a shocking level of intrusion on the child. A Swedish study with 13 women with congenital adrenal hyperplasia (CAH) suggests that service users feel highly dependent on the physicians. All of the women in the study reported that the main focus of their clinic appointments was "between their legs" (Engberg et al., 2016, p. 24). The power imbalance would make it difficult for people to question the medical process for fear of repercussions. Nevertheless, professional unease was evident among some pediatric specialists who, in the context of CAH, warned against "the repeated psychological insult caused by frequent genital examinations and operations" (Jääslekäinen et al., 2001, p. 73). However, such observations were often incidental in medical publications. The topic has never received dedicated medical or psychosocial investigation.

The gaze brings patients under control and enables experts to monopolize the process. While it is unproductive to blame individual doctors for a practice that reflects hegemonic biomedical culture, integral to which is "a process of objectification in which the individual patient or layperson was rendered largely invisible and obliged to be passive in the face of expert advice" (Crossley, 2000, p. 20), much can be learned from research with general population samples.

Research with large general population samples has shown that negative experiences of pelvic examinations are common, especially among younger women and those who have not given birth (Fiddes et al., 2003), albeit the effects are transitory for most people. Nurse practitioners have drawn attention not only to embarrassment and anxiety in girls having their first pelvic examination but also to potential feelings of inadequacy in the practitioner (McCarthy, 1997, p. 247). Research suggests that health professionals are not always adept at predicting women's feelings and expectations or dealing with their discomfort (Fiddes et al., 2003). Ethically informed discussions of intimate examinations across general medicine (Coldicott et al., 2003; Lesnik-Oberstein, 1982) suggest the need to maximize psychological safety for care providers as well as care users. Research has focused more on women than men, but this trend is changing (Fairbank, 2011). Professional conversations over the years have resulted in care protocols to prepare care users and provide clinicians with sensitive and nuanced training (Domar, 1986). Intersex medicine has much to gain from developments in other areas of medicine on how to take better care of clinicians and patients before, during and after pelvic examinations.

3.3 An "Optimal-Gender Policy"

Intersex surgery began to increase in the USA from the 1930s, due in part to the pioneering work of Hugh Hampton Young at Johns Hopkins Hospital (Chase, 1998). By late 1940s, most medical experts in the USA agreed that surgical decisions should be based on psychosexual and emotional rather than gonadal factors. A surgeon was quoted to go as far as saying that "the anatomic structure of the gonads should be the least determining factor" (Reis, 2009, p. 126). Other physicians were less sure. The vexing question of assigning "hermaphrodites" to the wrong sex persisted, and there was no coherent rationale to guide sex assignment methodically and consistently. The emergent work of John Money and his colleagues Joan and John Hampson was to provide medical specialists with an elegant solution. In this section, I draw on scholarly analyses that have become available in recent years. Of note is the book *Fuckology: Critical Essays on John Money's Diagnostic Concepts* that comprises six single-authored chapters by humanities scholars Lisa Downing, Iain Morland and Nikki Sullivan (2014).

Money's academic output spanned several decades. His work in intersex might have been pivotal in establishing his authority as a sexologist, but his interests were much wider and included transsexuality and the paraphilias. Detailed examination of Money's writing suggests an expansive intellect that engaged with multiple disciplines and standpoints, an intellect that enjoyed big words, new vocabularies and befuddling pedantry. His lecture in 2002 on paraphilia exemplified these characteristics, when he espoused his vision for a supposed different sexology (which turned out to be more of the same). Referenced as a "biomedical/social soup," Money's thesis called for:

> A developmental theory based on longitudinal, not cross-sectional studies. Such a theory will, of necessity, be not univariate, but multivariate. The variables will be genomic status, hormonal history (prenatal and postnatal); sexual brain cell functioning; history of toxic, infectious, or traumatic exposure; infantile pairbonding; juvenile troopbonding; juvenile sexual rehearsal play; sex education; adolescent sexual history; amative history in imagery; ideation and practice and so on. (quoted in Downing et al., 2014, p. 43)

Money is often credited for developing a so-called optimal-gender policy for intersex in the USA. The term was a replacement for the hitherto prevailing "true-sex policy" (Meyer-Bahlburg, 1999, p. 3455). The development had a multidisciplinary lead-up. Observations of intersex patients and a review of the literature up to the 1950s led experts at Johns Hopkins to conclude that gender assignment had not always followed a protocol. However, whichever gender was assigned in infancy, it usually prevailed in adulthood, regardless of biological sex markers. The idea of gender plasticity made sense when looking at the pool of information (from the professionals' point of view). Infants could be assigned to either gender of rearing based on expected optimal outcomes along reproductive, psychosexual and mental health dimensions.

Before Lawson Wilkins, often referred to as the father of pediatric endocrinology, demonstrated the effectiveness of cortisone on symptoms of CAH, which included progressive virilization in chromosomal females, his concern for the welfare of the children had led him to support the assignment of severely virilized XX children as boys (Feder, 2014, p. 26). The idea of gender plasticity was already in place. Money's subsequent psychosexual differentiation theory did not represent a pioneering departure *from*, as often implied in the literature, but an expansion *of* Wilkins' approach (based, presumably, on intuition). Money's approach to intersex, which took on board a collection of interesting ideas, did not look anything like a coherent developmental theory, rather an evolving case management protocol for ambiguous genitalia (Kessler, 1998).

Money joined Johns Hopkins (where feminizing surgery had already been developing) at the invitation of Wilkins (see Karkazis, 2008). The group of experts, which included psychiatrists Joan and John Hampson, was poised to settle the management of doubtful sex (Feder, 2014, p. 30). It would have been unthinkable, even for Money, to conceptualize a psychology that was unpalatable to medical experts, whose work had begun to define Johns Hopkins as a pioneering center for intersex management (Chase, 1998). The experts would have been looking for a psychology/sexology to complement and advance intersex medicine, not to contradict it and turn the clock back. Money might have aspired to science, which would have been a requirement at the institution, but he was no slave to epistemology and methodology. He strung together a bucket list of interesting ideas at the time. The ideas included the German ethologists' concept of *critical period* for *imprinting* and the Freudian notion of penile visibility in male gender development. He came up with a mixed account of gender development for intersex management. It posited that there is a window for gender assignment up until about 18 months of age. Money emphasized the role of the parents in augmenting gender development. For parents to carry out this role, they must be in no doubt as to whether their child was a boy or a girl. What would cast doubt would be genitals that are incongruent with the assigned gender. Money neither introduced nor disrupted the idea of surgery to normalize genital variations. He simply incorporated what was already being practiced, albeit not consistently, into his formulation as a matter of course and provided credibility for the practice to become consistent, indeed routine.

In one of several publications in 1955, the psychology/psychiatry trio reported the gender outcomes of 76 patients born with ambiguous genitalia (Money et al., 1955a). They observed that 30% had lived for more than two-thirds of their lives with external genital morphology that was incongruent with the assigned gender. They remarked about their patients as follows:

> For one reason or another, they did not receive surgical correction of their genital deformity in infancy, but lived with a contradictory genital appearance for at least five and for as many as forty-seven years. In all but one instance, the person had succeeded in coming to terms with his, or her anomaly, and had a gender role and orientation wholly consistent with assigned sex and rearing. (p. 307)

These observations suggest that, first of all, surgical sex assignment was not consistently practiced up until that point, that is, a good proportion of people had been missed – for one reason or another. Secondly, despite the gender-genital incongruity of these individuals who had missed out on surgical correction, all but four remained in their assigned gender. The team had no reason to consider surgical sexing essential for augmenting the assigned gender. This might have been a point worth driving home. Instead, a publication by Joan Hampson (1955) expressed concerns about the psychological difficulties of girls growing up with a large phallus. She referred to the testimony of "several patients" who apparently reported self-doubt and "teasing and questioning from others" on account of their genital variations. In that paper, Hampson's "best estimate" for the timing of clitorectomy was "as early as is consistent with surgical safety," which "serves additionally to remove parental doubt" (p. 271). Here was a piece of psychological guesswork that has proved remarkably resilient and still popular in intersex medicine, regardless of the ups and downs of Money's credibility in the decades to come.

Money's iteration of the idea of gender plasticity was in perfect dialogue with surgical notions of genital plasticity (an idea that is still very much alive). Children could be raised in whichever gender that was most amenable to surgical sex assignment (Downing et al., 2014, pp. 69–98). Here was an idea so self-evident to the medical community that it was to be denied proper theoretical and methodological scrutiny. Supportive evidence for Money's theory in the ensuing decades amounted to no more than "a handful of repeatedly cited cases" (Kessler, 1998, p. 15). However, it resonated with "contemporary ideas about gender, children, psychology and medicine" and attained the status of gospel among its practitioners (Kessler, 1998, p. 15). Every major city in the USA was to have an intersex clinic that would shoehorn nondimorphic bodies into dimorphic lives (Chase, 1998).

Where Money and the Hampsons' writing departed from preferred practices of their medical colleagues at the time, it was generally ignored. For example, they advised doctors to tell caretakers as well as children the truth. In one of their 1955 articles, the psych trio devoted large chunks of writing on disclosure to parents and patients about intersex. Their advice: "a proper vocabulary equips parents to talk straightforwardly with the child and to answer questions as the need arises." They elaborated:

> An hermaphroditic child needs only eyes and ears to know that the focus of medical attention is on his or her genitals, even if the hermaphroditism is concealed. Thus, far from burdening them with unnecessary worries, it is actually a lifting of the burdens of secret worries and doubts for the doctor to talk frankly with children. Truth is seldom as distressing as the mystery of the unknown. (Money et al., 1955b, p. 294)

Money et al. (1955b) went as far as to suggest the use of "sketches" if embryology was too difficult for laypersons to comprehend – a rather modern idea taken up decades later by peer support groups. In terms of fertility potential, the authors recommended: "If sterility is predictable, then it is preferable for a child to grow up with this knowledge rather than have it dramatically disclosed later in life" (p. 294). The authors suggested straightforward explanation as "a general policy" among care providers and ended their paper with the statement: "A clear and explicit understanding of basic principles is a prerequisite to frank and straightforward discussion" (p. 300). However, Money seemed to have changed his mind later. In relation to CAH, for example, considering the stigma, he later thought that it was preferable "to say nothing until wedding plans are under very serious consideration" (Money, 1968, p. 33, cited in Preves, 2003, p. 54). The mind changing may well reflect social conformity at Johns Hopkins and group think, a dangerous team characteristic whereby members converge toward rather than question each other's views.

In a strange article, Money and Lamacz (1987) drew attention to the harm of unbridled genital exposure and examinations. They cited the experiences of three girls whose exposure exemplified pediatric management of the time: One girl presented idiopathic precocious puberty and two genital variations. The authors made the observation that repeat genital exposure and examinations "may be experienced subjectively as nosocomial sexual abuse" (p. 713) and claimed that negative sequelae persisted into adulthood. The authors did not anchor their observation on psychological, bioethical and professional governance frameworks but situated their discussion, possibly strategically to warn doctors to act differently, on potential litigious implications.

Regarding childhood vaginoplasty, Money was of the opinion that vaginal absence was "of remarkably little concern to younger girls," "a psychologic issue only in early adult life" and was more manageable on a fully developed anatomy (cited in Downing et al., 2014, p. 79). All the same, vaginoplasty became a standard procedure for female-assigned infants. Regarding masculinizing surgery, Money was known to have been disparaging. For example, he was known to be critical of transsexual men for being "obsessed" with the idea of standing up to urinate. Referring to the result of phalloplasty as "a lump of meat," he suggested that transsexual men use a prosthesis for sexual activities to circumvent genital surgery (Downing et al., 2014, p. 80).

Medicine is a powerful system of socialization that exacts conformity as the price of participation. An important message of the Money debacle that is often missed is the implicit hierarchical relationship between medicine and psychology even on matters psychosocial. The nature of this relationship is rarely discussed in DSD. It is as important to stay curious about it today as it was in the Money era.

3.4   Size Matters

The Money publications of the 1950s may have helped to augment pediatric confidence in intersex management, as suggested by the tone of Lawson Wilkins' statement regarding the gender of rearing of infants with intersex variations: "When the diagnosis is made in early infancy, all types of female pseudohermaphrodites should be reared as females. In male pseudohermaphroditism the assignment of the gender role depends largely upon the degree of phallic development" (Wilkins, 1960, p. 846). With the hit and miss nature of earlier practices tidied away, visible genital variation in the newborn became a decidedly *social* emergency requiring crisis management but by *medical* doctors rather than social workers (Chase, 1998). A leading expert at the time explained: "Gender assignment and surgical correction must be done as early as possible to avoid subtle rejection of the child by the family, particularly if the patient's appearance is grossly discordant with the chromosomal or expected sex" (Donahoe, 1987, p. 1333). Note that the urgency refers not to physical health or survival, which is implicated in some intersex conditions, but the prevention of psychological harm. Doctors must mount an emergency *biomedical* response to avert anticipatory *psychological* problems. They must study the child's body and decide on a sex, which could not be just any sex but one that was "dictated entirely by the size of the phallus" (Donahoe et al., 1991, p. 537). It is fair to say that by the latter decades of the twentieth century, sex assignment had taken on unapologetic phallocentric and (hetero) sexist flavors. The commentary by the American Academy of Pediatrics (AAP) of 2000 contained positive aspects of care (see Feder, 2014). However, it also reiterated that the size of the phallus was "of paramount importance" in male sex assignment due to "the difficulty assessing the potential for penile growth" (AAP, 2000, p. 141).

   If doctors could rehabilitate the phallus to urinate from standing and be able to inseminate a woman, then it could be designated a penis, and the child could become a boy. If however the phallus was not very promising in that way, it would be designated a clitoris, and the child would have to be raised a girl, whose "offending shaft" (Randolf & Hung, 1970, p. 230) would be removed, along with the testes if present. Such grim predictions were at odds with an observational study by two urologists involving 12 men with a "micropenis" who had escaped social-surgical female sex assignment (Reilly & Woodhouse, 1989). The authors failed to observe the high levels of sexuality-related emotional and behavioral disturbance imagined by pediatric specialists of their days. While half of the men reported having been teased, all of them reported feeling male and experiencing erection and orgasm. Of the 12 men, 9 reported satisfaction with partnered or unpartnered sexual activities, and 7 were married or cohabiting. A contemporary case report involving 3 men with very small penises seeking counseling suggested that with support, couples were able to come to terms with genital variations and access positive sexual experiences (van Seters & Slob, 1988). These exceptions to contemporary professional narratives appear to have failed to capture medical imagination. There did not seem to be any appetite to investigate the alternative views.

Rather, gender assignment was to be guided by surgical expedience. Phalloplasty was crude and could not deliver a penis that met stereotypical male appearance and function. Girls and women on the other hand did not need anything to be built; they just needed their phallic tissue "subtracted" (Fausto-Sterling, 2000, p. 59). Specialists have been quoted to say, "You can make a hole but you can't build a pole" (Hendricks, 1993, p. 15). Female genitals are, in that sense, a receptacle. Female assignment became the norm and male assignment the exception, approximately in the ratio of 9:1 (Newman et al., 1992).

The genital anatomy was assessed using the Prader scale developed in the 1950s, initially to quantify the degree of genital masculinization of XX children with CAH and subsequently as a general tool for describing degrees of genital ambiguity. The genital anatomy is graded from 1 at one end for female-typical genitalia and 6 at the other end for male-typical genitalia including a penile urethra (see, e.g., Ogilvy-Stuart & Brain, 2004, p. 404). Figure 3.1 shows the satirical version called the Phall-O-Meter, produced by the Intersex Society of North America (ISNA) to poke fun at medical phallocentrism.

Nowadays, the external masculinisation score (EMS) is more likely to be used to assess genital phenotype when the presentation is anything other than female-typical (Ahmed et al., 2000). The EMS is a clinical scoring system based on the position of the gonads, stretched length of the phallus, presence of labioscrotal fusion and position of the urethral meatus to quantify the degree of "undervirilisation" in chromosomal males. More recently, the external genitalia score (EGS) has been developed as a gender-neutral alternative to the EMS (van der Straaten et al., 2020). The EGS

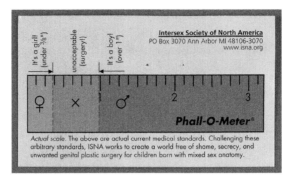

Figure 3.1   The satirical Phall-O-Meter produced by the ISNA. Reproduced with permission from Bo Laurent. A colour version of this figure can be found in the plate section.

takes account of the site of the urethral meatus and genital tubercle length in more detail, but it correlates well with the EMS.

Predicting the future adult's gender identity and sexual functioning from the size of a baby's phallus and the surgeon's ability to rearrange it has turned out to be highly problematic. Thus far, I have discussed professional reasoning and values in traditional medical management of intersex, the most controversial aspects of which are concealment of information and surgical "normalization" of genital variations that pose no threat to physical health. In the next chapter, I describe what normalization genital surgery is and discuss the evidence of benefits and costs from a psychosocial perspective.

3.5   Absence of Psychological Care

Given the extent to which pediatricians would go to protect intersex patients' mental health, the absence of psychological support made no sense. The Society of Pediatric Psychology was established within the American Psychological Association in 1968, and the *Journal of Pediatric Psychology* was founded eight years later. Psychological interests in pediatric conditions would have been evident by the 1970s. Yet there are numerous accounts of medical specialists in intersex failing to recommend psychological care for child, family and adult, when the needs would have been blindingly obvious (Davis & Feder, 2015). There are even accounts of patients being actively discouraged from seeking psychological help.

Psychological care is characterized by emotional safety to enable conversations to become increasingly honest and challenging. Through an ongoing dialogue, individuals develop awareness and insight about their strengths and concerns and make choices that are based on increased clarity and self-acceptance. Having been denied proper information about their variations, what would care users and their families be discussing with increasing candidness in psychological consultations? The absence of psychosocial support in the past may not have been incidental.

3.6 Implication for Psychological Practice

A number of factors coalesced to justify concealment and perpetuate sex-"normalizing" interventions. Medical discussions about sex assignment revolved around the infant's genitals, chromosomes, hormones and gonads, but with special emphasis on the potential for the child to become a cis-hetero-normative adult. Money's theory provided a convenient rationale that exonerated medical specialists from having to give a reason for a project that had begun before him and now continues without him. The widespread practice of surgical sex assignment in childhood has made it impossible to know about the physical, psychological, social and sexual realities of untreated genital variations. It is impossible to determine to what extent difficulties reported by adults are caused by their anatomical difference, other aspects of the diagnosis, the developmental interference, the imperfect results of surgery, poor psychological care, or some other factors. An important lesson from psychological failings in the Money era is the danger of psychological theories and practices being shaped by heteronormative values and complicit with ethically dubious medical practices.

CHAPTER 4

Adult Outcome of Childhood Genital Surgery

Childhood genital surgery has been a subject of intense debate for debate for almost three decades. In the more distant past, where discourses of diverse bodies and identities were less available, there was no conceivable alternative to respond to genital variations other than surgical "normalization." Care providers intervened with full conviction that surgery was in the best interest of the child. It was genuinely felt that the "normalized" genitalia would convince people (including the child) that the child was a boy or a girl, enable caretakers to accept and bond with the child and minimize problems with peers later. It was also felt that as an adult, the individual with "normalized" genitals would have the best chance for (heterosexual) pair bonding. These are cosmetic, functional, psychological and sexual outcomes. By definition they can only be verified by methodically following up children into adulthood, which means many years after the primary surgery. However, surgery was so self-evident that this kind of longitudinal research was not carried out. Furthermore, surgery was widespread, so that there would have been no comparison group available for research.

With hindsight, treatment benefits are not self-evident at all. Surgery is a technically and emotionally complex journey involving multiple operations, repeat hospital admissions and regular anatomical examinations to check results and note whether any further repair is required. It often is. From first-person accounts, the childhood surgery trajectory can have an enduring negative psychological impact on people who have been subjected to it.

Critics of childhood surgery have pointed out that young children are not preoccupied with their genital appearance, prepubertal girls do not menstruate, are not sexually active and have no need for a vagina, and prepubertal boys do not engage in penetrative sex. Therefore, surgery does not benefit the child. As far as augmenting gender identity is concerned, research shows that adults with sex variations are more likely than the general population to adopt nonnormative gender identities (Schweizer et al., 2014). For those who reassign gender and opt for reconstructive genital surgery, sensitive tissue that has been lost cannot be replaced. As for emotional benefits for caretakers, the impact on parental anxiety is mixed (Ellens et al., 2017).

The projected social harm of a bigger clitoris in a girl is underresearched, as is that of a boy who sits down to urinate. Although stigmatization is realistic (e.g., Meyer-Bahlburg et al., 2018), there is no evidence that surgery can prevent it. If anything, medical processes are stigmatizing in themselves (Meyer-Bahlburg et al., 2017). Noninvasive and psychological care programs should be developed, but none has been articulated and researched (Liao et al., 2015).

In an age where discourses of diverse bodies and identities are more available, one might wonder why surgery could not be delayed, if only to have more time to see how the child develops and whether the variation causes as much difficulty as feared. Chase (1998) suggested that young children are being operated on because they may resist surgery later, as did some of Hugh Hampton Young's patients. There have been examples of caretakers who resisted surgery for their children in the past (see, e.g., Dreger & Chase, 1999, pp. 83–89). However, professional anxiety about patients running away from surgery is unlikely to be the explanation for early surgery. Rather, caretakers who continue to struggle with children's genital variations are not presented with credible alternatives to manage the sense of threat.

Given the arguments, the process of informed consent must be detailed, rigorous and transparent. This means caretakers are guided over time toward a sound understanding of, first of all, what a surgical path actually entails. What is entailed is not just the primary surgery but a process that typically involves multiple operations, hospitalizations and examinations spanning a number of childhood years and potentially into adulthood too. Secondly, caretakers must be counseled on what makes such a care path controversial, what is known about the risks and benefits, and what is not known but could be important to the adult (Liao et al., 2018). These are the concerns of the current chapter, in which I provide a narrative summary of what is *feminizing* and *masculinizing* surgery and research with adults on a range of outcomes. Only the more substantial studies are included in the summary, whose purpose is to help psychological practitioners to understand that the focus of decision counseling must include the entire surgical trajectory and not just the primary surgery.

4.1 "Feminizing" Surgery

Once assigned female, unless caretakers refuse to give proxy consent, which used to be extremely rare but may be becoming less so, the clitoris deemed too big for a girl is usually reduced to a size deemed compatible with girlhood: "Infants raised as girls will usually require clitoral reduction which, with current techniques, will result not only in a normal-looking vulva but a functional clitoris" (AAP, 2000, p. 141). Although pediatric experts expressed few doubts that they could construct a sensate vulva to meet heterosexual requirements, it is not clear from the surgical literature what standards they had in mind. Clitoral measurements of newborn girls have been available since 1980 (Fausto-Sterling, 2000, p. 60), but the measurements are rarely cited in medical publications. Furthermore, "normal" female genitalia are highly variable in the general population (Lloyd et al., 2005). The diversity in vulval appearance is also unacknowledged in surgical publications. Rather than consult published measurements, surgeons presumably take a pragmatic stance and choose techniques that they know best to approximate an appearance that they deem normal.

Feminizing surgery to address hermaphroditism was identifiable in the nineteenth century (Dreger, 1998) but likely to date back to even earlier. Of the different clitoral operations, clitorectomy (amputation of the clitoris) may have had the longest history. It was performed throughout the nineteenth century as a cure for epilepsy, hysteria, insanity and masturbation in several European countries and North America. In intersex medicine, clitorectomy for female assigned children continued well into the 1960s (Fausto-Sterling, 2000, p. 61). In recent decades, girls have been more likely to undergo clitoral reduction or recession. Clitoral reduction involves cutting off most of the erectile tissue along the elongated phallus and sewing the glans and preserved nerve and blood supply (neurovascular bundle) back onto the clitoral stump. Clitoral recession involves pleating together the erectile tissue to shorten the clitoral shaft and hiding it under a fold of skin so that only the glans is visible. The clitoral skin may be used to create a clitoral hood and labia minora. Depending on the anatomical configuration of the child, some labioscrotal mass may be removed too.

The highly popular *one-stage feminizing genitoplasty* (Rink & Adams, 1998) means creating a vaginal opening at the same time, even though it has no anatomical purpose for the child and is considered to be the "most complex" component of the feminization package (DiSandro et al., 2015, p. 324). Again, it is uncertain what standard surgeons are aiming for. Is the neovagina meant to be proportionate to the body size of the infant and expected to grow proportionately with the rest of the child's body? Is it meant to be large enough to accommodate an imaginary adult penis in future? If the neovagina is meant to be a cosmetic device to reassure adults and further surgery has been in the plans all along, is not the one-stage promise a deception?

The type and extent of vaginal construction depends on the genital formation of the girl (Creighton et al., 2012). In congenital adrenal hyperplasia (CAH), for example, the operation may be a simple incision to connect the internal vagina to the surface (introitoplasty), or extensive dissection to separate the urethra and vagina and bring them to the surface of the perineum as two separate openings (urogenital sinus mobilization). Sometimes skin flaps are required to bridge the distance from the vagina to the perineum. These procedures risk urethrovaginal fistula, shrinkage (stenosis) of the neovagina and injury to the continence mechanism (DiSandro et al., 2015). The genital tissue may grow pubic hair inside the vagina at puberty. Postoperatively, the girl usually has to perform daily dilation to keep the neovagina open and, controversially, if too young to manage this, her adult caretakers might have to dilate the vagina.

For XY girls without a female-typical perineum, a segment of the gut is cut out to create a vagina (Creighton et al., 2012). Transplantation of gut to make a vaginal vault was first described in 1904 but soon ceased (Lima et al., 2010), presumably due to catastrophic consequences. Surgical techniques and safety, however, continued to improve, so that any permanent damage to vital function or loss of life was to become more rare, and gut vaginoplasty became available again in the 1990s. Some surgeons still prefer this procedure as first-line treatment for girls with vagina agenesis (e.g., Hensle et al., 2006; Lima et al., 2010).

Until recently, early gonadectomy was standard for XY girls to avoid the increased risk of cancer and for gender compatibility: "The testes should be removed soon after birth in infants with partial androgen insensitivity or testicular dysgenesis in whom a very small phallus mandates a female sex of rearing" (AAP, 2000, p. 141). Postgonadectomy, lifelong hormone replacement is required for physical health. Ongoing research suggests that the cancer risk is relatively small for some conditions but high for others (Ahmed et al., 2021; Cools et al., 2018; Lee et al., 2016). Depending on the diagnosis, more XY women with testes today are choosing to keep their testes in order to avoid having to take replacement hormones for their long-term health, but this would have been unusual before the 2000s.

Publications in feminizing surgery are mainly concerned with descriptions of operative techniques, sometimes with throwaway remarks alluding to high success rates and "normal" sensation and function without further elaboration. Studies that actually looked at outcome typically examined short-term physical effects from the providers' perspectives in small case series. The optimism was presumably maintained by an absence of complaint. Angela Moreno (1999) described being "put on show" in front of young residents before her clitoris was removed without her knowledge at age 12 years. She spent the next 10 years in "a haze of disordered eating and occasional depression" (p. 138). When she obtained her medical records in her twenties, she was shocked to see herself described in medical notes as having "tolerated [the surgery] well" (p. 138). Without probing into patients' and families' experiences, the confident tone in pediatric reports is unsurprising. Below is a brief overview of studies with adults who had undergone childhood feminizing genitoplasty.

One of the first studies that examined psychological variables from patients' perspectives involved 34 women with CAH, who were compared to 14 unaffected women in terms of sexual function (Dittman et al., 1992). The CAH group was less likely to have experienced partnered sexual activities and one-third of the sample reported anorgasmia. In a subsequent study, the sexual experiences of women with CAH were compared with those of women with insulin-dependent diabetes (May et al., 1996). The comparison group was chosen with a clear rationale: 1) both CAH and Type 1 diabetes are metabolic diseases involving regular medications and hospital visits, 2) both diagnoses are associated with potential sexual difficulties and 3) both groups had attended the same paediatric hospital as contemporaries. This study reported 41% anorgasmia in the CAH group compared to 12% in the diabetes group. Compared to the women with diabetes, the women with CAH were less sexually experienced (e.g., less likely to have masturbated), more avoidant of intimate relationships and, when in relationships, were likely to engage in sexual activities in order to test what their surgeons had done. The CAH group also reported more sexual anxiety, more communication difficulties, more preoccupation with coitus and, importantly, fewer attempts at problem-solving, such as trying everyday solutions like a lubricant to deal with vaginal discomfort. The authors interpreted the differences between the two clinical groups in terms of the different ways in which the two childhood conditions were managed. In contrast to the CAH group, the diabetes group understood their condition, had extensive and ongoing educational input and could openly discuss difficulties with their sexual partners. Interestingly, the CAH group disclosed feeling unable to discuss their sexual concerns with medical practitioners. Absence of complaints may have been taken by treatment providers to mean that sexual experiences were positive, as observed in an interview study with pediatric specialists (Kessler, 1998).

The formation of peer support groups, the emergence of intersex activism (see Chapter 5) and a wave of publications in the 1990s prompted gynecological interests in recalling adults who had been operated on in childhood. A report in the UK based on examinations of 14 girls with CAH with an average age of 13 years raised grave concerns about the multiple operations and the need for yet more work for all but one of the girls (Alizai et al., 1999). The authors reported fibrosis and scarring to be most evident in girls who had undergone "aggressive attempts at vaginal reconstruction in infancy." Their conclusion:

> These disappointing results, even in the hands of specialists, highlight the importance of late follow up and challenge the prevailing assumption that total correction can be achieved with a single stage operation in infancy. Although simple exteriorization of a low vagina can reasonably be combined with cosmetic correction of virilized external genitalia in infancy, we now believe that in some cases it may be best to defer definitive reconstruction of the intermediate or high vagina until after puberty. The psychological issues surrounding sexuality in these patients are inadequately researched and poorly understood. (Alizai et al., 1999, p. 1588)

The above observations contradicted the optimistic tone of pediatric literature up until that point. The report was swiftly followed by a more extensive gynecological evaluation, also in the UK, involving 44 adolescents and adults with CAH (Creighton et al., 2001). These clinicians replicated the observation that despite undergoing what was meant to be a one-stage feminizing genitoplasty, most of the girls and women had had multiple operations by the time they reached adolescence. Almost all of them required further surgery to permit menstrual flow or vaginal intercourse or both because of stenosis of the neovagina. The same group of clinicians subsequently recruited 28 women with mixed diagnoses associated with genital variations for a further study (Minto et al., 2003a). Both the surgery (n = 18) and no-surgery (n = 10) groups completed self-report measures of sexual function. Both groups reported sexual difficulties, but 25% of the clitoral surgery group reported anorgasmia compared to 0% of the no-surgery group. The next study by the same team involved assessing genital sensitivity of 22 women born with genital variations and 10 healthy controls using the GenitoSensory Analyzer®. Sensitivity was significantly reduced in the clinical sample. Impaired sensitivity was specific to the site where surgery had taken place and was clinically significant in its association with lower scores in self-reported sexual function (Crouch et al., 2008). The research group could not identify different outcomes for women who had undergone so-called nerve-sparing techniques compared to women who had had a total clitorectomy, although the numbers were too small to ascertain this comparison statistically.

The groundswell of ensuing studies included a Swedish gynecological evaluation and clinical interviews with 62 women with CAH and 62 age-matched controls. The researchers reported high rates of vaginal stenosis, reduced sexual function and delayed sexual debut (Nordenskjöld et al., 2008). A French study involving 35 women with CAH and a control group assessed sexual wellness using a self-report measure. Sexual difficulties were identified for the CAH group, with 81% of the sample reporting sexual pain (Gastaud et al., 2007). Where vaginoplasty fails (e.g., stenosis and scarring), the option of dilatation without surgery is generally not feasible. This means further surgery is required to enable menstrual flow and, if desired, coitus.

Taken together, cross-sectional research with adults suggests that post-surgery genital appearance is deemed by experts to be unacceptable for 28%–46% of the care users examined (Alizai et al., 1999; Creighton et al., 2001; Nordenskjöld et al., 2008). Evaluation by care users themselves and by their sexual partners is, lamentably, scant. Vaginal stenosis was identified in 36%–100% of patients. Repeat operations were the norm for children who underwent a supposedly one-stage intervention (Creighton et al., 2001; Gastaud et al., 2007; Krege et al., 2000). One study identified clitoral regrowth in 39% of patients (Donahoe & Gustafson, 1994). Repeat surgery to the clitoris and vagina can seriously compromise sensitivity, function and appearance. These effects say nothing about treatment experience, which is highlighted in psychosocial literature.

A problem for researchers who question childhood feminizing genitoplasty is the claim that techniques have evolved and that the documented poor results no longer apply, as expressed by the European Society for Paediatric Urology and the Society of Pediatric Urology of the USA in 2014: "It is critical to understand that the outcomes which one evaluates today result from surgery performed 20 or more years ago with techniques which are now considered obsolete. It does not guarantee superior results from modern techniques but one will have to wait another 15 years to evaluate current procedures" (Mouriquand et al., 2014, p. 9).

Some pediatric urologists may have interpreted the current debate as a signal to develop better techniques rather than cease the practice of childhood feminizing surgery. Having been slow to engage with the challenging voices of intersex activists, bioethicists, social scientists and medical providers who oppose the practice, they may have missed the opportunity to put their perspectives forward in human rights debates (see Chapter 5), which are being advanced in their absence.

4.2 "Masculinizing" Surgery

For children with intersex/ differences in sex development (DSD) who are assigned male, a central focus of surgical management is the hypospadiac presentations. Intersex/DSD diagnoses are more likely to be associated with proximal (as opposed to distal) hypospadias, which generally means that the individual has to sit to pass urine and is unable to have penetrative sex (due to curvature, or *chordee*) or, if heterosexual, is not able to inseminate a partner. Distal hypospadias in the absence of chordee is common in the general population and recognized by many surgeons as mainly a cosmetic concern that is not necessarily experienced as a burden (Dodds et al., 2008). Experts are far more likely to agree with each other that proximal hypospadias requires treatment because the problem is not just cosmetic but functional (Wood & Wilcox, 2022).

The hypospadias literature is vast. Over 300 techniques with a wide variety of modifications have been described (Wood et al., 2019), not least because the genital presentations are so highly variable. In many situations, the genitalia may be more female- than male-typical in appearance and structure. The scrotum can be more labia-like and the hypospadiac meatus may be located in the perineum. Additional procedures may be carried out for scrotal reconstruction. Esthetic results and sexual and reproductive functions become important to adults, so that methodical follow-up into adulthood is the proper way to evaluate to what extent childhood surgery achieves its "normalizing" goals. However, many reports are based on short-term assessment of prepubertal children by the treating clinicians. These are heavily critiqued from within the pediatric urology community (Braga et al., 2016).

Reports on complication rates and other outcomes are variable in terms of results and methodological robustness. The permutations within the broad statistics of 5%–70% complication rates are mind-boggling, but perhaps unsurprising given the variability in anatomical presentation and surgical techniques. Risk factors for complications include the original urethral characteristics, age of primary surgery, endocrine factors, the patient's wound-healing capacity, the surgeon's expertise (defined by number of cases treated per year and choice of techniques) and postoperative management (Wood et al., 2019). Postsurgical cosmesis and penile length are worse for patients with the more severe (proximal) hypospadias, which is also associated with higher incidences of postsurgical spraying, dribbling after voiding, and urinary stream deviation (Wood et al., 2019), as well as persistent curvature that tends to surface postpuberty and also sexual difficulties (Wood & Wilcox, 2022).

Unlike patients with proximal hypospadias who are now recognized to require long-term follow-up that examines urinary and sexual function and fertility, surgery for distal hypospadias is often portrayed in the literature as straightforward with good results and requiring only short-term follow-up (DiSandro et al., 2015). A recent report gravely challenges this assumption. The US group examined their prospectively maintained hypospadias database and identified all patients undergoing primary hypospadias surgery between 2 and 13 years of age in the period between 2007 and 2018 (Lucas et al., 2020). The research group defined complications as a need for an additional unplanned surgical procedure. For this largest single-center cohort of 1280 individuals, the complication rate was 10% for distal hypospadias. The median time it took for complications to be detected was 83 months post primary surgery. As expected, the complication rate for proximal hypospadias was much higher, at 54%, although the median time it took for complications to surface was considerably shorter, at 29 months. Overall, only 47% of the complications would have been detected within the first year following surgery. This means reports based on short-term follow-up risk missing more than half the complication rates.

Some of the findings of the above single-center report resonate with those of a review in New South Wales that examined a cohort of 3186 boys with hypospadias born in 1946 in a 20-year period up to 2010 (Schneuer et al., 2015). Of this cohort, 61% had undergone surgery with an overall 13% complication rate involving fistulas or strictures. While outcomes were undoubtedly worse for proximal hypospadias (33% complication rate), the report concluded that, overall, 52% of the complications occurred more than one year later.

A recent consensus by a group of European urologists concluded that care users will require multiple operations, and that a significant percentage will develop complications secondary to the operation(s) (Wood et al., 2019). The complexities have led some specialists to remark that while "creating more typical male genitalia in boys who were born with atypical genitalia seems like a noble idea, studies are lacking regarding long-term outcome and quality of life" (DiSandro et al., 2015, p. 327). It is noteworthy that, for these authors, the trend toward assigning more children as boys is automatically taken to mean more *masculinizing* surgery. These experts summed up the current state of the art of *masculinizing* surgery as follows: "Because of the high complication rate there have been many surgical techniques developed and many variations of those techniques, in order to find an operation that works better than what had been done in the past. However, that perfect operation is quite elusive" (DiSandro et al., 2015, p. 327).

Thus far, there is no agreement on which techniques might result in the lowest complication rates and fewest lifetime operations for any type of hypospadias. Today's providers at least agree that surgery for proximal hypospadias is fraught with difficulties and that, whatever the quality of the research, it is undeniable that there are many different types of complications that could take years to become evident. The pattern of findings invalidates short-term study designs in this field.

Medical management of hypospadias is referenced by an expert as "more art than science" that "consumes tremendous energy and yields humbling results" (Canning, 2015, p. 284). In his commentary, this expert urged all urologists to not just conduct follow-up assessments but to do so methodically, which means including evaluations by the caretaker and, if appropriate, the patient. Given the more or less linear relationship between length of follow-up and number and extent of complications, a plea was made for surgeons to resist publishing before they have achieved a median five-year follow-up on more than a hundred patients, so as to be able to segregate the more easily corrected distal hypospadias without chordee from the more difficult to correct proximal hypospadias with chordee. In patients' best interests, surgeons are urged to be "painfully honest" as they report outcomes as appraised by themselves, caretakers and patients (Canning, 2015, p. 285). The commentary reflects a build-up of frustration among some hypospadias surgeons who, for some years, have called for better research.

An international task force recently critiqued biased observational case series with limited generalizability (Braga et al., 2016). These experts produced a checklist of 20 items to improve validity and transparency in reporting outcome and in ways that studies can be compared across. A recent review of modern surgical techniques for proximal hypospadias identified cosmetic, urinary and sexual concerns as expected and reiterated the call to use established evaluation tools consistently to improve research quality (Gong & Cheng, 2017). Since surgery is at least partly motivated by anticipated social and sexual benefits, I would add that evaluation is psychologically informed. Until better research informs us otherwise, current knowledge poses a serious challenge to earlier optimism (Donahoe et al., 1991).

Given the complications, it is not surprising that many caretakers express a level of regret in giving proxy consent on behalf of their sons to have surgery. In one study, parental regret one year after surgery for distal hypospadias was expressed by 50% of the sample (Lorenzo et al., 2014). Expression of regret was associated with development of complications. A subsequent study that also focused on distal hypospadias followed up 323 caretakers (Ghidini et al., 2016). Close to 40% of caretakers expressed moderate-to-strong regret. In this study, regret was associated with an initial desire to avoid surgery in the first place, rather than with the surgical method or the development of complications. This finding suggests that at least some caretakers may not have had sufficient space to voice and explore their doubt before giving proxy consent for the child. The most recent study suggests that while a degree of parental regret was prevalent for 45% of the sample, only 6.2% expressed moderate to severe regret – a much lower rate than previously suggested (Bethell et al., 2020). Regression analyses identified that a distal meatus, a small glans and development of complications requiring repeat surgery were predictive of increased levels of regret.

The surgical trade-off for mild hypospadias is likely to differ markedly from the trade-off for proximal hypospadias. A recent systematic review made this point and concluded that caretakers' postintervention evaluation of their decision relating to proximal hypospadias is underresearched (Vavilov et al., 2020). The authors also identified myriad confounding variables including those relating to the original presentation (e.g., meatal location, small size glans) and psychosocial factors relating to decision-makers (e.g., parental educational level, decision conflict between caretakers, initial desire to avoid surgery).

It is human nature to justify one's decision, even when it becomes questionable with hindsight. The simplistic survey methods used in hypospadias regret studies are woefully inadequate for saying anything meaningful about such a complex psychological phenomenon as regret in consenting for another. Rather than conclude prematurely that caretaker regret is astronomically high based on limited assessment methods and bias toward distal hypospadias, we could interpret the above regret studies as indicative of a need to conduct psychologically informed investigations into caretakers' and providers' postintervention evaluation. In Section 4.3 I justify my call for psychological theories to inform such endeavors.

4.3   Theoretical Critique

Prospective, longitudinal research on physical, psychological and sexual health and harm as appraised by care users constitutes the only convincing evidence for surgery. However, by early adulthood, many care users would have left (or lost themselves to) pediatric services. This means pediatric surgeons responsible for the primary surgery are unable to learn from patients who have become of age. Absence of longitudinal data, especially from service users' perspectives, means that caretakers who give proxy consent to surgery on their child are not fully informed.

There would have been opportunities to prospectively and methodically record the anatomical, functional and psychological effects of the different components of the surgical trajectory from care users' perspectives. The information would enable today's decision-makers to weigh up the complex trade-offs. These opportunities are now lost. Retrospective case reviews are the norm in research with adults, but such methods are far from ideal. Nevertheless, findings from available studies suggest that multiple genital operations are the norm. Research has focused mainly on women with CAH. These studies have demonstrated poor cosmetic results and impaired genital sensitivity and sexual function. Many care users are left with ongoing sexual anxiety and communication difficulties and lack of psychological skills to negotiate social and sexual situations.

Despite the equivocal outcomes, research with select samples of adult clinic attendees has observed a relatively high rate of acceptance of own childhood surgery (see Meyer-Bahlburg, 2022). Patients are typically asked about their attitudes in a tick-box exercise, as if such responses were neutral or meaningful. In the recent review of 10 such reports between 2000 and 2021 that asked adult patients about their views of early genital surgery, the reviewer is rightly critical of the methodological weaknesses of the studies, not least the low participation rate and therefore poor generalizability (Meyer-Bahlburg, 2022). Nevertheless, the overall pattern of findings suggests that, with some variability between types of diagnoses, there is general support for early surgery among adults with lived experience.

If an equal number of patients with delayed or no surgery were available for research, such studies are likely to identify support of delayed or no surgery. The absence of a direct (delayed and no surgery) comparison group places a severe limit on understanding. My criticism of the simplistic studies above applies equally to studies looking at parental regret of hypospadias surgery on children. Survey methods, some more nuanced than others, can be useful for addressing certain questions. When applied to topics that are conflicted and controversial, research methods that squeeze out the social and dilemmatic nature of thought are of limited value. Such methods have long been criticized in the social sciences. Billig et al. (1988), for example, raised serious concerns about psychological research that treats participants as respondents in cognitive balance with coherent and fixed values. The authors suggested that the research participant is looked upon as a conflicted deliberator giving culturally contingent expressions. They went as far as suggesting that without conflict and dilemma, there could be no deliberation, argumentation or thought.

Adults' reflections on their childhood surgery are an important topic for research, but such an inquiry needs to be embedded in robust knowledge frameworks that enable researchers to tease out multiple and potentially conflicted perspectives and interpretations. It is important to bear in mind several questions here: 1) What does it mean for adults with variations to disavow decisions made in their interests by loving parents who have endured significant distress on their account? What would such disavowal mean for the research participants' family relationships? 2) Given the lack of alternative discursive resources with which to construct alternative meanings of genital variations, how do medicalized adults imagine what could have been or should have been? 3) Given the absence of a non-surgical pathway, even today, how do individuals and families envision another way to respond to genital variations?

Below I briefly mention three non-DSD studies, to indicate just how important it is for researchers to elicit meaningful expressions about receiving interventions. I do so with one purpose only – to make a case for future research to be less reductionist and more nuanced. Firstly, an interview study in the UK asked a group of young women about the effects of childhood female genital cutting (FGC) that their parents had endorsed (Parikh et al., 2020). Many of the participants, as in previous FGC research, did not make the connection between their current mental health and sexual difficulties with a childhood event long forgotten about. Furthermore, talking about their cutting as a problem created enormous dilemmas in how their families and community might be positioned in relation to nonpracticing families and communities. Secondly, I draw attention to a Norwegian qualitative study with women who had undergone clitoral reconstruction after FGC (Jordal et al., 2021). A mixture of perceived benefits and disappointment was identified in the research participants' accounts. However, even the disappointed women expressed gratitude for being given an operation, because it meant that their problem was being taken seriously. Finally, in a qualitative study involving women with cloacal anomalies, gratitude to the care providers was a barrier to expressing regret for having accepted treatments that had resulted in more complications (Liao et al., 2014).

The above reports and many other studies highlight the usefulness of a discursive or phenomenological paradigm in researching how people construct options, preferences and rights, what it means to have accepted treatment with mixed outcome, and how feelings of gratitude, disappointment, ambivalence and regret are strategically expressed for oneself and another. When researching phenomena that implicate one's relationships with one's own family and culture of belonging, such as those pertaining to attitudes to childhood surgery, then question, method and interpretation need to be guided by explicit knowledge frameworks that can make sense of research participants' expressions.

Theories have always been centrally important in psychosocial research and practice. Constrained by the biomedical framing, the nontheoretical nature of much of psychosocial research in DSD is of limited value to psychological practice. In Chapter 7, I argue for the central importance of psychological theories in research and practice in intersex/DSD and to hold in mind how power gives space to some expressions and restricts others.

4.4   Implications for Psychological Practice

Surgical sexing of children whose future identities are not yet known needs to be supported by evidence. This means methodical and ethical follow-up of children into adolescence and adulthood with detailed assessment of anatomical appearance and function, psychosocial well-being and sexual function. Without a rigorous approach to prospective longitudinal research, it is impossible to determine to what extent the current difficulties reported by adults are caused by the anatomical and functional difficulties that surgery has created or left behind, the developmental interference that they have been subjected to over the years, other aspects of the diagnosis, poor psychological care, or some other factors.

With all its imperfections, empirical research with adults has accumulated to highlight the potentially high human costs of childhood surgery. It is regrettable that the vast body of work comprising first-person accounts, empirical research and scholarly analyses involving experts in medicine, psychology and sociology is not taken more seriously in DSD medicine. The limitations of surgery are more likely to be acknowledged in contemporary medical publications. However, framed in the language of an *individualized* approach, the practice continues to evade questioning. There is still no concerted investment in conceptualizing and researching psychosocial care paths.

CHAPTER 5

Advocacy, Public Engagement and Healthcare Reform

From the mid-1990s, the visibility of intersex lives began to increase, initially via support and advocacy group publications such as $A^L T^A S$ by the Androgen Insensitivity Syndrome Support Group in the UK (AISSG UK) and "Hermaphrodites with Attitude" by the Intersex Society of North America (ISNA). Adult first-person accounts referenced difficult communications within the family and in peer and romantic relationships, and the psychological impact of harmful medical practices. A sense of loneliness, isolation and shame could be identified in almost every account, as well as dread of being discovered as having a sex development variation. Many individuals reported having believed that they were the only person in the world in the same situation. Caretakers recounted memories of grief and confusion when their child was diagnosed.

First-person accounts were read by a new generation of care providers who, unburdened by a past that needed defending, were eager to educate themselves about care user perspectives. Health professionals practicing in countries without support groups would adopt support group newsletters to pass on to their patients. Media interests followed. Mainstream newspaper and magazine articles, television documentaries, literary works and feature films that air intersex issues have been accumulating over the years. *Intersex*, as somatic traits, lived experience and personal identity, though still poorly understood, has at least perforated through the shroud of medical secrecy. Relationships within the advocacy movement and between advocacy groups and medicine have however become increasingly complex.

In this chapter, I draw on online dictionaries to define "advocacy" to mean action to influence policies within economic, political and social systems and institutions. Action may include public speaking, knowledge production, research and petitions, and negotiations with officials and organizations. In that sense, peer support is a form of advocacy. It involves producing educational material to dispel myths, facilitate research and negotiate better healthcare. Intersex activism is another form of advocacy that involves different approaches that may include confrontational and disruptive acts such as public protests, boycotts and rallies.

Although destigmatization and improvement to healthcare were goals shared among peer support and activism groups in different parts of the world, their focus, methods and affiliations were richly diverse, as were the identities of the actors involved. Some groups that were active in the 1990s have continued to thrive. Others have discontinued. New groups have emerged. In general, intersex activism is anchored in opposition to nonessential medical and surgical interventions that are driven by cultural norms of binary bodies, functions and identities. Peer support, on the other hand, tends to emphasize education and encourage interpersonal connection.

In all of the recent differences in sex development (DSD) care publications, service user involvement is becoming increasingly prominent. This is true for modern healthcare in general, not just DSD. The aim of the chapter is to provide a succinct summary for psychosocial practitioners and other clinicians who have not yet engaged proactively with any part of the advocacy movement. While it is important for all care providers to actively involve people with lived experience in aspects of service design, psychological care providers (PCPs) may particularly wish to consider the value of peer support and advocacy as a way out of shame and secrecy for their clients.

5.1   Patients' Rights

In many postindustrial nations, the right *to* healthcare is integral to an egalitarian ideology. Where health services are free at the point of care, the focus has shifted to equality *in* access. By contrast, in the USA, discussion of patient rights *in* medicine has been emphasized for longer, with the (equal) right *to* healthcare (or at least to healthcare insurance) lagging behind other major economies in the Global North.

Recognition of patients' rights in the USA had its broader precursor in the civil rights movement in the 1960s. Civil rights became a springboard for a range of social movements including gay, disability and women's rights. Patients' rights initially concentrated on institutional care settings, such as rights to respect and privacy, information requisite for informed consent, refusal of treatment and so forth. Right of access to medical records was added in the 1980s (see Annas, 1992). There are many stories of intersex people accessing their medical records and ascertaining past medical interventions in the 1990s (see, e.g., Davis & Feder, 2015). By the mid-1990s, patients' rights discussions were flourishing and visible throughout the healthcare system in many parts of the world, integral to the larger project of human rights. Patients' rights were concerned with a widening range of topics, with shifts in focus and language to reflect new and looming biotech advances that were bringing additional bioethical challenges. For example:

> Medical advances in the areas of life-prolonging technology, prenatal diagnosis, organ transplantation and artificial implants, and the increased specialization in medicine have all tended to increase the technological and decrease the human aspects of medical care. To maintain a balance in which decision making is shared and the patient retains the right and responsibility to make the ultimate decisions regarding personal care and medical treatment, explicit recognition and protection of the legal rights of patients are essential. (Annas, 1992, p. 2)

In the USA at least, patients' rights conversations had by the 1990s matured to a point that the status quo power relationship between care provider and user was being challenged. Patient-led movements sought to challenge medical authority by contesting disease categories and enhancing patient autonomy. Amid other achievements, these efforts set the scene for burgeoning "self-help" groups in the 1980s and 1990s. Care users of a range of health services got together for mutual support and to improve health literacy and research for patient benefits. Sharing stories was part of the culture. Many support groups had their own newsletters and information booklets. Stories of self-actualization in adversity have since inspired and educated care users and providers alike. These social changes provided the backdrop for intersex support groups.

5.2   Syndrome-Specific Peer Support

In the late 1980s, fledgling support groups for specific diagnoses began to form to facilitate mutual exchange and support, and to improve the language and information about specific syndromes. A number of clinicians in intersex medicine were involved in facilitating some of the early support work. Gary Warne, a pediatric endocrinologist, is often credited with having written one of the first books on congenital adrenal hyperplasia (CAH) with the family in mind, as well as a booklet on androgen insensitivity syndrome (AIS). He and other clinicians contributed to the formation of early peer support forums in Australia (see Warne, 2003).

By late 1990s, peer groups for AIS, CAH, Turner syndrome, Klinefelter syndrome and Mayer-Rokitansky-Küster-Hauser syndrome (MRKHS) had emerged in different regions of the world. Personal stories posted by individuals in newsletters and support group websites enabled virtual communities to form. The following story in 1997 shared by a member of the AISSG UK exemplified many care users' responses to the discovery of peer support. This individual expressed that she had "convulsed with sobbing" upon reading the story of another woman in the support group's newsletter $A^L I^A S$ (see Figure 5.1). She described her medical journey as one that haunted her from early teens to adulthood as follows:

> The image of being painted into a corner was vivid in my mind since the age of 12 or 13. It haunted me until age 36. I never saw any way out of the corner except by taking my life, until I came across the letter [from another AIS woman, in a medical journal, giving the support group contact details]. The letter wasn't just a release from a corner, it was a release from the prison that was my mind, a place where everything was locked shut inside and could find no freedom of expression.

Professional responses to first-person accounts like the above were mixed at first. Some health professionals responded positively by collaborating with care user forums, such as running Q&A sessions at their weekend gatherings to address concerns. Clinicians were often asked to assist in the production of accessible patient information. The willingness to be informed by patient experience had begun to be mobilized in select medical circles.

Support groups are typically started by individuals in isolation with the intent to bring together people who are similarly impacted. Mutual understanding and a sense of solidarity inspire the volunteers to develop predigested clinical information to improve health literacy, so that newly diagnosed people would not have to repeat the same negative experiences of trauma and isolation. The organizations are typically registered charities or nonprofit entities. In addition to providing support and education for the membership, groups may raise funds for (medical) research and conduct other philanthropic activities. Syndrome-specific groups vary in the types of activities and services that they offer. They may provide actual social gatherings or, nowadays, act as an online resource, or both. Activities often reflect the personal experience, capacity and skills of the founding individual(s) or a very small number of active and vocal members. Without organizational and funding structure, productivity can be down to the personal effort of a handful of people and therefore vulnerable to the changing personal circumstances of the individuals.

■ AIS SUPPORT GROUP ■   £2.50

AᴸIᴬS

VOLUME 1, NUMBER 1, SPRING 1995
© AIS Support Group UK

AᴸIᴬS No. 1

AIS Suppport Group (UK), PO Box 269, Banbury, Oxon, OX15 6YT, UK.

Tel: ____ _____ (for parent/patient *support/advice* only). General enquiries, literature requests (send SAE for list), subscription details etc. via the PO Box please – not by phone.

[Since this first issue was published we have grown. See **http://www.medhelp.org/www/ais** for details of overseas branches.]

About the Group

Welcome to the first newsletter (**AᴸIᴬS** – Learning   About **AIS**) of the AIS Support Group. It has been mailed to all the support group's contacts, including a number of clinicians.

The Androgen Insensitivity Syndrome Support Group was started in 1988 by the mother of a youngster (now 6 years old) with AIS, and was formalised in 1993. We believe it is the first support group for this condition.

This first issue is timed to coincide with the first parent/patient meeting of the group (See "First Group Meeting" on page 2.) and with a medical symposium on AIS to be held in April (See "RSM Symposium" on page 2.). It concentrates on the psychological aspects of AIS.

We hope it will help to break down some of the barriers of silence that have encouraged stigma and isolation amongst parents and sufferers. Future issues may cover topics of a more

medical nature such as early knowledge of AIS, incidence figures, carrier detection, pre-natal diagnosis, gonadectomy, HRT and osteoporosis, plastic surgery etc. and will contain additional contact addresses.

It should be emphasised that any medical details contained in the newsletter are not necessarily recommendations of the Support Group but are selected excerpts from the published literature on topics that parents seem to be asking about. Parents and patients should be guided by their physicians.

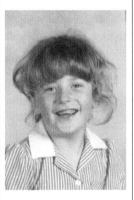

A factsheet for parents and adult patients, giving the basic medical facts about the condition is available from the group. Please ask for our full literature list and order form.

The Aims of the Group

To reduce the secrecy, stigma and taboo that has existed around AIS and other intersex states, by encouraging doctors, parents and society to be more open.

To encourage the provision of psychological support within the medical system, for young people with AIS and their parents.

To put parents and people with AIS in touch with others and to encourage them to seek support and information.

■

Figure 5.1   Front page of the first issue of *AᴸIᴬS*. Printed with permission from Margaret Simmonds, formerly AISSG UK. A colour version of this figure can be found in the plate section.

In her research with people with lived experience in the late 1990s, sociologist Sharon Preves (2003) recruited participants from as many as 16 North American intersex and related support, advocacy and educational organizations. She conducted 37 in-depth life history interviews with people aged 20 to 65 years and encountered diverse gender identities and sexual preferences among the individuals and groups (pp. 8–9). Some interviewees distanced themselves from the term intersex, albeit their bodies were thus medically classified at the time, and many identified unambiguously as female or male. Almost all of Preves' informants were college educated and the majority were Caucasian. It has been observed that intersex research in multicultural countries is drawn on white, middle-class experiences and intersex advocacy led by white middle-class people (Davis, 2015, p. 13). With that limitation in mind, Preves' informants provided useful accounts of medicalization. Despite their marked differences in identity and general outlook, all the research participants reported experiences of isolation, stigma and shame and searching for information, with several going as far as looking up medical textbooks in public and university libraries (Preves, 2003).

The need for community was so great that people with no peer group in their own country would travel across the seas to engage with others with the same variation. People who attended meetings of the AISSG UK, founded in 1990, subsequently founded 24 groups internationally (Baratz et al., 2014).

Peer support has brought huge relief to many individuals, as exemplified in the excerpt from the $A^L I^A S$ newsletter above. Groups are set up to be philanthropic rather than political. With a few exceptions, they tend not to pose a significant challenge to medical discourses, although it should be acknowledged that their very existence disrupts medical complacency in constructive ways. All the same, support providers have a difficult balance to tread. Even the seemingly simple act of predigesting complex diagnostic information (not to mention discussion of treatment choices) for lay audiences usually requires a level of values-based interpretation and judgment. Because of the sensitivity around how to represent a particular variation, even the most painstakingly balanced information can result in sweeping criticisms that could make support providers feel demotivated to continue with the thankless tasks. These circumstances render support groups vulnerable to fragmentation, as well as burnout for the one or two people trying their hardest to help others.

Syndrome-based peer support providers may not overtly challenge medicalization, neither are they duped into rubber-stamping medical views and recruiting participants for medical research without question. They connect with medical experts to encourage them to refer potential members. They participate in medical conversations in order to have a place at the table to advocate for their community. They recognize their ambiguous position as a lone (and sometimes token) patient or parent representative in medical corridors of power. Some of them may feel valued, others barely tolerated. On the other side of their thankless position are members of the group who complain that their leaders do not challenge medical authority enough. It is inevitable, even desirable, that some participants outgrow the anonymity and safety of syndrome-specific peer support, embrace an intersex identity and join or form activism-based networks.

There is a move toward generic intersex/DSD peer groups to address themes across all variations rather than particular syndromes. For example, although set up for AIS initially, the AISSG in the USA welcomed people with a wide range of variations, not just AIS. The name of the group was changed to AISDSD a few years ago to reflect the wider membership. In 2020 the name was changed again, to Interconnect. Likewise, AISNederland has become DSDNederland. The support organization dsdfamilies was founded by parents of children with a range of variations in the UK to provide information and support. Interconnected UK was formed in 2020 to do likewise. The first known intersex support group in Poland, Fundacja Interakcja, was launched in 2019. All of these groups aim to be inclusive of everyone with an innate sex variation. They are but a few examples of groups emerging worldwide that engage with a range of discourses and identities. It remains to be seen whether these newer support groups succeed in negotiating better care for their community and reframe variations in social terms.

5.3   Intersex Activism

At the same time that peer support groups were being formed worldwide, a US-based group began to experiment with other tactics. In 1996, at the first known public demonstration by intersex people, a group of activists who self-styled themselves as *Hermaphrodites with Attitude*, the name of the newsletter of the Intersex Society of North America, gathered outside the annual meeting of the American Academy of Pediatrics in Boston, Massachusetts (see Figure 5.2). The protest targeted the meeting of the Lawson Wilkins Pediatric Endocrine Society therein, for its continued support of *intersex genital mutilation*. Far from being closeted, the protestors actively courted media attention. They argued, publicly, that childhood surgery on medically benign genital variations violated their rights as

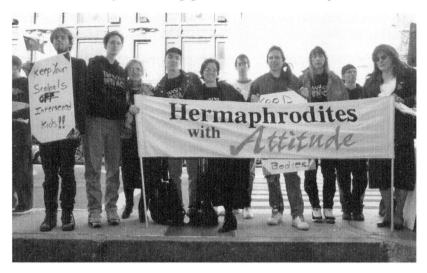

Figure 5.2   First known public demonstration by intersex people and allies. Printed with permission from Bo Laurent. A colour version of this figure can be found in the plate section.

children and subordinated their bodily integrity to heteronormative ideals to which they did not subscribe.

Founded in 1993, intersex people and nonintersex allies of the ISNA advocated for systemic changes to end shame, secrecy and childhood genital surgery. Their project was greatly facilitated by the mainstreaming of internet use. While intersex conditions are numerous, each is rare. With a geographically scattered small population that did not know about each other, it is hard to imagine how the group might have grown such a formidable presence in intersex medicine so quickly without the Internet. The Internet had the advantage of enabling individuals and families to share personal narratives anonymously. It enabled a geographically dispersed community to be built around mutual validation and collective resistance. The Internet also helped the organization to achieve media exposure. By early 2000, the ISNA website was receiving on average a thousand visitors every day. Five years later, the Society estimated that it had reached 30 million people through media coverage since its beginning (Downing et al., 2014, p. 193). A vibrant community outside medicine was developing a rival expertise in intersex based on an alternative language and perspective. The growing number of activists moved ISNA from its lonely beginning to an increasingly confident and cohesive organization that issued demands to the medical establishment. They clarified their position as follows:

- Intersexuality is primarily a problem of stigma and trauma, not gender
- Parents' distress must not be treated by surgery on the child
- Professional mental healthcare is essential
- Honest, complete disclosure is good medicine
- All children should be assigned as boy or girl, without early surgery

ISNA, which remained in existence until 2006, departed from syndrome-based support and framed all genital variations in social terms. While the organization engaged with medical discourses, it also mobilized feminist and bioethical critiques of medical management. In the Fall/Winter 1995/1996 issue of *Hermaphrodites with Attitude*, for example, the editors cited Suzanne Kessler's *Meanings of Genital Variability* presentation at the 1995 Annual Convention of the Society for the Scientific Study of Sexuality. The presentation argued that while genital differences are biologically identifiable, the meanings are socially constructed:

1. Your genitals signify neither of the two gender categories. We need to know what gender you are, therefore we must do further testing.
2. We know your gender. Your genitals signify the wrong gender. We must operate to make them conform to the right gender.
3. We know your gender. Your genitals, although not within the normal range for your gender now, will be in the future. We expect they will clarify on their own.
4. Your genitals are providing a clue that there is an underlying medical problem that needs to be addressed. We prescribe a nonsurgical treatment.
5. Your genitals are inferior (less functional, ugly). We pity you and suggest cosmetic/corrective surgery.
6. Your genitals are superior (more versatile, attractive). We envy yours and want ones like them.
7. Your genitals are just another body part that varies from person to person, like noses and ears, and it doesn't matter what they look like as long as they function well. We don't think very much about your genitals, or our own.
8. Your genitals signify something about your parents. They have misbehaved or are genetically unsuitable. They are embarrassed by you and your genitals.

Intersex activists and peer support participants share a culture of storytelling. Some of the accounts of intersex lives were elaborated in a special issue of the *Journal of Clinical Ethics*, edited as an anthology by ethicist and historian Alice Dreger (1999). It included an article by clinical psychologist and sex therapist Howard Devore, who grew up in what he called the surgical maelstrom and who described a childhood filled with "pain, surgery, skin grafts, and isolation" (Devore, 1999, p. 80). By the age of 40, Devore had had 16 genital operations. He observed that while medical specialists insisted that a child should not go to school with ambiguous genitals, ironically, they managed to create rather "strange-looking" genitals for the child. Devore reminded us that it is not just genitals that are scarred but also other body parts where tissue is taken from, a fact that should be acknowledged more often.

Based on her research in the late 1990s, Preves (2003) suggested that shame was the most pronounced feeling experienced in medical encounters. It would seem that the very intervention intended to protect patients from shame turned out to be a shaming experience after all. Preves quoted from the narrative of informant "Faye": "The point is the emotional damage you do by telling someone 'You're so fucking ugly that we wouldn't send you home to your parents the way you were.' I mean, give the parents some credit. Teach them. Help them to deal with the different child" (p. 78).

Other stories remind us that it is not just neonates and young children that get signed up to the kind of surgical maelstroms described by Devore (1999). Angela Moreno's intersex condition was not medically discovered until puberty, when the increased androgen production from her testes caused her to *masculinize*, resulting in a clitorectomy without her knowledge. She was told that she had ovarian cancer and her ovaries were removed. Her parents were told not to tell her what had happened (Moreno, 1999).

A compilation of stories of medical trauma by Davis and Feder (2015) included 18 narratives of people who had medical interventions in childhood and adolescence in the 1980s. The accounts included that of a founding member of the Swiss group Zwischengeschlecht. This group has been demonstrating against *intersex genital mutilation* in front of medical gatherings for years. The stories collated by Davis and Feder were of ruptured attachment and estrangement in families, social withdrawal, dissociation and escape into drugs, alcohol and self-harm. Families approach intersex in diverse circumstances, some better resourced than others. In my experience as a practitioner, I have come across individuals and families with mental health difficulties well before the intersex diagnosis. What is inexplicable in some of the first-person accounts is how

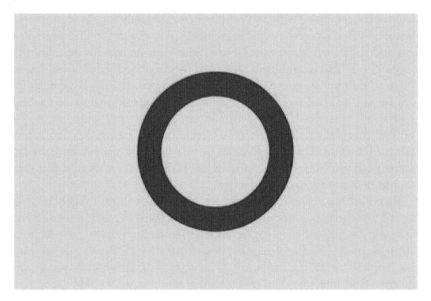

Figure 5.3   An intersex flag created by and reproduced with permission from Morgan Carpenter. A colour version of this figure can be found in the plate section.

health professionals could have missed the significant mental health needs despite multiple opportunities to ask how the patient is doing.

Intersex activism is not confined to English-speaking regions of the world. It is also prolific in Colombia, Malta, Germany, Portugal and Iceland. It is important to bear in mind that intersex activism is not a monolith. There are significant differences in perspective between regions, organizations and individuals. Some groups prioritize identity recognition. Others consider it harmful to insist on a separate identity based on biological characteristics and focus effort on changing medical practice and protecting bodily integrity of children.

In 2013, activist Morgan Carpenter created an intersex symbol of a golden yellow field with a simple, unadorned purple circle emblem in the middle that avoids referencing gender stereotypes (see Figure 5.3). Newer groups being formed are able to benefit from previous experiences and new communication technology. The variety of groups means that many participants can access and enjoy multiple advocacy cultures. Activist groups may be more or less effective in galvanizing their membership to create the impact that they desire. Smaller groups that consist of one or two people are less well resourced and more precarious. While destigmatization and patient-focused healthcare remain the explicit goals shared by all groups, divergence among advocates is inevitable. The different types of variations generate different pressing concerns. For example, MRKHS does not affect the external body and is less likely to attract interventions that infringe on child rights, while CAH and some XY conditions are associated with external genital variations and irrevocable childhood interventions.

As more actors with a range of identities become involved in intersex activism and more groups are being formed, the movement can feel confusing and at times antagonistic. Carpenter (2018a) tried to tease out some of the confusion:

> Some of this confusion arises from assumptions that to be LGBTI means to be old enough to have agency to affirm a sexual or gender identity. Available data suggests that most intersex people grow up to identify with sex assigned at birth (often described as cisgender), while very many of us are heterosexual. The word intersex bears the brunt of public misconceptions, including associations with being queer or transgender, but fundamental concerns about how bodies are regulated affect all intersex people irrespective of the words we use. (p. 32)

The most obvious schism in the world of advocacy is not across conditions but between the priorities of intersex-identified adults and those of parents of children with variations. Detailed analyses of intergroup relationships are available in Davis (2015), Karkazis (2008) and Preves (2005). Although these works are largely US-focused, some of the fissures within the advocacy movement are identifiable outside the USA. Thus far, close collaboration between gender-diverse adults and gender-normative caretakers is rare. Many caretakers are sympathetic to the interests of adult intersex communities. They are aware that one day their child could be part of such a community. However, they are otherwise preoccupied with the daily concerns relating to the health and wellbeing of their child and feel dependent on an alliance with medical specialists.

5.4   Mass Media

By the turn of this century, knowledge of intersex/DSD was no longer confined to the academy. Interests across contexts were evident in the proliferation of medical debates, social and psychological analyses, ethical discussions, legal interpretations, historicized accounts and, increasingly, the mass media. A barrier for some peer group providers to engage with

mainstream media was how to decipher legitimate interests from voyeurism and sensationalism. Despite the risks, media exposure seems to have
become more possible. As early as 1996, a documentary program called *XY
Women*, which was part of the BBC Dark Secrets series, was aired. The
program contrasted the experiences of two women with AIS. A helpline
number was given at the end of the program and enquirers were sent a
factsheet with contact details of AISSG UK. Many affected women subsequently spoke of how the program had enabled them to achieve a major
breakthrough in their lives by helping them to understand their bodies and
facilitating conversations with family members. A large number of newspaper and magazine articles, documentaries, podcasts, films and literary
works have accrued since then.

Some of the outputs were by intersex people working to change public
understanding using affordable contemporary small-scale broadcasting
technology. One of the first known documentaries about intersex lives is
Hermaphrodites Speak!, a 30-minute film in which several intersex people
discuss their lives and the medical practice changes that they wanted to see,
at the first ISNA retreat in 1997. Recent productions include freely
accessible online videos and visual art. *Orchids, My Intersex Adventure* is
Australian activist Phoebe Hart's 2010 documentary that explores various
social scenarios faced by intersex individuals. *Intersexion*, a film researched
and presented by New Zealander activist Mani Mitchell, set out to
demystify intersex by looking at how people with nonbinary bodies
negotiate childhood, adolescence and adulthood in the social sphere and
included interviews with professionals. The Interface Project (interfacepro-
ject.org) involves people of all ages and identities, each offering a brief
synopsis of their journey, and ends with the motto "No Body Is
Shameful."

Intersex is also featured in mainstream broadcasts. *How Do Intersex
People Navigate Life and the Medical System?* was the title of an Insight
program by the Specialist Broadcasting Service in Australia in 2017.
Participants in the television program included several intersex advocates
as well as parents and clinicians, who debated about childhood surgery.
A decade prior to that, in 2007, several US intersex activists engaged with
Oprah Winfrey and her audience in an episode entitled "Growing Up
Intersex." Some of the activists subsequently participated alongside ethicists, medical doctors and clinical psychologists in the BBC documentary
Me, My Sex and I, aired in 2011. The year before, the American documentary *XXXY* explored intersex people and medical professionals' opin-
ions on intersex surgery. These are but a few mainstream television

productions that have been accumulating since the 1990s bringing intersex issues into the public domain.

Intersex is featured in a number of literary works, the most celebrated of which is the 2002 novel *Middlesex*, which was awarded the Pulitzer Prize among its many distinctions. In the novel, the protagonist has a condition that would be medically considered a 46,XY DSD today (see Chapter 2). The novel stimulated many conversations about intersex in the general public. In the 2013 novel *Golden Boy*, the protagonist has a different rare condition, which last century's medical scientists would have called true hermaphroditism and today's doctors are more likely to call 46,XX ovo-testicular DSD (see Chapter 2). The novel was well received by intersex activists across the globe. A recent review has identified 14 film works on the topic (De Clercq, 2022) including *Both*, a 2005 North American–Peruvian drama by an intersex director. It tells a story of a stunt double on a journey of discovery of her intersex variation and the surrounding secrecy in the family.

It is difficult to evaluate the effects of mass media interventions, for example whether the exposure makes it more or even less possible to talk about innate sex variations in the social domain. Representations that encourage voyeurism are clearly harmful, but there are other risks of media exposure, such as the foregrounding of medicalizing and exoticizing perspectives of intersex (Enzendorfer & Haller, 2020). There is evidence that even media exposure aimed to raise awareness can have stigmatizing effects. Some young people with variations have reported unhelpful experiences of listening to intersex being misrepresented in informal talk among friends and colleagues after a television program (Brömdal et al., 2017; Lundberg et al., 2021). These reports resonate with observations in my clinical practice. Intersex is increasingly in the public domain. The effects on people with lived experience are likely to be variable depending on many factors.

5.5   Human Rights

Human rights efforts worldwide are focused upon childhood surgical sex assignment involving *feminizing* or *masculinizing* genital surgery and routine gonadectomy that do not address biomedical concerns. In 2013, a new German law required caretakers to register their child with nondimorphic sex characteristics in a temporary third category, to allow more time for one or the other legal gender to be assigned. The background to this is that caretakers in Germany only have one week to register the birth of the baby as female or male. This could put caretakers under undue pressure to make quick decisions on sex-normalizing interventions. The legal move with the intention to reduce surgical sex assignment can, however, backfire. While the intention was to give caretakers time to consider their options, the law is discriminatory because children with variations are made an exception in society. Caretakers being prohibited from registering their child in the usual way may feel under even more pressure to have social and surgical sex assignment lined up in order to register the birth as female or male. Movement toward a third gender represents a departure from pioneering intersex activists, who argued for legal gender assignment in line with cultural norms but without interventions to align the child's body to the assigned gender.

Speaking from an Australian context, Carpenter (2018b) drew attention to the contradictions between medical and legal constructions. The former constructs intersex bodies as "disordered" female or male, while law and society construct intersex people as neither female nor male. Intersex per se does not give rise to the contradiction but the constructed meaning of intersex does. Neither medical nor sociolegal models allow for individual self-determination. In the Darlington Statement of 2017, Australian and New Zealander activists called for human rights affirming oversight of relevant medical interventions and standards of care and criminal prohibition of deferrable medical interventions on children who cannot consent for themselves (AISSG Australia et al., 2017). The group urged health professionals to bring their practice in line with Australian human rights norms. A case was made for people with lived experience to be properly funded to support their communities, because many intersex people with a history of unwanted interventions and medical display have difficulties in trusting professional services.

The Gender Identity, Gender Expression and Sex Characteristics Act of Malta in 2015 was the first national law to end "non-vital" childhood genital surgery and prohibited "any sex assignment treatment and/or surgical intervention on the sex characteristics of a minor" (Malta, 2015). Medical intervention driven by "social factors without the consent of the minor" represents violation of the law. Maltese caretakers may consent to such treatments only in "exceptional circumstances" that cannot be "driven by social factors." The step taken in Malta represented a triumph for intersex activism (see Figure 5.4, a commemorative photograph of the participants present at a Maltese conference in 2013).

Activists work in their own national contexts and collaborate internationally. Groups such as InterACT and Zwischengeschlecht have been effective in putting childhood surgical sexing on the agendas of high-profile international human rights organizations such as Amnesty, the European Union (EU) and the United Nations (UN). In 2014, for example, the UN Human

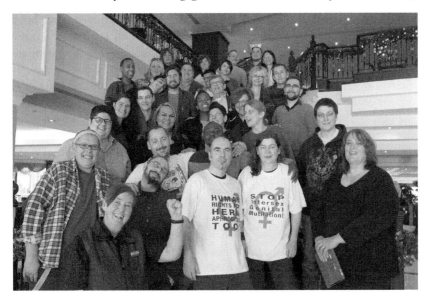

Figure 5.4   Intersex activists in Malta, 2013. Printed with permission from Morgan Carpenter. A colour version of this figure can be found in the plate section.

Rights Council published a report that identifies surgical interventions on intersex minors alongside other examples of torture (Mendez, 2014). A year later, a UN factsheet declared that member states should recognize the risk of abuse engendered by unnecessary surgery and treatment on intersex children (UN, 2015). Nongovernmental agencies increasingly recognize intersex surgery on minors as an infringement of human rights but allow that some interventions are medically essential. For example, Amnesty International reporting on medical practices in Germany and Denmark drew attention to a common urogenital sinus as an example trait where there is "a clear medical necessity for surgery" (Amnesty International, 2017, p. 26). Based on extensive research in the USA, Human Rights Watch launched its written and video reports to advocate against all surgical procedures that seek to alter the gonads, genitals or internal sex organs of children with atypical sex characteristics too young to participate in the decision, when those procedures both carry a meaningful risk of harm and can be safely deferred (Human Rights Watch, 2017). As for Amnesty in the same year, the report noted that "[t]here are sometimes health issues among children with intersex conditions that do, indisputably, require surgical intervention, such as the removal of cancerous gonads" (p. 95).

Taken together, human rights bodies have not typically called for a cessation of all medical interventions but condemned those that are socially driven. Activists recognize that parents of children with sex variations are faced with the agonizing choice as to whether or not to consent to sex alteration surgery on their child. The information provided by medical experts alone could mean that parents are not always fully informed about the potential physical and psychological risks. The UN Convention of the Rights of the Child (Article 5) sets out the role and duty of parents in decision-making processes and in ways that do not assume decisions to be a straightforward situation of expressing an individual's personal preference (Mills & Thompson, 2020, p. 547).

5.6   Healthcare Reform

Early medical responses to challenges by intersex advocates were predictable. First-person accounts of pain, sorrow and bravery were initially marginalized as those of a minority for whom treatment had failed. Medical providers were noted to have referred to the challengers as "green-wellied loonies" and "zealots" (cited by Morland, 2009, p. 195). Before the turn of this century, however, synergistic care user actions were visible everywhere including Europe, Japan, Australia and New Zealand.

Instead of being relegated to picketing medical conventions, care advocates were soon invited to join in medical conversations. In 2000, ISNA's founder Cheryl Chase was invited to speak at the meeting of the Lawson Wilkins Pediatric Endocrine Society. In 2002, the first joint care provider and user meeting in the UK took place in London. About one-third of the hundred some delegates were care users and two-thirds health professionals. The sessions were cochaired by users and providers, and the program sought to balance both perspectives (Creighton et al., 2004). The AISDSD of the USA (now renamed Interconnect) has for some years collaborated with a number of DSD teams on accredited medical education events on intersex/DSD. Care user representation is now standard in DSD conferences and healthcare polices in Anglophone and Western European nations. Collaboration between experts by profession and experts by lived experience has travelled further afield in recent years. "Is It a Boy or a Girl? The Limits of the Male-Female Binary" was the title of the first interdisciplinary symposium on intersexuality held in Hong Kong, Special Administrative Region of the People's Republic of China, in 2018. The program featured presentations by an intersex activist, a government lawyer, a pediatric endocrinologist and two psychologists (see Figure 5.5). What struck a Chinese medical

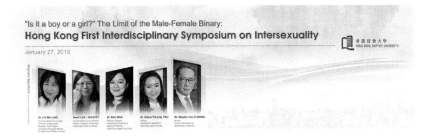

Figure 5.5   First Interdisciplinary Symposium on Intersexuality in Hong Kong. Printed with permission from Elaine Tsui. A colour version of this figure can be found in the plate section.

delegation in the audience was not the program but the unwavering public presence of Chinese intersex activist Small Luk (Elaine Tsui, personal communication). First-person accounts in public had until that point been unimaginable for the astounded medical experts.

As discussed in Chapter 2, "The Consensus Statement on the Management of Intersex Disorders" in 2006 was the first international consensus paper and an outcome of an invitation-only meeting that took place in Chicago (Lee et al., 2006). The document was not constructed as a clinical guideline, rather as a response to a troubled and troubling area of medicine and a strategic development to facilitate basic science research on the horizon. It was the first care standard document that unequivocally placed intersex variations on the same platform as other congenital disorders. Service users could, for the first time in history, supposedly expect the same benefits of evidence-based interventions and the same protection from unethical practices. Optimal clinical management is said to comprise the following (p. e490):

1.   Gender assignment must be avoided before expert evaluation in newborns
2.   Evaluation and long-term management must be performed at a center with an experienced multidisciplinary team
3.   All individuals should receive a gender assignment
4.   Open communication with patients and families is essential, and participation in decision-making is encouraged
5.   Patient and family concerns should be respected and addressed in strict confidence

Among the concerns addressed, truth telling is explicitly endorsed. Disclosure concerning karyotype, gonadal status and prospects for future fertility is said to be "a collaborative, ongoing action that requires a flexible individual-based approach" (p. e293). Furthermore, diagnostic and treatment information for children is to be "a recurrent gradual process of increasing sophistication that is commensurate with changing cognitive and psychological development" (p. e293). Communication is understood as diagnostic education, that is, an offer of expert information to the patient. This master narrative of intersex/DSD is, however, problematic from a psychological point of view and further discussed in Chapter 6.

The role of advocacy groups in healthcare policies was formally acknowledged. Input from peer groups is said to be useful for improving service delivery as well as for the individual patient. The consensus states (p. e496):

- Peer support ends isolation and stigma, providing a context in which conditions are put into perspective and intimate issues of concern can be discussed safely with someone who has "been there."
- Children who form relationships with peers and affected adults early in their lives benefit from a feeling of normalcy early on, with support in place well before adolescence. Adolescents often resist attempts to introduce them to peer support.
- Support groups can help families and consumers find the best quality care.

In terms of psychological input, the consensus statement suggested that mental health staff with expertise in DSD promote positive adaptation and facilitate team decisions about gender assignment and reassignment, timing of surgery, and sex-hormone replacement. Psychosocial screening tools could be deployed to identify risk for maladaptive coping in the family. Recent research shows that many specialist teams working with DSD services draw on a level of psychological expertise (Pasterski et al., 2010). There remain, however, fundamental gaps in psychological understanding in the field.

The tone relating to childhood surgery for genital variations was ambivalent, but surgery is placed within a multidisciplinary framework with an explicit mandate to collaborate with caretakers. Surgical practice is to be influenced by team discussions and founded on the best clinical and scientific evidence, taking into account user preferences and circumstances. The consensus statement recommended no surgery for girls diagnosed with CAH whose clitoris is only slightly or moderately bigger than average until they can contribute to decision-making. Surgery was to be reserved only for girls whose clitoris is deemed much larger than socially acceptable, provided caretakers fully appreciated the potential risks. These suggestions sound like stale wine rebottled with new labels, because experts without the benefit of half a century of hindsight were suggesting exactly the same back in the 1950s. In 1955, psychiatrist Joan Hampson explained that "psychologic difficulties consequent on growing up with a large phallus should not be underestimated" but that "when the clitoris is not strikingly hypertrophied, remaining fairly inconspicuous and almost concealed between the labia majora, there seems to be no need to do anything" (Hampson, 1955, p. 271). Because orgasmic function and erectile sensations may be impaired by clitoral surgery, the consensus statement suggested that surgical procedures should be anatomically based to preserve erectile function and innervation of the clitoris, and that the emphasis should be on functional outcome rather than a strictly cosmetic appearance. This too is not saying anything new, given the persistent absence of evidence to suggest that any surgical technique could leave clitoral sensitivity unaltered.

The most notable achievement of the Chicago consensus is the widespread professional uptake of the term disorder of sex development. Since Chicago, additional national and international updates have followed (Ahmed et al., 2021; Cools et al., 2018; Lee et al., 2016). These publications reflect the rapid advances in biogenetic research rather than development of nontechnical aspects of healthcare. For example, nonsurgical care paths have remained a low priority in DSD services. Unsurprisingly, the groups most satisfied with so-called healthcare reforms are biomedical scientists.

Intersex activists continue to protest at medical venues and work with human rights agencies to press for the kind of healthcare reforms that they wish to see. By 2020, two US hospitals had issued a statement to stop childhood genital surgery, albeit with caveats. However, at the time of writing, the UK's National Health Service's draft proposal to decommission childhood feminizing surgery remains halted without explanation. In Australia, no hospital has suspended surgery but the first of eight territories is expected to publish a public consultation on draft legislation in 2022 with a primary focus on informed consent. These changes are brought about by intersex activism outside medicine rather than progress within medicine.

5.7   Implication for Psychological Practice

First-person accounts suggest that, ironically, the most distressing aspects of medical management are often the very interventions intended to alleviate distress. Overwhelmed by grief and confusion, caretakers of children with variations understandably seek to increase certainty. Having little information on how their child may fare in the social world, any intervention with the promise of normalcy will always look as if it would deliver more certainty. Psychosocial practitioners can support caretakers to work productively with the dilemmatic situation. However, the effectiveness of this input is often systemically constrained. These constraints are discussed in Chapter 6.

As well as understanding medical discourses, psychosocial practitioners are required to engage with arguments put forward by intersex advocacy groups. The advocacy movement has come to an interesting time. Many groups exist around the world deploying a range of approaches to tackle different aspects inspired by the leaders' experiences, values, skills and capacity. Some groups are focused on support and education, some work with medical experts to shape services toward patient-centered care, some engage with the mass media to educate the public and some lobby human rights agencies to regulate medical power. Together, the different strands of advocacy work in different regions of the world will continue to bring pressure on societies to develop responses that transcend medicine.

CHAPTER 6

The New Care Standard

As discussed in Chapter 5, many people with lived experience of sex variations have decolonized themselves, reclaimed their expertise and reframed their concerns in terms of rights and citizenship. In recognition of past problems, various practice changes were put forward, as intersex medicine entered into an age of consensus. The Chicago consensus of 2006 is not the only consensus statement. Although the various consensus statements are sometimes referenced as international and even global, they reflect the workings of mainly invited Anglo-European pediatric experts. The publications disseminate the latest biomedical research and make recommendations for implementation. While *patient-centered care* (PCC) is talked about, and this language has been jumped up to *holistic* care in more recent publications (e.g., Cools et al., 2018) without any explanation of the difference, the coverage of nonbiomedical contributions in the care documents is much more vague (see Chapter 8).

A recent study asked adults, caretakers and health professionals how they would define optimal service delivery and clinical outcomes (Suorsa-Johnson et al., 2021). The themes identified dovetail almost exactly with those that have already been put forward in medical publications, including multidisciplinary teams, roles and expectations, knowledge of the diagnosis, physical health, complex decision-making, social support and acceptance. Rhetoric of the new care standard has seeped into provider consciousness and is diligently recycled but usually with limited discussion as to how the aspirations are potentially conflicted. Thus the technological recommendations are being put forward without detailed consideration of non-medical expertise.

In the West at least, there is broad verbal agreement that healthcare should be delivered by a multidisciplinary team (MDT) along PCC principles. It is true that many pediatric specialists and scientists have brought their specialist skills to provide a one-stop service for children with variations, but this in itself does not qualify the providers as a team. If they should function as a team that reflects multidisciplinary characteristics, it does not automatically render the service patient-centered.

Since the late 1990s, childhood genital surgery has rarely been talked about in contemporary medical publications without being referenced as a dilemma. Rather than articulating what makes it a dilemma, discussion is typically outsourced to *centers of excellence*, as if they have the answers (e.g., DiSandro et al., 2015, p. 325). What are these so-called centers of excellence? How do they work? Research with health professionals provides useful insights on how differences in sex development (DSD) experts interpret patient needs and their respective roles. I draw attention to the SENS project (katravels.wixsite.com), which included interviewing 32 European DSD experts. This work is in dialogue with past and current analyses of health professionals' talk in the USA. Works in the USA began with Suzanne Kessler's (1998) groundbreaking analysis of conversations with several professionals. Ten years later, an extensive analysis of conversations with dozens of informants including 19 health professionals by Katrina Karkazis (2008) became available. This work was followed by Ellen Feder's (2014) study, which included 12 health professionals. Georgiann Davis' project involved a range of participants including 10 medical informants. In her publication in 2015, she expressed skepticism about the MDT as "an uncontested space in which medical professionals can assert their expertise and enhance their authority" (p. 77). An ongoing piece of work by Stefan Timmermans and coworkers (2018) involves 31 recordings of parent–clinician interactions. These studies have provided cumulative insights into how clinicians interpret service provision for DSD.

6.1 Patient-Centered Care

In her conversations with clinical experts in intersex in the 1980s, Kessler's (1998) observations of the power relationships between clinicians and caretakers resonated with medical paternalism at the time. She remarked that parents were almost entirely dependent on medical specialists to interpret the meaning of genital variations for them: "Parents are provided with a comprehensive treatment plan involving medication and surgery that is presented as an imperative and nonnegotiable. The medical view is the authoritative view, and the parents adopt it, adding to it their own private concerns" (p. 97). Kessler's observation of medical power was far from unusual at that time. Since then, medical power has been increasingly questioned in all areas of healthcare and patient rights increasingly voiced.

Demands for PCC are founded on the broad principles of patient rights but to specifically address the provider–user power imbalance in an increasingly technology-driven world. The PCC terminology has, however, been bandied around in many clinical contexts, including DSD services, with limited clarification as to what changes stakeholders are willing to commit to. PCC has been said to be "most commonly understood for what it is not – technology centred, doctor centred, hospital centred, and disease centred" (Stewart, 2001, p. 444). Furthermore, in consumerist economies, where medical providers can advertise directly to consumers to sell treatment in the absence of physical illness, a simplistic interpretation of PCC can be misappropriated by provider industries, with the potential to harm consumers. The boundary between patient-centeredness and treatment- and profit-centeredness can be dangerously blurred. Moira Stewart (2001), a professor of family medicine, clarified what PCC is:

> Patients want patient centred care which (a) explores the patients' main reason for the visit, concerns, and need for information; (b) seeks an integrated understanding of the patients' world – that is, their whole person, emotional needs, and life issues; (c) finds common ground on what the problem is and mutually agrees on management; (d) enhances prevention and health promotion; and (e) enhances the continuing relationship between the patient and the doctor. (p. 444)

Stewart's ideas are reflected in the definition of PCC in the *Clinical Guideline for the Management of Disorders of Sex Development* developed by a consortium involving the outgoing Intersex Society of North America (ISNA) (Consortium on the Management of Disorders of Sex Development, 2006a). The care document privileged the long-term physical, psychological, and sexual wellbeing of the patient. Citing professional literatures, it defined PCC for intersex/DSD as follows:

1. Provide medical and surgical care when dealing with a complication that represents a real and present threat to the patient's physical wellbeing.
2. Recognize that what is normal for one individual may not be what is normal for others; care providers should not seek to force the patient into a social norm (e.g., for phallic size or gender-typical behaviors) that may harm the patient.
3. Minimize the potential for the patient and family to feel ashamed, stigmatized or overly obsessed with genital appearance; avoid the use of stigmatizing terminology (like "pseudohermaphroditism") and medical photography; promote openness (the opposite of shame)

and positive connection with others; avoid a "parade of white coats" and repetitive genital exams, especially those involving measurements of genitalia.

4. Delay elective surgical and hormonal treatments until the patient can actively participate in decision-making about how their own body will look, feel, and function; when surgery and hormone treatments are considered, healthcare professionals must ask themselves whether they are truly needed for the benefit of the child or are being offered to allay parental distress; mental health professionals can help assess this.

5. Respect parents by addressing their concerns and distress empathetically, honestly and directly; if parents need mental health care, this means helping them obtain it.

6. Directly address the child's psychosocial distress (if any) with the efforts of psychosocial professionals and peer support.

7. Always tell the truth to the family and the child; answer questions promptly and honestly, which includes being open about the patient's medical history and about clinical uncertainty where it exists.

As humanities scholar Iain Morland (2009) discussed, PCC as put forward by the Consortium on the Management of Disorders of Sex Development (2006a) above represents the kind of progressive paternalism that did not necessarily follow on from intersex narratives up until that point. Morland acknowledged the importance of replacing surgery-centeredness with patient-centeredness as a necessary project for ISNA. He nevertheless found it problematic. Citing social research, he suggested that some patients may resist being "centered" by their healthcare providers. They may "desire neither to make decisions about their treatment, nor even to be fully informed about their treatment options" (p. 202). Further citing research with adults who consciously capitulate to medical authority in consenting to genital surgery, he questioned whether patient-centeredness is indeed the wish of all intersex patients (p. 203). Morland's insight is admirable and deserves closer attention. The focus of this chapter however is to query implementation of the positive care values being professed in professional literature.

PCC has been routinely mentioned in DSD publications in recent years, but there are major obstacles in implementing the concept in the aforementioned spirit. The contemporary biogenetic framing of DSD means that narratives of intersex are intrinsically pathology-centered and the care process technology-bound. See for example the below proclamation by "Dr D," a medical informant in Davis' study (2015): "Saying DSD makes it absolutely clear as a bell . . . . You have an enzyme disorder in this pathway or you have a structural disorder from that pathway, this is an accidental birth defect and you were born without this part. It makes it so much easier and less threatening" (p. 68). One might ask less threatening compared to what and, importantly, for whom. The idea that telling someone that they have "an accidental birth defect" and that they were born without certain body parts is "less threatening" is almost wild.

In DSD services, which are almost all located in tertiary children's hospitals, the concept of PCC is further complicated by the fact that life-changing decisions are made not by the actual patient but the surrogate – a third party. If PCC means honoring the preference of surrogates, then almost all actual patients would be surgically "normalized," as this is something considered "obvious and necessary" by almost all caretakers (Crissman et al., 2011, p. 4). On the other hand, if the open future of the patient is prioritized, then PCC may compel clinicians to subvert surrogates' wishes and delay any irrevocable elective interventions until the child is old enough to participate in decision-making (Timmermans et al., 2018). These dilemmas are typically glossed over in DSD publications.

6.2 Multidisciplinary Team

Team functioning in all walks of life – from manufacturing to the military – has such far-reaching consequences on humanity that a vast volume of research and analyses has accumulated over the years. The assumption that a team is a collection of people is pervasive and applied so liberally that many studies that claim to analyze team function have in fact studied "pseudo-like groups" instead (West & Lyubovnikova, 2013, p. 134). This is problematic for team scientists, whose task it is to study characteristics of team effectiveness and how to foster them.

A UK medical regulatory body echoed team scientists' understanding by stating that merely working in close proximity does not qualify healthcare providers as a team. Rather, a team means "a small number of people with complementary skills who are committed to a common purpose, performance goals and approach for which they hold each other mutually accountable" (Royal College of Physicians, 2017, p. 3). Team members are meant to share goals, be interdependent in their productivity and affect the results through their interactions with one another.

The journal *American Psychologist* dedicated a special issue to team science by drawing from all areas of psychology on team process and outcome in a variety of contexts. The article by Rosen et al. (2018) focused specifically on research into healthcare teams. The authors reviewed relevant articles published between 2000 and 2017 to "synthesize the evidence examining teams and teamwork in healthcare delivery settings in order to characterize the current state of the science" (p. 433). While this type of research tends to concentrate in emergency medicine and critical care, where medical errors can have the most profound consequences, useful lessons can be learned for all healthcare teams. According to this review, communication failure is a common finding in research. Furthermore, communication is found to be typically unsystematic and fragmented between disciplines.

In any one healthcare institution, there are many teams, including management, finance and clinical teams. Clinical teams may be unidisciplinary (e.g., a team of community midwives) or multidisciplinary (e.g., a team of physicians, dieticians or exercise specialists). An MDT is characterized by the aforementioned characteristics of joint purpose and interdependence *and* draws from multiple disciplines "to explore problems outside of normal boundaries and reach solutions based on a new understanding of complex situations" (NHS England, 2014, p. 12). Multidisciplinary working is taken to mean "using knowledge, skills and best practice from multiple disciplines and across service provider boundaries (e.g., health, social care or voluntary and private sector providers) to redefine, re-scope and reframe health and social care delivery issues and reach solutions based on an improved collective understanding of complex patient need(s)" (NHS England, 2014, p. 12). These characteristics are far from evident in psychosocial research with DSD experts.

Although the concept of MDT was endorsed in Chicago, there was no more clarity on how services should be held to account than in the Money era when different disciplines were also working alongside each other. MDTs are resource-intensive. Each meeting could take hours involving a large number of senior clinicians. Yet there is little discussion on format and content that would determine how multidisciplinary collaboration is achieved, what might cause it to fail and what would be the impact on patients. In an extensive piece of research involving 400 primary healthcare teams in the UK, shared objectives were the biggest single factor in team effectiveness (Borrill et al., 2000). Shared objectives are of strategic interest to policy makers for their impact on mortality and morbidity over and above disease and treatment effects (Ball et al., 2003; Bellomo et al., 2004). Yet the topic of joint purpose and how to move toward it is rarely emphasized in seminal publications in DSD.

No discussion of the effects of team process on user experience and treatment outcome is evident in DSD publications. Clinical activities appear to be left to run on parallel lines, producing fragmented user experiences with attendant material and emotional costs to patients and caretakers. Imagine the scenario described by a clinician: "[I]t's a bit like a play, I guess, and centre stage is the family, and people will come in and leave the stage as needed. ... I'm very aware that parents get bombarded by all these people ..." (Liao & Roen, 2021, p. 207). Pediatric clinical psychologist Franco D'Alberton (2010) posited that patient safety is likely to mirror team safety. In other words, if team members do not feel safe to bring a different focus into discussion or express an alternative viewpoint, then it is unlikely that caretakers would feel free to do the same. The inability to voice differences is referenced as *group think*, a phenomenon antithetical to patient safety and to be avoided. Healthcare management even encourages "whistleblowing" to break up such a destructive team characteristic. In DSD, medical providers assume control of the process. It is therefore incumbent on these professionals to break down team hierarchy and encourage alternative voices and debate.

Team scientists make a distinction between task work and teamwork. Both are required. The former involves clinical procedures, skills and drills. The latter refers to nontechnical competencies, which are defined as intentional listening, translation of information coming from disciplines with highly specialized languages and speaking up deliberately in contexts in which psychological safety may be low and hierarchical norms strong (Rosen et al., 2018). Research suggests that DSD professionals are highly skilled in task work. However, they rarely cite clear examples of teamwork. We know from team research that being held jointly to account is characteristic of high-functioning teams. It follows that clarity of purpose of DSD teams is negotiated, made explicit, reviewed and updated. Thus far, training in these nontechnical competencies is not identifiable in research interviews with health professionals.

If future DSD services are committed to integrated MDT care, perhaps the very first step is to take mutual responsibility to debate their higher purpose. Research also suggests that team members need to familiarize with and integrate each other's contributions. Team leadership is generally assumed to rest with medical specialists, but leadership skills are not intrinsic to any one discipline. Letting go of hierarchical norms, team leadership might rest with the most effective facilitator who can galvanize members to collaborate to materialize agreed standards of care. Such a person may well be a medical specialist, but could also be a manager, or another kind of clinical expert, such as those with a background in nursing, clinical genetics, psychology, social work or some other discipline.

Thus far, there is no evidence that DSD services are characterized by core attributes of high-functioning teams. Future research into the quality of DSD care should directly observe MDT meetings, examine care plans, find out how services collect data on patient experiences and ask care providers about their well-being, job satisfaction, external and internal pressures and how they would like to be supported in their own and their patients' interests.

6.2.1　Under Application of Psychological Expertise

Given the unresolved dilemma of life-changing interventions on minors for *psychosocial* benefits, it is reasonable to expect initial clinical encounters to be characterized by a strong psychosocial presence. A freedom of information exercise in the UK (where the National Health Service [NHS] is obligated to answer questions posed by the public) reported that endocrinologists and urologists were the only specialists present in all MDTs (Garland et al., 2021). An international survey observed that during the initial evaluation period, a child psychologist was available for face-to-face discussion with parents in only 53% of so-called centers of excellence (Kyriakou et al., 2016). A recent scoping review of studies that address MDT mechanisms looked at team composition, models of collaboration and ethical principles (Gramc et al., 2021). The review confirmed that team members are mainly medical professionals working separately. The consistent absence of psychological expertise (especially at the most strategic points of the care process) is notably paralleled by the consistent presence of surgical expertise, often in the first family meeting, which is said to be necessary for the purpose of reaching a diagnosis.

Thus far the DSD nosology includes more than 50 variations in urogenital differentiation. Pediatric experts speak of "ordering stacks of diagnostic tests" to scrutinize all possible biological signifiers of sex (Davis, 2015, p. 78) in order to decide whether the child should inhabit a female or male reality. They struggle with uncertainty in the absence of a "crystal ball" (Liao & Roen, 2021, p. 206). Even when there is diagnostic clarity, the test results can be so complicated that clinicians find it daunting to have to explain to caretakers. They hesitate to talk to caretakers about the child's future, because "nobody really knows what the news is" (Liao & Roen, 2021, p. 207). In the words of the sociologist Limor Meoded Danon (2022): "[W]e are now witnessing the ongoing global genetic scanning of DSD variations" but, "as more sequencing takes place and additional genetic variants are discovered, uncertainty and confusion regarding the findings increase" (p. 224).

Situations of uncertainty and tension are precisely the kind of scenarios for which psychological care providers are intensively selected and trained. Their very existence in DSD services is to create a containing environment and engage all parties in honest if difficult and, at times, perhaps heartbreaking conversations. Yet research suggests that pediatric experts are floored by the idea of a psychological practitioner taking a leading role in care provision before they have finished their work. See, for example, the following exchange between the interviewer "I" and a pediatric endocrinologist "PE" in the SENS study (Liao & Roen, 2021, p. 210):

I: ... are there any cases where you think, "Actually having the psychologist do some work here."

PE: As an alternative to ... what?

I: Maybe, maybe more relevant actually than, than intervening on a medical level?

PE: ... I can't think of a specific example but I'm sure there, there are examples where, we're not medically intervening. Ah, and the, the sole intervention is giving psychological support. Ah, but I think that would be the exception rather than the rule .... I just can't think of a scenario at the moment where we, we'd say, you know if they had ah, significant DSD ah .... You know, there are a whole bunch of patients here who've had surgery at, early in life who clearly don't need anything else done out here, where the only management might be psychological, actually.

By positioning psychologists in the periphery, remedial input could come tragically late. A nurse specialist in the same study reflected on a scenario all too familiar to intersex survivors:

Um, I, one example I can give is ... a boy who ... had so many surgeries that, um, he became, told me he became really depressed and he was self-harming. Um, self-harming enough to be cutting his own penis ... he got some psychological support, but again he only, he, he dipped in and out of it and didn't stay, I think he only went for maybe one or two sessions after ... we had organised some support for him ... that's where I, I, I ... I don't know that we could do better. (p. 208)

Research that has identified gaps in psychosocial care (e.g., Bennecke et al., 2015; Chivers et al., 2017; Ernst, Liao, et al., 2018) stands in contrast to a survey of 60 European DSD centers that suggested the opposite, that psychological input for families was available in 95% of the participating centers, but that uptake was noted to be as low as 57% (Pasterski et al., 2010). The discrepancy may be due to methodological differences. Superficial questioning would mean that even a token psychological presence would enable so-called centers of excellence to tick a box. Alternatively, the intense biomedical process could unintentionally undermine psychological engagement even if psychosocial providers were present. If the psychologist or social worker is positioned as someone outside the team or someone whose input is only needed when a patient or family shows signs of distress, then it is understandable that caretakers would not appreciate the value of psychological input in communication and decision-making.

By constructing DSD protocols around biomedical requirements, medical specialists are the only providers who interact with patients and families at strategic time points. This means that medical specialists must have a clear grasp of what whole-person care means, what every team member's contributions are and how to socialize care users into engaging with the entire service. But research has identified worrying trends in medical specialists' grasp of psychological input. Medical professionals have discussed psychological input in terms of an occasional review, as being more relevant when they themselves have finished their work and when the patient or family members needed mental health treatment (Liao & Roen, 2021). As a case in point, when asked how the team's psychologist might support the family considering hypospadias surgery, hypospadias repair was considered by medical providers as so routine and unproblematic that input from the team psychologist was not usually required (Roen & Hegarty, 2018). In other words, psychologists, if present at all, are positioned at the end of the medical paths or only when difficulties arise, when they should be held accountable for the psychological oversight of the entire care process.

Medical communication about DSD can be overwhelming not just for caretakers but also for adolescents and adults. Research with young people suggests that they would often switch off and become disinterested in order to minimize interaction with health professionals, sometimes as a way to protect themselves (Sanders & Carter, 2015). Young people have spoken about feeling angry and frustrated in the medical process and described situations where neither the parent present nor the medical provider recognized their distress. These are examples of failure in socializing service users to engage with psychological care. This failure, alongside the other team factors mentioned above, may account for disengagement among care users even when psychological expertise was available (Pasterski et al., 2010).

6.3   Medical Framing

The literature tells us that the child with a variation is an emergency patient, that caretakers comply with intensive scrutiny of the child, that they interact with the surgeon from the beginning, that they are given fast-paced and voluminous and esoteric information that is difficult to digest, that they sustain high emotions for long periods and that there is no psychological oversight of the process. What are the effects of the synergistic enactment of medicalizing events within the care protocol, the exclusive focus on the variation rather than the person and the exclusively biomedical way of knowing and talking about the situation?

The potential for pathology-centered communication to shoehorn decision-making toward medical intervention is highlighted in a vignette study (Streuli et al., 2013). In the study, medical students were instructed to imagine that they had a child with a genital variation. The participants were randomly assigned to two experimental groups. The medical framing group was exposed to a video with an actor claiming to be a medical doctor who explained about the child's condition and the possibility of surgery. The second group was exposed to a video with the same actor claiming to be a psychologist who explained about the child's condition using less medicalizing language. Participants in the medical framing group were three times as likely as the other group to express a preference for genital surgery for the child. What is sobering is that both groups claimed to have made up their mind without undue influence. Medical framing can substantially inflate the probability of medical courses of action. This idea is not new. In Erving Goffman's (1974) formulation, a frame locates, perceives, identifies and labels phenomena. It provides individuals with a structure within which to understand events.

6.3.1   *Continuation of Childhood Genital Surgery*

As part of the SENS project, 23 European health professionals took part in a pencil and paper exercise by locating DSD interventions along a continuum ranging from medically essential at one pole to nonessential at the other pole (Hegarty et al., 2021). They were invited to talk about their choice. A notable observation was the difficulty of the task for the majority of participants. Their conflicted accounts reflected significant struggles to provide humane solutions to people in distress and manage risks of violating the rights of the child. To explain what makes an intervention medically essential, clinicians drew vaguely on popular understandings of child development, psychosocial concerns, and choice. Clinical discussions were often anchored on the physical feature rather than the different forms of existence that the child may grow to inhabit. Communication unfailingly deployed a biogenetic language.

As part of the diagnostic process, it is often necessary for a surgeon to examine the anatomy. However, meeting with the surgical team right at the beginning can be highly meaningful for service users. Jeffrey L. Marsh (2006), a craniofacial surgeon, stated the obvious, that surgeons are not wellness doctors and that people do not speak with a surgeon to discuss their well-being. Rather, there is a mutual expectation to discuss the possibility of fixing a body part. Furthermore, surgeons characteristically express their contribution as correcting a problem or reconstructing a body part but rarely qualify the language with the word partially, even though it is rare for an operation to be so perfect that there is no trace of the original feature. The mismatch between expectation and outcome tends to surface after the operation. Marsh expressed that in close to three and a half decades of academic learning and teaching and clinical practice, there had been no formal discussion of these important transaction variables (p. 122).

Marsh's remark is in dialogue with Crissman et al.'s (2011) observation that the parents they interviewed frequently used the word fix to describe how they understood surgery. These authors also noted parents' faith in the medical team, as per the example excerpt below:

> We really never had to make a decision … the doctors told us what was gonna need to be done … . I wanted them to do the best that they can for my son. So umm, anything they asked for or wanted to do, I was ok with it. (p. 5)

The above quote is almost identical to the one below from a recent UK study with parents who had chosen to have their daughter's clitoris surgically reduced (Alderson et al., 2022), whereby a parent said:

> I think I just took their advice and said, well, you know, "what do you think needs doing?," and I just took the surgeon's advice on that.

"Dr Cypress," a psychologist informant in Feder's (2014) study, spoke about the effects of a medical protocol that (inadvertently) positions surgery as psychology by proxy:

> [The parents] want to take [the clitoral enlargement] out. I say, well, this is not urgent medically, and my colleague says the parents feel urgency, and now is the time to address it. Delaying [clitoral surgery] becomes a hard sell when somebody [else] is saying, "I can take it out tomorrow. When do you want to come in?" (pp. 143–144)

Parents are increasingly cited as the source of pressure to conduct surgery and clinicians increasingly experience their own presentation of information as factual and neutral, absent of any framing effect. A clinician below described an example of having to actively resist parental pressure:

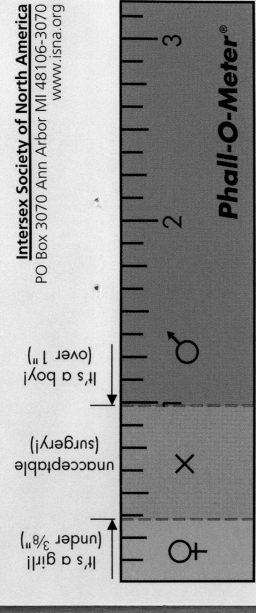

Figure 3.1 The satirical Phall-O-Meter produced by the ISNA. Reproduced with permission from Bo Laurent

■ AIS SUPPORT GROUP ■

£2.50

A^{L}I^{A}S

VOLUME 1, NUMBER 1, SPRING 1995

© AIS Support Group UK

A^{L}I^{A}S No. 1

AIS Suppport Group (UK), PO Box 269, Banbury, Oxon, OX15 6YT, UK.

Tel: _____ _____ (for parent/patient *support/advice* only). General enquiries, literature requests (send SAE for list), subscription details etc. via the PO Box please – not by phone.

[Since this first issue was published we have grown. See **http:// www.medhelp.org/www/ais** for details of overseas branches.]

About the Group

Welcome to the first newsletter (**A^{L}I^{A}S** – Learning About **AIS**) of the AIS Support Group. It has been mailed to all the support group's contacts, including a number of clinicians.

The Androgen Insensitivity Syndrome Support Group was started in 1988 by the mother of a youngster (now 6 years old) with AIS, and was formalised in 1993. We believe it is the first support group for this condition.

This first issue is timed to coincide with the first parent/patient meeting of the group (See "First Group Meeting" on page 2.) and with a medical symposium on AIS to be held in April (See "RSM Symposium" on page 2.). It concentrates on the psychological aspects of AIS.

We hope it will help to break down some of the barriers of silence that have encouraged stigma and isolation amongst parents and sufferers. Future issues may cover topics of a more

medical nature such as early knowledge of AIS, incidence figures, carrier detection, pre-natal diagnosis, gonadectomy, HRT and osteoporosis, plastic surgery etc. and will contain additional contact addresses.

It should be emphasised that any medical details contained in the newsletter are not necessarily recommendations of the Support Group but are selected excerpts from the published literature on topics that parents seem to be asking about. Parents and patients should be guided by their physicians.

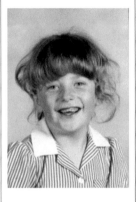

A factsheet for parents and adult patients, giving the basic medical facts about the condition is available from the group. Please ask for our full literature list and order form.

CONTENTS

The Aims of the Group

To reduce the secrecy, stigma and taboo that has existed around AIS and other intersex states, by encouraging doctors, parents and society to be more open.

To encourage the provision of psychological support within the medical system, for young people with AIS and their parents.

To put parents and people with AIS in touch with others and to encourage them to seek support and information.

■

Figure 5.1   Front page of the first issue of *A^{L}I^{A}S* – Printed with permission from Margaret Simmonds, formerly AISSG UK

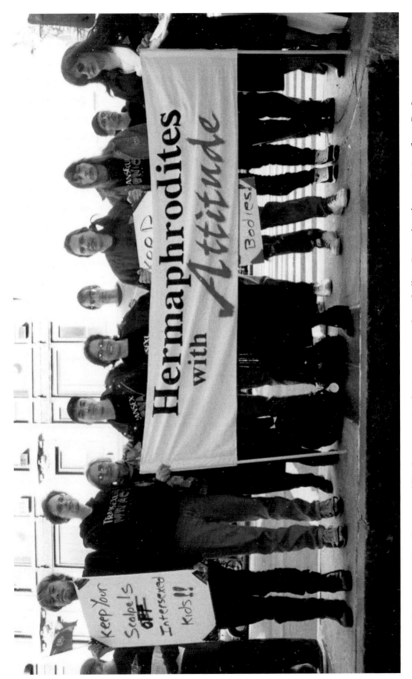

Figure 5.2   First known public demonstration by intersex people and allies. Printed with permission from Bo Laurent

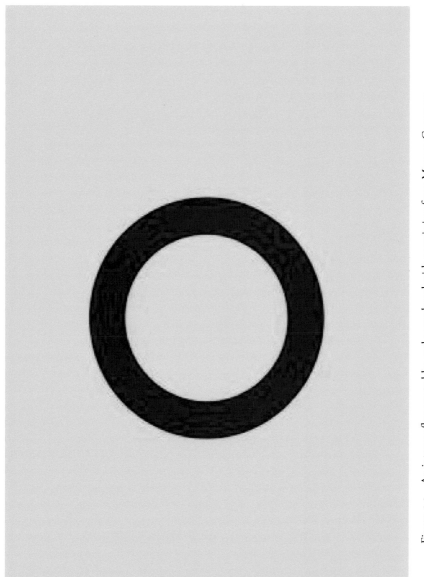

Figure 5.3   An intersex flag created by and reproduced with permission from Morgan Carpenter

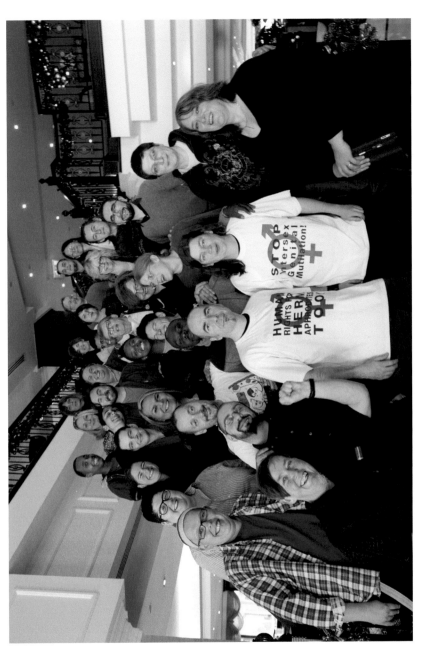

Figure 5.4 Intersex activists in Malta, 2013. Reprinted with permission from Morgan Carpenter

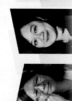

Figure 5.5   First Interdisciplinary Symposium on Intersexuality in Hong Kong. Printed with permission from Elaine Tsui

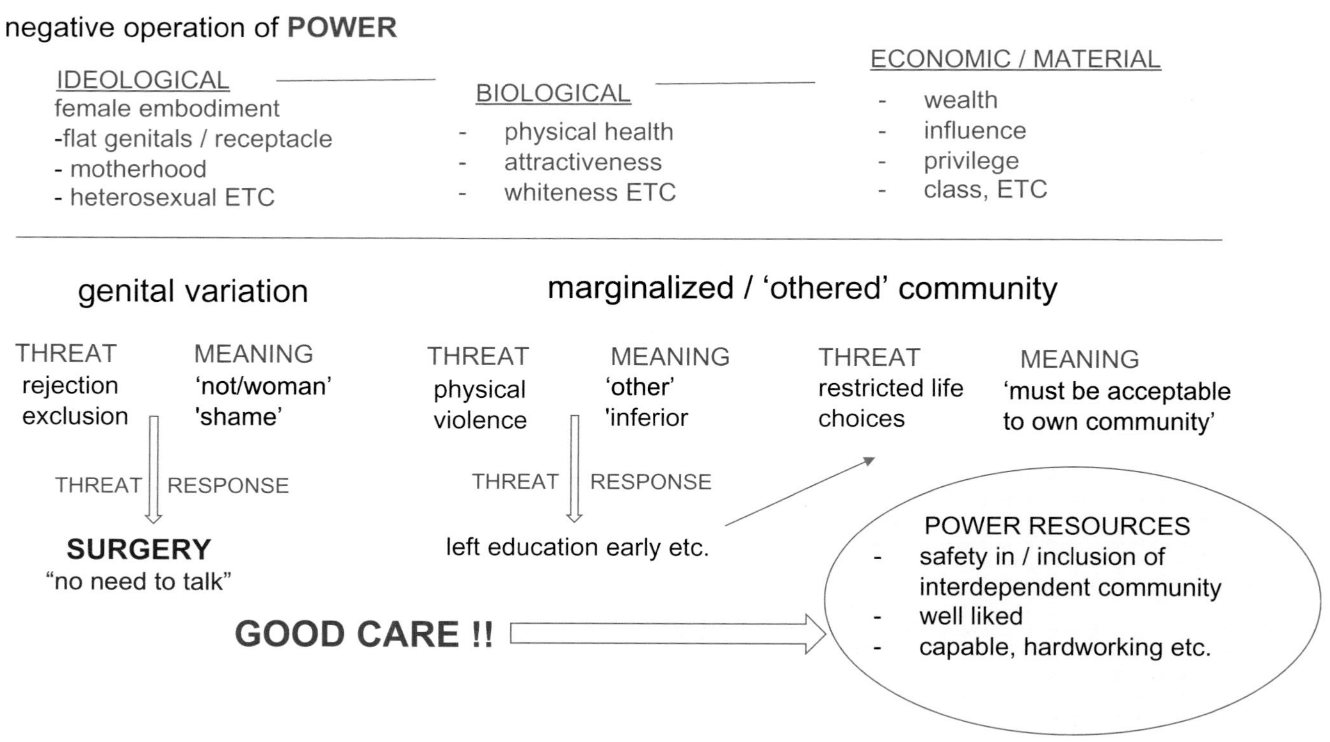

negative operation of **POWER**

IDEOLOGICAL
female embodiment
-flat genitals / receptacle
- motherhood
- heterosexual ETC

BIOLOGICAL
- physical health
- attractiveness
- whiteness ETC

ECONOMIC / MATERIAL
- wealth
- influence
- privilege
- class, ETC

genital variation

marginalized / 'othered' community

THREAT
rejection
exclusion

MEANING
'not/woman'
'shame'

THREAT   RESPONSE

SURGERY
"no need to talk"

THREAT
physical
violence

MEANING
'other'
'inferior'

THREAT   RESPONSE

left education early etc.

THREAT
restricted life
choices

MEANING
'must be acceptable
to own community'

POWER RESOURCES
- safety in / inclusion of
  interdependent community
- well liked
- capable, hardworking etc.

GOOD CARE !!

Figure 9.1   Formulation chart for Hetty

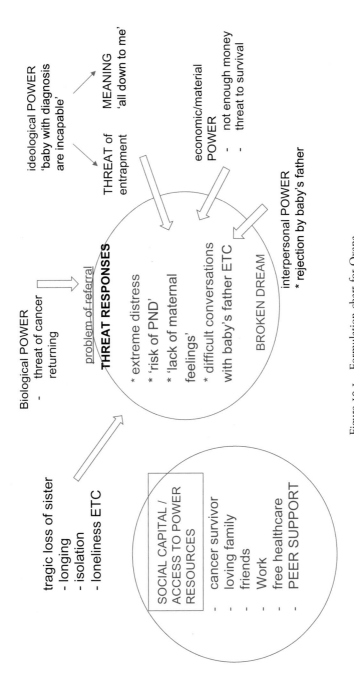

Figure 10.1 Formulation chart for Oxana

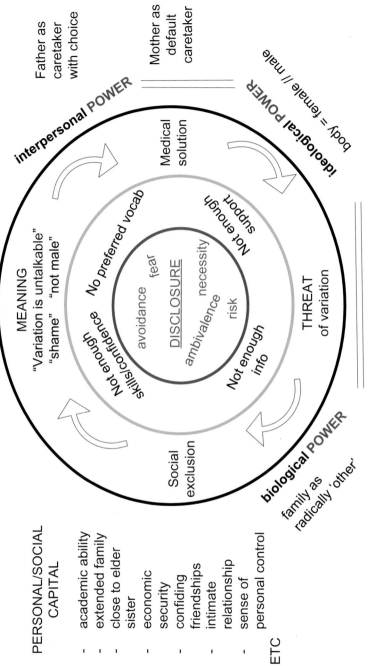

Figure 12.1   Formulation chart for Kereem

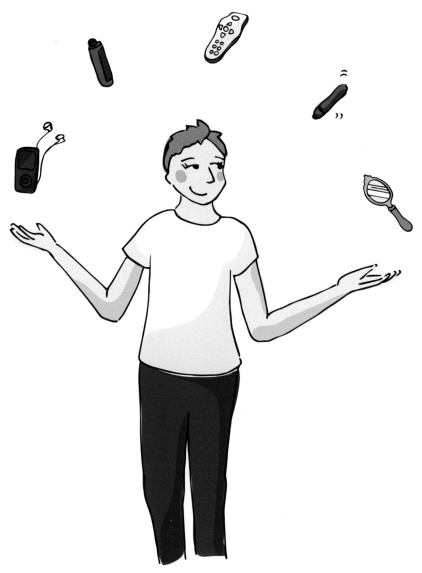

Figure 13.1   Making it fun (*Top Ten Tips for Dilation*). Printed with permission from dsdfamilies.org

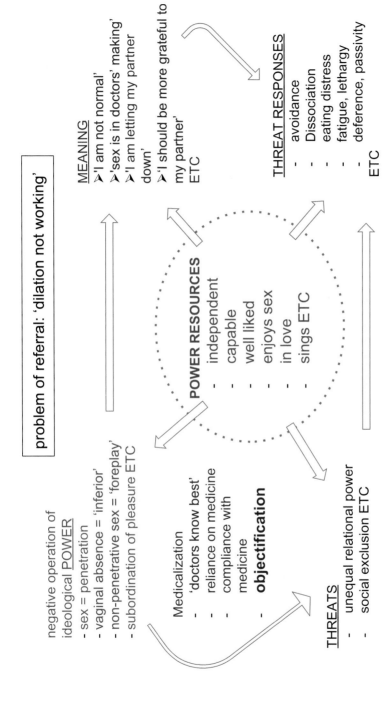

problem of referral: 'dilation not working'

negative operation of
ideological POWER
- sex = penetration
- vaginal absence = 'inferior'
- non-penetrative sex = 'foreplay'
- subordination of pleasure ETC

Medicalization
- 'doctors know best'
- reliance on medicine
- compliance with
  medicine
- **objectification**

THREATS
- unequal relational power
- social exclusion ETC

POWER RESOURCES
- independent
- capable
- well liked
- enjoys sex
- in love
- sings ETC

MEANING
➢'I am not normal'
➢'sex is in doctors' making'
➢'I am letting my partner
down'
➢'I should be more grateful to
my partner'
ETC

THREAT RESPONSES
- avoidance
- Dissociation
- eating distress
- fatigue, lethargy
- deference, passivity
- ETC

Figure 13.2 Formulation chart for Tess

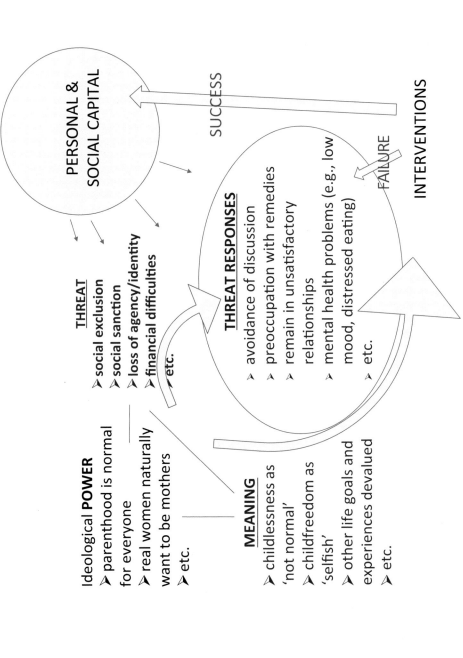

Figure 14.1   A Power Threat Meaning understanding of fertility distress

I am the one who says "we don't have to do this" if you have a very mild hypospadias … the parents' expectation is that really they want something to be done and I say "well this is very mild" "it is only cosmetics" and "there will be, could be a long journey with this, with operations and we can't ask the boy." (Roen & Hegarty, 2018, p. 975)

Timmermans et al.'s (2018) analysis of recorded doctor–patient interactions shows that merely by presenting genital surgery as *possible* and outcomes as *uncertain*, clinicians can inadvertently steer caretakers toward intervention. They described an example of a mother who had expressed a wish for her son to have hypospadias surgery. In this scenario, the urologist felt obligated to mention the view of "an ethicist who doesn't speak for all ethicists" and who had apparently suggested that parents should "just let boys sit to pee like girls" (p. 529). The disqualification of the ethicist and the construction of sitting down to urinate as being "like girls" is highly leading.

What is becoming clearer is that there is significant variability between services in how caretakers are counseled about *feminizing* and *masculizing* surgery for the child. Some caretakers report being told to take time to decide about surgery and explore alternative ways to address concerns about the child's variation (D'Alberton, 2010; Lundberg et al., 2017). Other caretakers, however, remember that delaying surgery as a real possibility was only ever vaguely acknowledged, if at all (Sanders et al., 2008).

At a strategic level, the absence of national and regional data on the prevalence of surgery is indefensible. Whatever opinion one holds in relation to childhood surgery, such information is indispensable. Various sources of information converge to suggest that uptake of childhood surgery is high. In a multicenter study in the USA, for example, all but one of the caretakers in the research sample had opted for genitoplasty for their female and male assigned children (Ellens et al., 2017). British and Swedish health professionals in the SENS study have alluded to an extremely high uptake even for the mildest hypospadias (Roen & Hegarty, 2018).

In a 2010 European survey, half of the participating DSD teams self-reported a reduction in clitoral surgery, a claim that the researchers did not verify (Pasterski et al., 2010). Scrutiny of NHS data in the United Kingdom indicated that the prevalence of clitoral surgery had not changed since the Chicago consensus in 2006, though concomitant vaginal surgery had decreased somewhat in frequency (Michala et al., 2014). The discrepancy between self-reports and statistics chimes with the SENS study, whereby clinicians described themselves as being far more conservative than their imaginary colleagues but also implied that they would perform surgery if caretakers should insist, if reluctantly.

In the last few years, Boston Children's Hospital and the Ann and Robert H. Lurie Children's Hospital of Chicago have made a public declaration they would stop performing certain cosmetic genital surgeries on children with DSD. Even with caveats, these movements represent a triumph for intersex advocacy. From a psychological point of view, knowing how caretakers struggle in the social context, it is disappointing that no alternative care path has been put forward to arm caretakers with skills and confidence to cope with the potentially substantial challenges.

6.4   Minoritization-Informed Care

The impact of medicalization, psychological disengagement and fragmented patient experience requires ongoing research. Meanwhile, conversation is needed to redevelop MDT processes in order to engage patients, families and health professionals psychologically, in accordance with declarations of PCC and holistic care. Given the historic difficulties, DSD services could consult trauma-informed care for inspiration (Marsac et al., 2016; Purkey et al., 2018; Raja et al., 2015). Whether an event (or process) is traumatic depends not just on the event itself but by the culturally supplied meanings conferred on these experiences, the level of safety of the environment that the person is in, how much support is available and how able is the person in coping. The effects of traumatic experiences may be short-lived or prolonged. In general, however, trauma disproportionately affects marginalized populations and is bound up with social inequalities and hierarchical norms.

In the story "Circles and Squares" in Chapter 1, the character "Jude" is portrayed as having dissociated in part of her medical journey. A difficult moment for her family is when a group of animated biomedical specialists debated enthusiastically with each other about a scientific paper by her bedside. "Jude" is a fictional character, but her experiences are far from fictitious. Being cognizant of medical power means recognizing how power is enacted, not by intention but by enactment of the pathology-based language of sex variations, the energy of the collective professional presence and the physical positioning of the patient as inert and docile. These configurations would not be seen in a trauma-informed service.

Trauma, however, is not the default presentation in sex development services today, at least in my experience. However, all service users are minoritized by their bodily differences, which are still not talkable in the social sphere. Therefore, the idea of minoritization-informed care is more inclusive of most service users. Being minoritization-informed would require the service and hosting organization to be trained (Goldstein et al., 2018) to recognize potential and actual minoritization distress in clients, families and staff, examine what is potentially marginalizing in the care process and fully integrate knowledge about minoritization-based distress into policies and procedures. It may overlap and is compatible with agency-based care that is inspired by the social model of health that emerged from disability theory (Crocetti et al., 2020). Such a service is characterized by:

- A safe therapeutic environment
- An understanding that disengagement and, at times, seemingly self-destructive practices are a way of coping with extreme distress
- A focus on strengths rather than deficits by asking questions such as: How have you managed to survive up to this point? What are you most proud of?
- An expression of hope from the provider that the client can address past and current difficulties with support and nurturing input
- The cultivation of resilience and resistance as part of skills training, including building healthy strategies for coping with difficult feelings
- A vision of what recovery might look like for the client

6.5 Implication for Psychological Practice

The demands of modern healthcare require diverse expertise. In many areas of clinical practice, there is a lack of integration of professional roles and contributions. These problems have far-reaching implications on patient experiences and outcomes. The less positive aspects of DSD team function identified in psychosocial research are not unique to DSD but are part of the larger fabric of human–technology conflict in modern medicine. Nevertheless, these patterns need to be addressed. Research in DSD has identified marginalization of psychosocial expertise in service configuration, even when it comes to intervening medically on psychosocial concerns. Psychological practitioners in DSD can expect to be conflicted in how they integrate their own professional values with a technology-bound protocol that intensifies medicalization of rather than demedicalizes sex variations. Without a mandate to reshape the care process as equal partners, pediatric psychologists inhabit an ambiguous if not treacherous space that implicates them in medical interventions currently framed as human rights abuse (Hegarty et al., 2021).

Critical psychology provides practitioners and academics with tools to examine power relationships, language and norms on service configuration and user experience. When the former European Network for Psychosocial Studies in Intersex/Diverse Sex Development (EuroPSI) was launched in 2014 for practitioners and academics to develop mutually enriching conversations, dozens of psychosocial experts made significant personal sacrifices to connect with each other and peer supporters outside the medical sphere. I suggest that there is a deep need for exchanges on psychosocial perspectives. EuroPSI has recently been redeveloped to become the Psychosocial Studies in Intersex International (PSI-I), which was relaunched online in 2021. Opportunities for psychosocial professionals, who are themselves minoritized within DSD medicine, to connect with peers and participate in critical conversations are improving. The rich exchanges may seep into our professional consciousness to collectively advance ethical and psychosocially informed care in future.

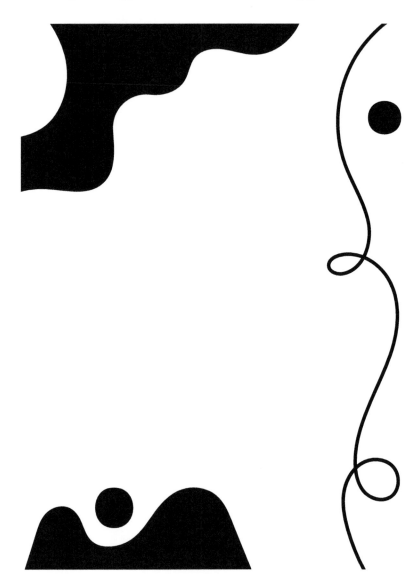

Introductory Notes

Psychological care providers (PCPs) have a wide variety of thinking tools and practice techniques to draw on, and some are more useful and relevant than others for this service context. Chapter 7 starts with a discussion of the strengths and weaknesses of key theoretical frameworks in healthcare psychology. A major weakness of individualistic psychological models is their lack of capacity to address structural factors in psychological wellness and distress.

I introduce aspects of the Power Threat Meaning Framework (Johnstone & Boyle, 2018) and provide examples of how to draw from its theoretical richness to think systemically about what sex variations pose to individuals and families and how the variations are responded to in the social context . The Framework provides the theoretical backbone for some of the practice vignettes in the final section of the book (Chapters 9–14).

Chapter 8 begins by highlighting a lack of clarity about the role of PCPs in sex development services. It suggests that researchers and practitioners make a collective effort in future to develop more clarity about roles and responsibilities and encourage theoretical debate. The chapter proceeds to outline the psychological consultation process that is generic and familiar to most PCPs. An initial assessment template is suggested and used in some of the practice vignettes. Chapter 8 proceeds to outline the more popular psychotherapeutic interventions.

In summary, this section serves as a reminder that the work of PCPs is always anchored in explicit knowledge frameworks. It provides a discussion of conceptual understandings that are familiar to many PCPs. The section further outlines some of the therapeutic tools available to PCPs. Importantly however, it draws attention to the vague and at times conflicted roles and responsibilities of specialist PCPs in the field. Thus far the dilemmas are rarely discussed. Future conversations about psychosocial approaches are strongly encouraged.

CHAPTER 7

Psychological Practice
Epistemic Considerations

In a collection of first-person accounts (Davis & Feder, 2015), the majority of intersex survivors referenced psychological therapy as a safe space to tell their stories and be listened to. For most of the adults, psychological input was accessed (eventually) through individual effort outside intersex medicine. The kind of psychological care mentioned by many intersex survivors relates to remedial therapies to help people identify and resolve problems of living. In order to do this kind of work, all psychological care providers (PCPs) draw on theoretical tools to make sense of needs and patterns of difficulties. The question is, what are the robust theoretical tools that are appropriate for working with people with variations? Thus far, there has been no sustained conversation on what ought to be the most important topic for PCPs. The conversational gap is being addressed in this chapter. Although this chapter and the next are not specific to sex development, they have to be included in a book whose aim is to develop the role of PCPs.

As I am a clinical and health psychologist, I can but focus on familiar frameworks within my own discipline. I preempt my discussion of the frameworks by briefly comparing four examples of psychosocial research in the field. In doing so, I hope to suggest to all PCPs that research and practice are informed by assumptions and values and that by rendering them explicit, they can be debated and refined.

I next summarize the prevailing psychological theories in clinical practice. I first discuss *psychosomatic* theorizing of the relationship between physical health and psychological well-being. I then discuss the *biopsychosocial model*. Because it has become the cornerstone of healthcare psychology in the Anglophone world and increasingly bandied around in differences in sex development (DSD), it is important to grapple with its strengths and limitations.

In the final section of the chapter, I introduce the Power Threat Meaning Framework (PTMF), which places the social context, in particular different forms of power, at the point of analysis (Johnstone & Boyle, 2018). The PTMF does not represent an epistemological departure from critical intersex studies, but it offers more tools to enable PCPs to bring issues of power into the healthcare context. As a meta framework, the PTMF has the potential to enable all support providers – professional and peer – to articulate the way in which wider social factors shape individual experience and choice. Space does not permit a full presentation of the PTMF here. I encourage interested readers to make use of the generous materials online to deepen their understanding. For the purpose of this book, I draw attention to the facets that are most directly relevant for making sense of the recurring themes in the field of sex development.

7.1   Recognizing Epistemic Assumptions

In response to epistemological concerns raised by social scientists regarding psychosocial research in DSD (Liao & Simmonds, 2014; Roen & Lundberg, 2020), I discuss four example studies in this part of the chapter. My objective here is to highlight how different assumptions in research can shift the landscape of psychological knowledge (and ultimately shape commissioners and policy makers' interpretation of psychological care in sex development services). The purpose of the exercise is to encourage all PCPs to discern the value of all research rather than accept research findings at face value.

Consider the research question: What proportion of people with DSD (or their caretakers) suffers from *psychopathology*? This is a prolific theme in DSD and elsewhere. The starting point here is an assumption that there is such a thing as pathological lived experiences, that the researchers know how to categorize and measure them, that the process is objective and neutral and that there are no repercussions on the people that they are measuring.

I first draw attention to a Swedish study that undertook a retrospective psychiatric survey of 335 girls and women with congenital adrenal hyperplasia (CAH) based on Swedish national register data for people born between 1915 and 2010 (Engberg et al., 2015). Women with CAH were observed to be twice as likely as a control sample to have a psychiatric disorder, twice as likely to have stress-related and adjustment disorders and almost three times more likely to have a record of alcohol misuse. The authors attributed the higher prevalence of unhappiness in the CAH group to genetic and biochemical variables. In other words, it is the patients' biological destiny to struggle with mental health problems. This may not have been the researcher's intended goal, but it is the logical conclusion of the assumptions, examined or unexamined, that underpin the research.

The implied psychosomatic causality, a framework that I critique in Section 7.2, reduces complex human experiences to biology. Although all human experiences are mediated by our biology, the rules that govern bodily functioning are not the same as the rules that govern thinking, feeling and (in)action. Biological factors afford and delimit life experiences, but so does our access to education, work, leisure, healthcare, relationships and love. Sex variations are shaped by genetics, but it is what the variations signify to the heavily scripted social world that triggers cascading psychosocial effects on lived experience. The Swedish study is emblematic of the kind of research that understands psychological distress as arising from within the person and exonerates the disempowering social context, if inadvertently. Such an outcome may not reflect the intention of the researchers, and often, the implications of our work are not available to us at the time.

The second example I discuss is a Dutch study that compared 130 people with mixed DSD diagnoses and a reference group of 372 people with fibromyalgia (de Neve-Enthoven et al., 2016). An assumption of this study is that DSD is comparable to a diffuse soft-tissue chronic pain condition associated with movement restrictions, fatigue, mental health problems and, often, high utility of medical treatment. But difficulties articulated by DSD populations do not match such a profile. Having chosen a control group that makes very little sense, the researchers contrived to use an array of measures including subjective fatigue and psychopathology without providing a rationale. They concluded that the DSD participants "reported good psychosocial wellbeing" and that "they generally reported a good [health-related quality of life], no serious emotional problems ... compared to reference groups" (p. 60). A different interpretation is that an opportunistic fishing exercise turned up a spurious catch.

Now compare the above study with the third example, a psychosocial study involving young people with exstrophy conditions (Wilson et al., 2004). This study set out to learn about the young people's ambitions. Although the study identified normative scores on self-esteem and other psychometric tests and also positive self-narratives, the authors did not conclude that exstrophy is therefore unproblematic. Rather, they inquired into specific problems that are potentially associated with exstrophy conditions. Most of the sample reported experiences of being bullied, with one-third severely so. But the participants also gave information on how they coped and the importance of being pragmatic and carrying on with their life goals. Encouragingly, five of the seven participants were currently in tertiary education and studying acting and drama. There were also participants who wished to become healthcare professionals. In this study, the young people were invited to voice their struggles with exstrophy without having their mental health reduced to a score on a rating scale. They were also invited to showcase their strengths. Here, the researchers began with the assumption that there are many facets to how people experience physical health problems and, while the authors made use of psychometric scales, they were the masters of rather than slaves to their tools. Above all, they did not confuse psychology with psychopathology or psychometry.

My final example is a German study with a small and biased sample of people with mixed DSD diagnoses (Schützmann et al., 2009). The study reported an unprecedented level of *psychopathology* (e.g., 59% suicidality). The authors reflected that due to methodological weaknesses, no claim of generalizability could be made. One might wonder, therefore, what was the point of the exercise. The point, I surmise, was to document the casualties of medical management, in order to challenge the status quo. This study could reflect what Tuck (2009) referred to as *damage-centered* research (p. 409). The assumption is that by accumulating evidence of suffering, people in power are made accountable. But, Tuck explained, this kind of reasoning is flawed and reinforces a one-dimensional notion of people as ruined and helpless. Tuck called on communities, researchers and educators to reconsider the repercussions of encouraging an entire community to understand themselves as broken.

If the above reports were taken at face value, DSD teams might buy in psychosocial input to help people cope with their diseases (Engberg et al., 2015), treat psychiatric corollaries of medical management (Schützmann et al., 2009) or appreciate clients as agentic and capable like everybody else but having highly specific psychosocial care needs (Wilson et al., 2004). Having explained the importance of discerning assumptions and values embedded in research, in Section 7.2 I describe prevailing psychological theories, all of which expose certain truth claims and obscure others.

7.2   Psychosomatic Theories

In a range of healthcare contexts, clients with physical health problems without identifiable medical causes are often referred to PCPs as the last resort. Where a medical cause cannot be found, it is not common for referrers to make psychosomatic assumptions. In this section, I briefly discuss psychosomatic formulations.

Psychoanalytic ideas of *somatization, hypochondriasis* and *hysterical conversion* have been highly influential in interpreting bodily experiences that cannot be (fully) medically explained, at least at a point in time. For example, psychoanalytic therapy used to be offered to women who could not conceive. A latent conflict relating to the maternal role was said to underpin complaints of infertility, so that infertility "should always be treated as a psychosomatic entirety" (Wischmann, 2003, p. 485). The decoding of unconscious defenses against childhood fantasies and traumas was claimed to have led to a change in the female patients' experience of femininity and ability to have children (Leuzinger-Bohleber, 2001). It is notable that this kind of theorizing is almost always applied to women, but then cultural values are recognizable in all psychological theories.

Ideas of repressed feelings giving rise to somatic symptoms have seeded a body of research to look for the impact that emotional release may have on somatic symptoms. However, research did not identify clear support for the hypothesis that medically unexplained somatic symptoms are caused by a failure to display emotions (e.g., Schilte et al., 2001).

Knowledge of stress physiology was soon to liberate psychosomatic theories from notions of unconscious drives. The work began with the observation that noxious stimuli could cause the formation of acute erosions in the digestive tract of rats (Selye, 1956). The work with animals was a precursor to a body of experimental research in human stress responses spanning several decades. The body of work culminated in stress being defined in terms of sympathetic arousal and disruptions to the physiological homoeostasis.

Stress is understood as an environmental event that triggers physiological changes to enable the individual to escape from the stressor. Different stressors, which include positive (e.g., a new relationship) and negative (e.g., a relationship break-up) events, are understood to carry differential weight in terms of potential capacity to tax the response system (Holmes & Rahe, 1967). The weighting system reflected the assumption that, first of all, stress can be studied objectively and, secondly, linear relationships can be identified between the size of the stressor (stimulus) and the scale of the impact (response). Clearly, impact is variable and context-dependent, and a transactional model of stress emerged to incorporate subjective appraisal into the formulation (Lazarus, 1996). *Primary* appraisal refers to whether an event is perceived as benign or harmful and *secondary* to the individual's assessment of whether they are adequately prepared or resourced to cope. Research has subsequently attempted to identify psychological factors that mediated subjective appraisal of stress and its attendant impact on health outcome.

Whatever the strengths and weaknesses of the stimulus-appraisal-response framework, it has contributed to the development of a range of stress reduction interventions. This development is significant for the growing acceptance of psychological contributions to improve outcome in chronic disease. The introduction of the biopsychosocial model in the 1970s fitted with a growing field of research seeking a language that legitimizes a psychosocial presence in medicine.

7.3   The Biopsychosocial Model

By the early 1980s, the rise of health psychology, a term evolved from several previous incantations including psychological medicine, psychosomatic medicine, medical psychology and behavioral medicine, had begun its long marriage to the biopsychosocial model (BPSM). The BPSM is bandied around not just in clinical and health psychology but a range of disciplines. Its importance is taken for granted by PCPs in sex development services. Therefore, it is important to briefly summarize what it is.

A premise of the BPSM is that disease trajectories cannot be understood merely in terms of an underlying physical deviation from normal bodily function. Rather, biological, psychological and social factors are all relevant to illness (and wellness). Biopsychosocial was a term coined by Engel (1977), in an attempt to develop a new *medical* model (my emphasis). Research to identify psychological factors in physical health outcome spread to an increasing range of chronic conditions including respiratory diseases (e.g., asthma), digestive tract problems (e.g., inflammatory bowel syndrome), skin disorders (e.g., psoriasis), metabolic diseases (e.g., diabetes), chronic pain syndromes (e.g., lower back pain) and disputed diagnoses such as chronic fatigue and fibromyalgia. Factors being researched include personality types, which supposedly predispose individuals to various diseases.

As health psychology in Anglophone nations expanded its remit from chronic disease to take on public health (i.e., prevention), psychological research in health-related behaviors, such as smoking, eating, drinking and exercising habits exploded. Staunch claims to a pivotal role in population-based interventions were mobilized within health psychology to shed its mental health heritage and augment a separate professional identity from clinical psychology. The lynchpin was the claim to identify and modify lifestyle (behavioral) factors to help entire populations to be healthier. Divisions of health psychology were formed in the USA and UK and psychological experts would stake their reputation in behavior change interventions.

Although behavioral factors are at the heart of Anglophone health psychology, investigations almost always rely on proxies in the form of self-reported beliefs and attitudes (cognitions). In other words, rather than observe actual eating and drinking behaviors in people's familiar settings, the researcher might ask how confident the research participants are about changing their eating behavior (self-efficacy). Health psychology was on a mission to construct core models of health cognitions as a basis for understanding health behaviours (Murray, 2017, p. 15). A major achievement of this endeavor was the tacit acknowledgment in medicine that patients are not passive followers of medical knowledge and may actually act in opposition to clinical advice. In other words, information per se is rarely enough to produce behavior change in order to improve or maintain health. It is now extremely rare for a physician to show images of diseased lungs and expect people to stop smoking cigarettes.

Health-related cognitions may have been a reasonable way to start, but the bulk of health psychology research does not seem to have moved past them. The growing list of psychological constructs loosely termed social cognitions includes self-efficacy, locus of control, health value, dispositional optimism, hardiness and resilience. These constructs are assumed to be static personal attributes that are eminently reducible to pencil and paper tests. It is fair to say that almost any construct put forward for testing (and which ends up in a publication) attracts some correlational evidence, usually in terms of its association with another construct. Mainstream health psychology literature to date is, in Crossley's (2000) words, saturated with statistical associations of "flimsy constructs that sideslip across each other with minimal effort to integrate into a coherence account" (pp. 63–75).

Practical constraints in research into real-life sickness and wellness and the need for a scientific veneer have rendered home testing of health and illness cognitions irresistible, as evident in the plethora of psychometric scales that exist in the market. Cross-sectional correlational studies are the norm in the literature, sometimes involving large batteries of pencil and paper tests. Research is largely with convenient white middle-class samples, and authors usually recommend that the next project should be more socially inclusive, rather than taking responsibility themselves to access "hard to reach" communities. Despite significant methodological limitations especially in relation to sampling, lack of generalizability is rarely emphasized. With a few exceptions of robust theory-driven strands of work, the bulk of mainstream health psychology literature is a kaleidoscope of at times interesting but more often unsatisfactory proxies for lived experience.

The language of the BPSM has enabled health psychology to claim a departure from psychosomatic medicine and move away from linear causality toward interactive hypotheses. However, critics question whether the BPSM is just another disingenuous euphemism for psychosomatic medicine (Crossley, 2000). Healthcare psychologists may have sold themselves short by routinely citing the BPSM as their conceptual platform, usually without explaining what the model is and how it enhances explanatory or predictive power. It is an interesting phenomenon in its own right that the loose BPSM template should have become the rhetorical mainstay of health psychology (Stam, 2015). It is doubtful if Engel could have predicted such a bumper crop when he planted the seeds in 1977.

7.4   A Systemic Focus

It has been the life's work of the epidemiologist Professor Sir Michael Marmot and a large team of multidisciplinary experts to evidence that healthy and happy lives are largely founded on favorable social conditions (Marmot, 2015), not cognitions. Some healthcare psychologists take structural factors seriously rather than allow them to be obscured by an individualistic focus. As an example, building on research that links health literacy to health inequalities, the English Longitudinal Study of Ageing showcases what healthcare psychology research can achieve, when it highlights the impact of social inequalities in health. The study identified that one in three adults over the age of 65 in England had difficulty in understanding basic health-related written information. Reduced understanding is associated with a higher risk of death over five years, even after accounting for socioeconomic circumstances and baseline health (Bostock & Steptoe, 2012). This is a sobering message for individualistic psychological theories. I bring this project into focus here to argue the case for psychological theories to take account of structural factors. But it is also worth mentioning, by the by, that no research in DSD has examined the effects of health literacy, even though the health literacy demands are huge. It is also worth mentioning there has also been very little interest in the health and well-being of senior citizens with variations.

Dissatisfaction with assumptions in mainstream health psychology has contributed to increased interests in critical health psychology, whose proponents suggest that every theory and method is a human construction that allows for some things to be seen and done and other things to be overlooked and unavailable. The obscuring of structural inequalities means that sometimes, an individual may be judged for eating too many donuts, when their zip code is the strongest predictor of their morbidity and mortality.

Interestingly, the worldview of critical health psychologists is aptly captured by the words of the historian, ethicist and activist in intersex Alice Dreger (1998): "Figure out how someone organizes his world, and you will see how he sees his world. You will also see how the organization system likely arranges the world as to reinforce that system maker's idea of the world – how what seems important gains in importance, and what seems unimportant fades from view" (p. 140).

Scrutinizing who benefits from existing social norms and who is displaced by them is precisely the kind of sensemaking that enables psychological practice with minoritized communities to be poignant and relevant. By attending to norms, values and expectations about physical appearance, gender roles and sexual expressions and considering how the ideas are propagated and reproduced, PCPs working in sex development can begin to unpick how people with variations and their families are disadvantaged, not by observable force, but by the power of language and its enactment. By talking about variations in ways that are complicit with the cultural idealization of binary bodies, health professionals are joining with social power to displace their patients. In a world made up of two kinds of people, their patients are not supposed to exist and the ongoing crisis of meaning is framed as a medical problem requiring treatment. In the rest of the chapter, I argue that PCPs engage with the concept of power as they make sense of how variations in sex development are responded to, past and present.

7.5 Understanding Ideological Power

Power is an abstract idea, yet the word brings on an immediate sense of urgency. Dictionaries define it in diverse ways, as energy, as physical strength, as ability to act, as privilege and influence and as capacity to control. In terms of how power operates on lives, the late clinical psychologist David Smail (cited in Boyle, 2020, p. 5) argued that we are all located in a field of power in such a way that we do not get to choose or decide how to relate to power outside of its influence.

Power may operate at variable distances from a person, but it is always mediated proximally. Take an everyday example of stereotypic gendered division of domestic responsibilities in a standard heterosexual household. The woman in the household may believe that being female, she is *naturally* more capable at *multitasking* than her male partner and chooses to do the lion's share. Her extensive labor is *proximally* experienced as her personal aptitude, preference and choice. Overworked and overwhelmed, she may seek medication to curb her anxiety. Social constructions of gender roles operate *distally*, making it harder for the woman to see that her experience is culturally primed and actively steered by discourse (common understanding). Gender inequalities are worked into social stereotypes and fogged up by discourses. The discourses are not experienced as social constructions but as truths by which lives should be lived. The greater in influence, the more distal power is.

The Power Threat Meaning Framework (PTMF), which I explain more fully below, is a conceptual resource that PCPs and their service users can draw on. Coproduced by psychological service providers and users, the framework brings together strands of critical thinking including feminism, social constructionism and critical theory into a coherent model to address human distress by taking into account social injustice. Because the majority of practitioners are unused to some of the ideas, the main publication is thorough and detailed (it stands at 190 000 words). A further disadvantage is that it is deeply anchored in mental health, social care and the justice system. Translation into practice at the grass roots is in its infancy even for these services. Outside these services, it is up to individual practitioners to explore it for their interests and needs. I draw on the overview (Johnstone & Boyle, 2018) and a recent introductory text (Boyle & Johnstone, 2020) to describe aspects of the framework that I consider most directly relevant for psychological practice in sex development services.

The PTMF is in essence a theorization of the operation of different forms of power (both proximal and distal) and the moderation of its impact by personal and social resources available to an individual. The forms of power include economic and material (e.g., control of resources), biological (e.g., possession of physical strength) and interpersonal (e.g., ability to withhold love). The PTMF suggests that ideological is the least obvious and least acknowledged form of power. I especially focus on ideological power in this chapter for its profound impact on how sex variations are responded to.

An ideology is a set of beliefs that are not easily open to proof or disproof but exerts influence through the use of language and meaning. Take for example the Western belief that thinness is more attractive than fatness. It is not to be argued with. It just is. People are culturally primed to not only scrutinize their own size but other people's sizes in order to make size-based social judgments and see how they and other people may fit within the social order. Distress of the person in the *wrong* size is framed as the individual's problem rather than as a problem of the wider culture that maintains unrealistic ideals, perhaps to serve various industries, or to control women, who are affected the most by antifat discourses.

We are aware that in sex development, how a bodily feature is talked about has cascading social and psychological effects for the individual. These effects, in turn, reinscribe, reproduce and reinforce a particular version of truth and suppress other understandings. Consider the example of a larger clitoris. It could be thought of as a rare gift to be enjoyed. However, the medical language for this is *clitoral hypertrophy* and *clitoromegaly*, because it is incompatible with the idealized female form. But, giving the larger clitoris a meaning of aberration can pose a meaning-based threat to the woman. As not-woman, her core needs for acceptance and inclusion may be threatened. Having tools to unpick how power creates meaning-based threats and how people construct threat responses in order to survive can enhance PCPs' capacity for anti-oppressive practices.

I introduce the PTMF here because I believe that it provides a different language for making sense of lived experience and because it has the potential to offer service users and providers, peer supporters, champions and activists a shared epistemological home to connect and collaborate with each other. I discuss the PTMF in more detail below but preempt discussion by stating that it

1. does not privilege the psychotherapies over and above other remedial approaches involving art, music, nutrition, exercise, peer support and community activism
2. encourages ways of understanding and responding to human distress that are not peculiar to Western lenses and respects the many creative ways of supporting people through varied forms of narrative and healing practices across cultures
3. offers professional and peer providers and other agencies a sense-making system to approach human struggles
4. facilitates clients, families, groups and communities to tell their stories
5. identifies possibilities for problem-solving and challenging the status quo.

In the following discussion, I bring in a few direct examples from sex development to explain the dynamic interplay between power, threat, meaning and threat responses. Aspects of the discussion are revisited in some of the practice vignettes in the ensuing chapters of this book.

7.5.1   *Power Threat Meaning in Sex Development*

Idealization of binary sex and gender and heterosexuality underpins many ongoing difficulties reported by people with variations. Consider a young woman without a uterus growing up and living in a gender-normative community. Dominant discourses of female embodiment ("all women bear children") construct her as "not-woman" and "unworthy" and may threaten her prospect of marriage. Threat (e.g., inability to produce children) is commonly associated with meanings such as exclusion, shame, humiliation, entrapment, inferiority and worthlessness. Acceptance of controversial physical interventions, for example, is often based on such meanings. One might ask, why not just change the meaning. This is not so simple. Meaning, though deeply felt within a person, is already given in the social sphere and not in the person's control. I further explain before returning to the woman.

Picture an infant who interacts with the world with available bodily capacities (subject to social rules). As the child grows up hearing, seeing, touching, tasting and moving in the material world, the child acquires language, rules and experiences mediated by language. The child's learning is internalized and becomes inner speech and metacognitive tools with which to produce meaning. Meaning is additionally flavored by memories and feelings. For example, being ignored by an unfriendly receptionist in a public place may trigger sensations of being neglected by a caretaker and produce an angry reaction. Personal meaning is, therefore, highly complex and never truly personal but largely a social given. It can be negotiated, but only up to a point.

The meaning of inferiority and unworthiness of an absent uterus in a woman is culturally supplied. The meaning threatens the aforementioned woman's core need for a purposeful life that, in her case, is centered on marriage and biological motherhood. Pressure is put upon her to respond in order to survive. How this woman responds to the situation depends on her access to power resources (e.g., abilities, education, family, community, wealth and spirituality). Therefore, survival strategies will differ markedly from one woman to another. For example, a woman with access to personal abilities, education and training may grow her life in such a way that leads to personal independence and autonomy. She may not feel fulfilled by such a life, but her material survival is at least not threatened. Consider another woman with the same variation but whose access to power resources is much more restricted. This woman may respond to the threat by social withdrawal. She may end up being medicated, even institutionalized, because her difficulties are not being understood in ways that take account of power. I have produced two extreme examples of threat responses to make a point here. In reality, there are, of course, many more shades to how a person responds to meaning-based threat.

Safety and inclusion is a core human need. The threat to core needs for inclusion is evident in the many teenage girls with vaginal agenesis who tell me that they cannot go to social spaces with friends until doctors have given them a vagina. This may seem strange, because a vagina is not required for enjoying a movie with friends. However, integral to the dominant ideology of female embodiment is the idea that every woman has a vagina that can accommodate an erect penis. From the young person's point of view, every social occasion at that age may have some potential for romantic attraction. Before surgery, the young heterosexual woman would be going out to meet potential male partners as a "not-woman." Such meanings, though externally produced as explained above, are felt deep within. By staying at home, she will not be "found out"; she is safe from threat. However, she may be lonely and isolated. Vaginal surgery, where available, might be considered a power resource that eliminates the threat of social exclusion. But surgery may also be experienced as painful and shaming. Many women say that even after vaginal construction, they do not feel entitled to relationships and live in fear of being "found out."

One PCP may work productively with the young woman using a cognitive behavioral therapy program to reduce her anxiety and enable her to become available for coitus. Another PCP, using a different sense-making framework, may engage the same client to deconstruct the self-diminishing understanding of herself as inferior, and to imagine new ways of thinking about her body and selfhood. Yet another PCP may do both. None of these three PCPs is right or wrong. After all, what transpires in therapy is largely determined by the client (based on my practice experience). What is important is that all three PCPs are aware of the ideas that are influencing their work and the ideas that their work is serving.

So far, I have talked about responses to threat that are characterized by fear and shame. But threat can be insidious yet not at all obvious. Consider a man with Klinefelter syndrome who is subjected to a diffuse combination of pointed admiration about his height and affectionate teasing about his breast tissue. The individual may wish for these interactions to stop but, by raising the issue, he may upset his friends, or they may tease him even harder. He may find himself avoiding certain activities and venues and experience the avoidance as a personal preference (e.g., "I was born an introvert, that's why I don't socialize much").

People can experience ongoing low-level and diffuse threat without being fully aware of the impact. I have worked with many women with Turner syndrome who ask for help with social anxiety, which they believe to be intrinsic to the diagnosis. But their anxiety about social spaces may be an entirely rational response to having been patted on the head like a child and teased about their stature, usually warmly and affectionately (e.g., being told that they are "small but perfectly formed"). On one hand, they are accepted and embraced; on the other, they are aligned to their physical difference rather than their talent and personality. This kind of double-edged experience is difficult to articulate but can lead to shame and social withdrawal.

Threat response may be active beyond the time of the experience of negative operation of power in the past. Consider the many adults with variations who avoid medical services to the detriment of their health. They may tell themselves that they are too busy or that they are well and do not need to see a doctor. Their avoidance may be linked to childhood experiences of feeling frightened and out of control in hospitals, experiences that they have forgotten about. Even if they remember, their negative experiences are socially sanctioned and therefore not understood as threat and not linked to the threat response (avoidance of doctors).

Disempowered people often disavow their experience of threat, because acknowledging it can feel dangerous, stigmatizing and shaming. Consider an adult whose childhood surgery has been damaging but nevertheless believes that their parents or doctors had made the right decision. First of all, the client may not make the link between their current sexual problems and the forgotten experiences of pain, fear and humiliation during repeat hospitalizations in the past. Secondly, the idea of parental culpability is emotionally overwhelming and too dilemmatic. The PTMF's treatise on ideological power enables PCPs to tease out how power has operated on all of the actors involved, including the parents and the doctors. It suggests that the reframing of sex variations within DSD medicine is the enduring way to challenge negative meaning and reduce the need for threat-based responses.

How people respond to the threat of ideological power may actually stop them from feeling safe in the long run. Research suggests that "normalizing" interventions on children rarely make families feel secure. Most caretakers continue to feel too threatened to discuss variations with close friends and relatives and the child in question (Crissman et al., 2011;

Lundberg et al., 2017). Adult women who have had vaginal construction may remain sexually anxious and avoidant (Boyle et al., 2005). The action taken by caretakers and adults, caught up in a crisis of meaning, needs to be understood as part of a constellation of responses to the threat of ideological power rather than in terms of individual culpability.

7.5.2 Anti-oppressive Psychological Practice

An empathic and receptive mode of inquiry into the client's distress does not imply a tacit confirmation of their premise. For example, we can empathize and validate their feeling of unworthiness without subscribing to the "truth" that they are not entitled to relationships until doctors can make them more "normal." Otherwise there would hardly be any point in therapy. On the left-hand side of Table 7.1, I suggest an example of what standard psychological inquiry, informed by common constructs in

Table 7.1. *Standard and PTMF-informed psychological conversations*

Example standard conversation that taps into familiar psychological constructs	Example PTMF-informed conversation
• "What is the name of your diagnosis?" [Disease identity] • "What information have you been given about it?" [Health education] • "What are your beliefs about the cause, timeline, cure. . .?" [Illness perceptions] • "How does your condition affect you and other people?" [Impact] • "How much control do you have about what happens next?" [Self-efficacy] • "What can you and other people do to cope?" [Social support] • "What are the benefits and barriers of following your care plan?" [Treatment adherence]	• "How has the process been for you?" [How is POWER operating in your life?] • "What has been said about your body?" [What kind of THREAT does the situation pose?] • "How do you make sense of it all?" [What MEANING do these experiences have for you?] • "How are you responding to the challenges?" [What kinds of THREAT RESPONSE are you using?] • "What do you see as your strengths – your abilities, the family, community, peer and advocacy groups, people with a different view to offer. . .?" [What access to POWER RESOURCES do you have?] • "How does all this fit together? What stories would you like to be able to tell?" [Your STORY]

healthcare psychology, may look like. On the right-hand side of Table 7.1, I suggest how an orientation to power may steer conversations with care users. There is merit in both and in many other frameworks not covered in this chapter and book. What is important is to stay alive to power, influence and minoritization.

Health professionals are trained to account for the service user's situation in individualistic terms – their genes, hormones, personality, helplessness or noncompliance. This way of accounting for care users' distress can, however, make PCPs complicit with oppressive discourses of individual culpability and blame. The PTMF can help PCPs to distance themselves from this kind of blame-the-victim stance that exonerates the negative operation of power. Instead, PCPs can engage the care user to do some detective work around systemic factors and challenge ideological power, if in a limited way. The care user may nevertheless proceed with a nonevidenced "normalizing" intervention, but it is still preferable to suggest that there are other ways to think about their situation.

Engaging with power will make psychological practice harder and less popular. It will involve asking difficult questions, such as: How do people find purpose in life when culturally constructed femininity milestones such as marriage and children are closed off? What kind of meaning could be conferred on a smaller penis that does not urinate from a standing position in order for it to be valued and enjoyed? How can sexual intimacy be constructed if coitus is not possible? What kind of language is needed to moderate meaning so that caretakers can talk to children about their variations without flinching and bracing? How can PCPs engage the DSD team to name their fears, so that the unwanted emotions do not drive the (usually unspoken) agenda that something must be done?

A formulation that takes account of power may be a work in progress, at best, in the currently restricted view of sex variations. Even so, it can be part of a vision in which a larger range of remedial approaches can be tried, approaches that 1) move away from notions of individual choice and culpability, 2) do not see professional thought and action as separate from social goals, 3) replace notions of neutrality with articulation of biases, 4) pivot around an idea so as to look at it from all possible sides and 5) are cognizant of anti-oppressive perspectives, especially those that are well hidden.

Anti-oppressive psychological practice needs to be preintegrated into an anti-oppressive service model. For example, a service that misunderstands the PCP as an emotion repository, refers patients when the medical path is too distressing, views psychological expertise as an option when medicine has run out of steam and masks technocentrism by paying lip service to holistic care will run counter to anti-oppressive ideals in healthcare.

7.6 Summary

The biomedical paradigm has led to major advances in medicine, science and technology; it works – but for understanding the rules that govern bodily functions, not for understanding the rules that govern subjectivities mediated by dominant social discourses that control meaning. What is crucially missing in the various psychological formulations about DSD-related distress is engagement with issues of power. By making power explicit, the PCP renders visible what is invisible, changes the meaning of a scenario and offers new ways of constructing conversations and solutions. It invites everyone concerned to understand that what goes on in DSD medicine is not a reflection of the truth about sex variations but a consequence of what the variations are made out to be – something that is neither natural nor inevitable. A focus on power helps us to understand the normative choices made by service users not as a reflection of their weakness but as a threat response that could help, or not. Such a focus shifts how we talk about sex variations, interventions and decisions.

The PTMF provides a set of tools that enable PCPs to coexamine with clients impacted by bodily variations the power structures that subordinate positive meanings of different bodies. As a meta framework, it can be a way to engage all parties to challenge socially excluding and discriminatory ideas of body and identity. As such it is compatible with and can help to progress a wide range of professional–peer collaborations to expand on the currently delimiting views of sex variations.

CHAPTER 8

Psychological Practice
Process Considerations

Psychological care in sex development has been widely endorsed since the 1990s. It is clearly acknowledged in the Chicago consensus (Lee et al., 2006). On the face of it, such broad endorsement is positive. In reality, research has identified gaps in psychological care (Bennecke et al., 2015; Ernst, Liao, et al., 2018), absence of psychological expertise at strategic points in the process (Garland et al., 2021; Gramc et al., 2021; Liao & Roen, 2021) and a restricted view of psychological contributions (Liao & Roen, 2021). In Chapter 6, I account for this pattern of findings systemically, that is, in terms of conflicting narratives in differences in sex development (DSD) publications. Holistic care and biogenetic framing, for example, are spoken of in the same breath, as if they are an easy fit. Are they?

Unlike medical specialists with strong academic-clinical networks for mutual learning and dissemination, psychosocial care providers (PCPs) in sex development services exist in ultralow numbers and work in isolation. They are bereft of effective clinical networks to facilitate their professional development. In future, their relevant professional bodies would need to address workforce development, so that service users can expect a consistent standard of psychological care, at least within national boundaries. Because the workforce is small in each nation and the core psychosocial concerns are broadly shared across nations (e.g., communication, relationship, identity, sex), there are strong arguments for international collaboration to develop best practice. In recognition of the need for isolated PCPs and researchers to connect, the Psychosocial Studies in Intersex International (PSI-I) was launched in 2021. Depending on the priorities of the membership, the network can potentially create a platform for PCPs to identify common concerns, review relevant research, disseminate best practice and design models for postqualification training and supervision.

Until then, it is up to PCPs to individually interpret the wide psychosocial brief in medical publications. In the absence of a collective vision, they are likely to fall back on the usual ways of receiving and acting on referrals by colleagues. The standard response to a referral can be summarized as comprising the following components: 1) agreeing on the purpose of referral with the client, 2) establishing rapport and building relationships, 3) assessing psychological needs, 4) developing a formulation and care plan and 5) doing the work and evaluating the outcome. These processes are the subject matter of this chapter, which begins with a brief summary of the context.

8.1 A Wide Brief

I examine key DSD care documents for their psychological content from a service design point of view. Table 8.1 represents my categorization of recognizable concepts in the psychosocial segments of the Chicago consensus (Lee et al., 2006) and three subsequent national and international care documents (Ahmed et al., 2021; Cools et al., 2018; Lee et al., 2016). Some of the concepts in Table 8.1 are *problems* of referral (e.g., "sexual aversion," "lack of arousability"), some are *remedial* interventions (e.g., "collaboration," "group work") and some are *outcomes* of remedial interventions (e.g., "acceptance," "resilience"). There are also concepts that could be taken to mean problem, process *and* outcome (e.g., "communication skills"). These ideas have face value but are yet to be operationalized for consistent implementation and evaluation.

Some of the recommendations in Table 8.1 are evidence-based and some experience-based while others reflect common sense. Taken together, the brief is wide but lacks details. Take the often-mentioned concepts of resilience and acceptance, for example. In DSD services, does resilience mean coping with the medical process? And does acceptance count if it is conditional on "normalization"?

The clinical skills required to implement the respective recommendations are on the right-hand column of Table 8.1. The skills set is vast and certainly unrealistic for a single practitioner. Many of the skills require specialists who work with adults, yet lifespan care is typically designed in pediatrics. PCPs specialize in working with different age groups. Just as a psychosexual therapist would not typically have the knowledge and skills to assess children cognitively, so pediatric psychologists would not typically be able to work skillfully with couples with sexual concerns. Yet both types of work are grouped under the role of PCPs in sex development services. Substantial translation is needed to define methods and outcomes before the plethora of concepts in the various care documents can be prioritized and integrated into prevailing service structures in which PCPs work. Meanwhile, I discuss generic psychosocial practice concepts with the DSD service user in mind.

Table 8.1. *Psychological concepts in recent DSD care documents*

Publications	References to psychosocial roles, tasks, methods, concepts	Psychological knowledge and skills
Lee et al. (2006) All DSDs Lifespan	**Patient and family well-being** • Disclosure associated with enhanced psychosocial adaptation • Cognitive and psychological development of children • Post-traumatic stress disorder • Participation in peer support **Assessment** • Screening tools (e.g., for maladaptive coping in family) • Comprehensive psychological evaluation • Psychological assessment targeting gender identity **Gender** • Atypical gender role behavior not always an indicator for gender reassignment • Explore feeling about gender over a period of time • Expert input for gender change **Sexuality and relationships** • Definition of "quality of life" to incorporate falling in love, dating, attraction, ability to develop intimate relationships, sexual functioning, opportunity to marry and raise children • Sexual aversion • Lack of arousability (does not equal low libido) • Fear of rejection, avoidance of intimate relationships • Medical shame and stigma (e.g., repeat genital scrutiny) • Sex therapy	◦ Psychology of gender development ◦ Psychometrics (selection, interpretation, limitations, risk of misuse, communication of results and how they are incorporated into care plans and/or child adult safeguarding, rationale for timing of retesting and interpretation of difference) ◦ Decision theories ◦ Systemic psychotherapies ◦ Relationship and sex therapies ◦ Person-centered counseling ◦ Cognitive and behavioral approaches (including behavioral goal planning) ◦ Eye movement desensitization and reprocessing

Conceptual issues

- Psychology as "brain gender"
- Psychology as "catch all" concept (anything not medical)

Conceptual weaknesses in recent research

- Simplistic, linear, causal links from biology to psychology
- Overdependence on psychometrics
- Well-being seen as fixed when it is likely to fluctuate across events (e.g., initial diagnosis, ending of an intimate relationship)
- Influences of social context obscured

Psychological difficulties identified in psychosocial research to date

- Variability in satisfaction with binary gender
- Variability in satisfaction with DSD terminology
- Fear of devaluation, relationship nonentitlement
- Negative body image, functional sexual difficulties, preoccupation with heterosexual intercourse
- Barriers to communication about variations, social isolation
- Dilemmatic decisions on normalizing surgery
- Variability in appraisal of own childhood medical interventions

Conceptual developments in future

- DSD well-being research to dialogue with "minority stress" research
- Research to be theoretically explicit
- Research to engage with a broader methodological base such as better use of qualitative methods
- Research participants to define own challenges and articulate emotions

- Epistemology
- Psychometrics (selection, interpretation, limitations, risk of misuse with social minorities)
- Qualitative methods
- Feminist/discursive psychology and gender studies
- Social psychology
- Minority stress frameworks
- Organizational development
- Healthcare psychology models
- Decision theories
- Systemic psychotherapies
- Relationship and sex therapies
- Cognitive and behavioral approaches (including behavioral goal planning)
- Person-centered counseling
- Goal planning
- Group dynamics and facilitation
- Pedagogies

Table 8.1. (*cont.*)

Publications	References to psychosocial roles, tasks, methods, concepts	Psychological knowledge and skills
	• Make sense of lived experiences by drawing on communication, organizational development, social studies and applied healthcare psychology literatures	
	Example topics for new research	
	• Parental awareness of management options	
	• Consequences of decision-making due to inadequate information and preparation	
	• Relationships between self-disclosure and psychological well-being	
	• Impact of advocacy groups to mitigate psychological distress	
	Example practices in	
	• Groupwork drawing on cognitive and narrative approaches (e.g., for women with MRKHS and TS);	
	• Communication skills training	
	• Team training	
Cools et al. (2018) All DSDs Lifespan	**Sex and gender**	◦ Psychology of gender development
	• Nonbinary	◦ Feminist/discursive psychology and gender studies
	• Resilience	◦ Decision theories
	• Gender expressions (e.g., juvenile play style, core gender identity) not always aligned; gender contentedness as ultimate goal	◦ Systemic psychotherapies
	• Language	◦ Relationship and sex therapies
	Collaboration with peer support groups including participation of appropriately trained peers in the decision-making process or in multidisciplinary team	◦ Cognitive and behavioral approaches (including behavioral goal planning)
		◦ Person-centered counseling
		◦ Pedagogies
		◦ Intercultural competence

Communication skills in social sphere

Decision-making on (provisional) gender role and medical and judicial options

Trade-offs in fertility research and experimentation

Psychologial counseling (e.g., personal attitudes, life experiences, cultural and religious background and socioeconomic factors in coping and acceptance)

Parents
- Orientation to psychological tasks
- Psychoeducation
- Decision-making
- Bonding

Emotional containment
- Anxiety or distress relating to uncertainty
- Present and future worries

Psychological needs assessment at multiple time points
- Diagnosis
- Medical interventions
- Transfer from pediatric to adult care
- Gender transition

Team
- Communication skills training for MDT members
- Consultancy on assessing patient/parent care experiences

Encourage participation in peer support

Acceptance

○ Attachment theories
○ Decision theories
○ Parent-infant psychology
○ Systemic psychotherapies
○ Cognitive-behavioral approaches (including behavioral goal planning and "third wave" therapies)
○ Pedagogies

Ahmed et al. (2021)
All DSDs
Initial evaluation (birth and adolescence)

8.2   Relationship to Help

Agreeing on the purpose of referral means creating opportunities for service users to voice what the referral means for them rather than acting on its face value. I suggest that every assessment begins with an exploration of *relationship to help* to clarify mutual assumptions about the referral – what is it for, whom is it for and so on.

Service users are not passive recipients of "treatment" but chief agents of change. Active participation is strongly implicated in psychosocial intervention outcome (Sparks et al., 2008). It has even been argued that psychological therapy merely facilitates a process that is already taking place in the help seeker (Orlinsky, 2009). These observations compel the PCP to be curious about how a care user approaches the helping relationship. Professional education for PCPs differs markedly in the extent to which trainees are supported to reflect on their own constructions of psychological help. Systemic psychotherapists are mostly likely to be encouraged to adopt a curiosity stance in relation to respective (rather than necessarily mutual) beliefs and assumptions about the helping process and to acknowledge the expertise of the other.

Reder and Fredman's (1996) account on *relationship to help* explains how users and providers hold certain beliefs about the healthcare process. The beliefs may be held quizzically, or very strongly to significantly alter client engagement and outcome. What does it mean to the care user, for example, to talk to a total stranger about intimate concerns without any certainty of being able to resolve the concerns? Reder and Fredman invited PCPs to reflect on how they and care users might be positioned in each other's storylines. The process of *hypothesizing* in advance of the first meeting has been introduced to encourage PCPs to be alive to the possibility that their constructions may differ from those of the client.

Take the example of a newly diagnosed teenager who describes having panic attacks and catastrophizing about the future. The PCP may assume that the teenager wants help to stop catastrophizing because this maintains a state of hyperarousal and gives rise to panic attacks. However, the teenager may have rather different beliefs about their needs. Whether we frame service users' discourses, stories and beliefs as resources or obstacles can profoundly alter how they experience us. A therapist's *irreverence* to their own *prejudices* (biased constructions) makes it more possible to juxtapose contradictory ideas in consultation, while their *excessive loyalty* to a specific idea risks alienating the client (Cecchin et al., 1993). When holding difficult conversations with disparate ideas, however, the PCP does not blend contradictory viewpoints but creates *bridging* conversations instead.

Consider a couple who seek to win the PCP over to their decision for their son to have hypospadias surgery, when the PCP thinks the meeting should focus on the caretakers' emotional containment first. A bridging or coconstructing conversation could start with the agreement that all parties are committed to the child's well-being, for example: "[Jason] is loved and accepted. We all want him to stay happy. This is what brought us together, to think how Jason can stay a happy child."

Depending how integrated DSD services are, psychosocial care may fit more or less meaningfully with the overall process. Team integration will affect the meaning drawn by caretakers and care users of a referral to a PCP. A *relationship to help* inquiry can tease out meaning. For example, the PCP could ask caretakers of a child with variations: "Whose idea was it that we meet today?" and "If Dr. Gurney [endocrinologist] were in the room with us, what would they want us to talk about?" Likewise, for an adolescent service user, the referral may have been triggered not by the young person but their caretakers or doctors. The PCP could ask, "What did you have to give up in order to be here?" If the young person shows ambivalence, the PCP could ask, "Who (else) should be here (instead)?" These questions demonstrate respect for the young person whose willingness is not taken for granted. They gather multiple perspectives including those of people who are physically absent but are nevertheless influencing the interaction.

The PCP can also elicit conflicted discourses in multidisciplinary team (MDT) discussions in the same way. Questions such as "What does the family want us to appreciate the most about their situation?" brings the family into the room even though they are physically absent. Questions such as "Which one of us is the most and the least enthusiastic about the idea being proposed?" enable differences to be voiced. Consider an everyday example here. Suppose it is the team decision to repeat the pelvic imaging of the child. To the DSD team, it is a minor inconvenience. To the caretakers, such action could carry a meaning that the child's body is a giant puzzle that even experts cannot decipher. By centering the child and caretakers in team discussions, clinicians are more able to reflect together on the performative effects of their action and speech.

There are limits to all psychological approaches, the effects of which are either constrained or enhanced by the fit between practitioner and context. Consider the family in Chapter 1 with the child "Lulu" who is scheduled to have feminizing genitoplasty. The parents' assumption is that "psychology" is for people without the emotional capacity to make decisions. Since the couple have already gone through a rigorous decision process involving trusted doctors and peers, the mother "Karla" minimizes psychosocial input as a "rubber-stamping" exercise. We know from research that "psychology" is sometimes positioned as a hoop to jump through (Liao & Roen, 2021). Suppose the psychologist complies with this brief to get the parents to think about their decision, when the decision has already been made? The interaction could be fraught and may not serve anyone. In such instances, the team is the "patient." Therefore, the consultation needs to be with/for the team about aspects of the care process that can entrap the PCP and service user in a paradox.

I discuss in Chapter 6 the importance for DSD services to be minoritization-informed. This means that, at times, the PCP has to take a stance rather than hide behind the concept of therapeutic neutrality. Family therapist Lynn Hoffman (1990) told a story of how she had become strongly critical of therapists' abdication of social responsibilities when oppressive cultural norms are being enforced. She referenced such neutrality as "a particularly offensive kind of ecological fascism" (p. 5) whereby an individual's right is sacrificed for the sake of the system remaining intact. On the other hand, taking the moral high ground and imposing one's political values on care users, for example by telling them that genital surgery will mutilate their child, represents an abuse of power.

Humanizing caretakers and advocating for the patient when it comes to controversial interventions requires a confident knowledge of research (see Chapter 4) and exceptional interaction skills on the part of a PCP, who must be able to count on the team's support. Collective failure on the part of the team to socialize families to an ethos of whole-person care will undermine the intention of the PCP to work ethically.

Relationship to help is a useful concept for navigating tense conversations. It is not a panacea that prevents workers from feeling uncomfortable in family consultation, for example when decisions are made with irrevocable impact on children who cannot speak for themselves. Nevertheless, it is an art well worth cultivating. It helps if the practitioner can project the qualities that psychological care users value. The practitioner–client relationship is the focus of Section 8.3.

8.3   Practitioner Qualities

Perceived quality of the therapeutic relationship is considered the second most important predictor of positive therapy outcome, after client variables (which may include engagement, commitment, complexity of the presenting problems and so on). The generic observation is corroborated by a small study with women with congenital adrenal hyperplasia (CAH), which suggested that the therapeutic alliance is of primary importance and that therapist traits and skills were more salient than having specific knowledge of and experience in CAH (Malouf et al., 2010). But what provider qualities are helpful for cultivating a strong therapeutic alliance?

In an interesting project, 10 therapists were carefully selected from a large pool of people to be interviewed so that the researchers could identify their common attributes (Jennings & Skovholt, 1999). The 10 individuals were chosen because professional colleagues had repeatedly nominated them for being exceptional. The following personal qualities were identified in this group of "master therapists," who 1) valued ongoing learning from experience and building knowledge; 2) were open to ambiguities and complexities of living; 3) were self-aware, nondefensive and open to feedback; 4) valued authenticity and honesty; 5) were able to relate strongly to others; and 6) were caring and empathic and believed that the client could change. The researchers wondered if they had merely tapped into qualities that would enable the individuals to function well in any line of work. In a different study, the following adjectives were used to describe the attributes of a model therapist: truth-telling, compassionate, kind, trustworthy, adaptable in wanting the best for the other, free of envy, encouraging, humble and optimistic about the human condition (Aveline, 2005).

Therapy research is succinctly summarized in *The Therapy Relationship: A Special Kind of Friendship*, a fascinating account by Richard Hallam (2015), who drew attention to the similarity between attributes that therapy users seek and attributes that people usually look for in a friend. In other words, PCPs can expect to be judged by their clients against friendship norms. This idea may astonish some PCPs, whose training has instilled in them the importance of *professional distance*, a concept that is poorly defined and, it would seem, somewhat superfluous to service users. Provided that the care user is open to input, willing to experiment and proactive on their own behalf, Hallam suggested that the idea of the therapist as a friend was not so terrible and certainly preferable to the idea of the therapist as a healer, which positions the help seeker as being broken in some way.

Effective psychological input is mobilized by relationships. The trusting relationship enables the care user to rethink their worst fears, assume position as an equal partner in decision-making and, in case of variations in sex development, question cultural norms that do not serve them well. Such work makes demands on the overall DSD service to centrally position the psychosocial care path.

It is the job of PCPs in any service to listen to first-hand accounts of fear, shame, trauma, loneliness, relationship breakup, self-harm and suicidality and to remain hopeful about the client's capacity to improve aspects of their lives. PCPs are said to be prone to perfectionism and being easily disappointed with themselves when the client's problem is unresolved (Hallam, 2015). Meanwhile, they cannot hold their own lives constant and may also experience relationship breakups and terrifying diagnoses that have parallels with their clients' situations. Because they tend to work in isolation with limited or no organizational support, they cannot be excused from work for long periods, even in the face of a personal tragedy. A study with therapists and their clients reported that 27% of therapists were practicing in a "disengaged" manner and 10% in a distressed mode (Zeeck et al., 2012).

There has been no dedicated inquiry into clinicians' realities, whether psychosocial, nursing or medical, of working in sex development services. My own experience suggests that professional networking and camaraderie exist for biomedical clinicians but are precarious for PCPs and nurses. PCPs are generally appreciated in their respective services but differ in how their expertise is positioned (Liao & Roen, 2021). They may differ markedly from each other in terms of seniority, knowledge and skills and percentage time dedicated to sex development work. Those appointed at an early stage of their career due to budgetary constraints may struggle to voice their need for further training. However, even highly experienced PCPs can benefit from restorative supervision and professional development. An important conversation for supervision is in therapist self-disclosure (Section 8.3.1).

8.3.1   Therapist Self-Disclosure

Historically, influenced by some psychoanalytic traditions, therapists were trained to be a neutral and anonymous medium, a blank screen on which the client's nonconscious transferential feelings are projected. These feelings are interpreted and the client gains self and relational awareness as therapy progresses. For therapists who cling to this orthodoxy, self-disclosure is still a taboo subject. Other therapists, however, expect to do the opposite, to render transparent their values and assumptions in ways that signify mutual respect and reduce the inequality in the therapeutic encounter.

Therapy is an interpersonal process, so that some self-disclosure, even if incidental, is inevitable. This may explain why over 90% of practitioners report that they disclose personal information about themselves to their clients at least occasionally (Henretty & Levitt, 2010). Therapist self-disclosure (TSD) can be as small as admitting to having watched the same TV show or read the same book, or it can be more substantial. Deliberate TSD to clients is not a blanket benevolent and efficacious act. It is a complicated subject and by nature context dependent. An evidence-based review led its authors to suggest that TSD can be a helpful therapeutic skill (Knox & Hill, 2003). They concluded:

> When used sparingly, when containing nonthreatening and moderately intimate content and when done in the service of the client, therapist self-disclosure can help establish and enhance a therapeutic relationship, model appropriate disclosure, reassure and support clients, and facilitate gains in insight and action. We thus encourage therapists to consider using therapist self-disclosure, always, of course, mindful of the impact of their interventions on clients. (p. 538)

Many practitioners working with minoritized clients (e.g., refugees, asylum seekers, women, people of color and LGBTQ+ clients) argue that it is important to name the power imbalance in the therapeutic space by being explicit about how they position themselves in relation to clients' identities and allegiances. However, TSD is not just a case of giving clients a choice to work with similarly identified therapists. Indeed, many clients do not seek this. Rather, TSD considerations compel care providers to examine their relationship to social diversity and recognize how this can influence language and interaction.

However, TSD decisions must always take account of professional boundaries. It is the therapist's job to serve the client; the client is not there to meet the therapist's emotional needs. That said, many therapists would admit that their dedication to interpersonal work is partly driven by their own needs for emotional engagement. This is not necessarily negative, but boundaries may be crossed. For example, a therapist may assume that the client shares their liberal views and become unguarded in expressing these views. This can inhibit the client's expressions. Knox and Hill (2003) recommended checking impact directly with the client with questions such as "How does my telling you this affect you?" (p. 537).

The centrality of decisions about "coming out" has led many therapists to state that practitioners who work with LGBTQ+ clients (e.g., in mental health, sexual health and substance programs) should be prepared to disclose their own sex/gender identities (see Henretty & Levitt, 2010). Sex development services however, are not to be confused with LGBTQ+ services, where gender dissatisfaction is not the rule. Indeed, much of the psychological struggle among service users is the perceived incompatibility between their gender-normativity and their sex characteristics. Nevertheless, it makes sense that all DSD clinicians examine their attitudes to nonheteronormative embodiment.

8.4   Assessment

A needs assessment is a standard response to a referral. It is an interactive process that identifies and names the concern(s) to be addressed and gathers information about the service user's personal strengths and social context. The method is driven by purpose, acceptability and preference. While I emphasize the clinical interview in my practice, many PCPs also make use of screening tools (e.g., Ernst, Gardner, et al., 2018; Sandberg et al., 2017), which are in keeping with suggestions in some of the DSD care statements (see Table 8.1).

The example interview format in Table 8.2 comprises a series of landing points, any of which may be developed to a greater or lesser extent, depending on who the service user is, the concerns being addressed and the PCP's interests and knowledge frameworks. The conversation does not have to follow the sequence in the template and is likely to roll back and forth in reality. The practice vignettes in Chapters 9, 10, 12 and 13 make use of the assessment template in Table 8.2.

I typically begin the process of inquiry by exploring the service user's relationship to help. The client may be the family (child with variation, caretakers, siblings, grandparents) or the adult with variation who is present with or without a partner. The conversation could move to reflect on general health and well-being, any current challenges and any significant life event that may have a bearing on the situation being addressed. This segment of the assessment is also a useful opportunity to ask service users how they would define health and well-being, which can inform the goal of any remedial intervention.

Generally, a discussion of health and well-being can lead smoothly onto personal strengths, such as education, work, family and other factors that can affect capacity for autonomy such as housing, finance and access to healthcare. Such information is crucial for conceptualizing what is feasible. Example prompts about coping capacities are: When difficulties arose in the past, what strengths did you bring to the situation? How did you use to take care of yourself in tough times? How do you want others to know how you are feeling? Who are your most likely champions? What gets in the way of you using support? What's one thing you would like to do for yourself that you are not doing yet?

Table 8.2. *An example assessment template*

Inquiry domains	Caretaker(s) with a child with a variation (Example areas to cover)	Adolescent/adult with a variation (Example areas to cover)
Goal of assessment	– Who is referring whom for what reason – What would care users like to get from the consultation	– Who is referring whom for what reason – What would care users like to get from the consultation
Relationship to help	– Who are in the system – Relationship with specialist services and community providers – Patterns of engagement with services	– Who are in the system – Relationship with specialist services and community providers – Patterns of engagement with services
General health and psychological well-being	– Current physical health and well-being – Past physical health and well-being	– Current physical health – Current and past psychological/mental health
Personal strengths and needs	– Caretakers' psychosocial skills (e.g., communication, emotion regulation) – Caretakers' hopes and fears – Caretakers' access to confiding relationships – Caretaker–child and siblings–child relationships – Child's school performance, interests, peer relationships – Caretaker and/or child hopes and fears	– Psychosocial skills (e.g., communication, emotion regulation) – Family relationships (e.g., closeness and distances) – Peer relationships – Capacity for independence – Education, work, creativity, interests – Hopes and fears
Understanding of variation and treatment past/present	– Factual knowledge – Understanding of immediate and long-term MDT care plan for child – Knowledge of respective roles of providers involved	– Factual knowledge – Understanding of immediate and long-term MDT care plan for self – Knowledge of respective roles of providers involved
Emotional responses to variation and/or treatment(s)	– Emotional reactions – Immediate and future concerns	– Emotional reactions – Immediate and future concerns
Social and cultural aspects	– Family relationships – Community support – Access to confiding relationships	– Family relationships – Community support – Access to confiding relationships

Table 8.2. (*cont.*)

Inquiry domains	Caretaker(s) with a child with a variation (Example areas to cover)	Adolescent/adult with a variation (Example areas to cover)
Gender and sexuality	– Cultural and religious identities – Knowledge of education and support resources and capacity to navigate resources – Caretakers' attitudes to diversity – Child's gender expressions	– Cultural and religious identities – Knowledge of education and support resources; and capacity to navigate – Sex/gender identity – Attitudes, preferences – Sexual experiences – Current relationship

The family may be a single- or two-parent household, stepfamily with shared care of the child and foster or adoptive parent with or without support of an extended family. Capacity of the caretakers and any concern relating to inter-generational attachment and conflict are taken into account. The family structure and the nature of relationships can take time to map out. The amount of probing that is appropriate will vary between service users but should routinely include developmental milestones of the child, support from schools and the family doctor and the family's willingness to engage with peer support at any point.

Social factors such as the wider culture, spiritual beliefs and diversity of the neighborhood can make a significant difference to the level of threat posed by sex variation. When inquiring about cultural factors, it is important not to use the word cultural as a euphemism for the Global South. Culture refers to shared beliefs, habits, customs and common understandings that shape a collective sense of being (Johnstone & Boyle, 2018, p. 67). Therefore, the word also references socially privileged subcultures in Anglo-European nations.

There is scope for the PCP to draw on any theoretical orientation in the process of inquiry. Should they choose to draw on the Power Threat Meaning Framework (PTMF) (see Chapter 7), they are likely to engage the client in detailed exploration of how sex variation is talked about, what is threatening, what power resources are available to meet the challenges ahead and to which extent medical solutions have worked as a survival strategy or a form of entrapment.

The initial assessment may be followed by a more specialist assessment, a remedial intervention or triaging to other services. Depending on the service remit, the PCP might work therapeutically to support a caretaker, provide a behavioral assessment with a toddler, explore identity with a teenager, provide sex therapy with a couple or refer on for peer support or a community service. These decisions should be informed by a good enough understanding of what needs addressing and how.

8.5   Formulation

A formulation is a shared and evolving "best guess" that places the client's life history, events and sense making within theories, research and experiences frameworks familiar to the practitioner. Sense-making frameworks are by nature speculative and should therefore be open to discussion. Psychological formulation aims to offer a working model of the presenting concerns that the client wishes to address. Rather than reducing complex thoughts and feelings to a linear causality, a psychological formulation aims to help the client to comprehend where the challenging situation may have stemmed from, how the negative cycle is maintained and how this understanding relates to the care plan. It is a map that enables the client to predict how the situation may progress if one or two of the variables were altered. The best guess is often revised as new information emerges.

Key elements of a formulation include 1) a rich description of the presenting concern(s), 2) possible precipitating factors in the distant and recent past (distal and proximal antecedents), 3) factors that may or may not have been involved in the initial development of the presenting concern but are contributing to its maintenance and 4) resources available to the person to modify the maintenance factors. In other words, a formulation may start with a story but usually moves beyond description. It is a theory-informed account of how the distal and proximal factors relate meaningfully to the concern being addressed. It provides a tentative, working explanation of the emergence and maintenance of the situation that needs addressing and highlights potential steps for positive shifts.

Theories are rich resources that PCPs draw on to make sense of a challenging situation and see more clearly what is required to introduce movement to the situation in ways that serve the client. It is a generic skill acquired in training by PCPs of all persuasions but often neglected in favor of meeting overflowing work demands in practice. In Chapter 7, I argue that the PTMF (Johnstone & Boyle, 2018) is a useful meta framework that positions challenges in sex development as cultural and ideological. However, having a meta understanding does not render a cross-sectional micro formulation, for example, of the role of specific thoughts and feelings that underpin a major decision, as less valuable. Each PCP has their own style and preferences. In the practice vignettes in Chapters 9–14, it is clear that a sociological dimension speaks more closely to me. However, an intrapersonal understanding, which some PCPs are more comfortable with, is no less valid. What is important is that all PCPs in this field return to the rigors of formulation, to routinely build and share a working model and arouse psychological engagement.

8.6 Psychological Interventions

PCPs in DSD medicine may not be in a position to provide a full program of therapy because the tertiary environment is not set up to facilitate ongoing care. Although they tend to work along a "consultation" model around a specific problem rather than a "therapy" model that privileges personal growth, it is nevertheless powered by therapeutic expertise. I therefore offer a flavor of the popular psychotherapies below.

Some of the therapies are further developed in the practice vignettes in Chapters 9–14. That said, this book is light on therapy and, instead, emphasizes engagement with issues of power. While it is important to invite thoughts and emotions and values and to work with them, as per conventional therapy, it is worth asking where do the thoughts and feelings come from, and what is sustaining the values?

My categorization of the common therapeutic approaches below is unorthodox. I refer to approaches that emphasize (but are not exclusively focused on) storytelling (e.g., narrative therapy, existential psychotherapy, family therapy) as *dialogical*, approaches that emphasize skills development (e.g., the cognitive and behavioral therapies) as *dialectical* and approaches to increase capacity to focus on the here and now rather than past and future (e.g., mindfulness) as *mind–body* practices. All of these approaches can be with a person, a couple or a group. Group-based interventions with adults that incorporate a mixture of techniques have been shown to be promising (Chadwick et al., 2014; Weijenborg & ter Kuile, 2000). However, groups are not feasible for services with a small throughput. Sex therapy, which I discuss in Chapter 13, may consist of elements of all three types of approaches.

As well as the myriad methods that exist, a PCP may be trained to orientate to one or more of the following briefs: 1) alleviation of "symptoms" (illness orientation), 2) increase in personal effectiveness (deficit orientation), 3) fostering a meaningful sense of self (growth orientation) or 4) taking safety measures (safeguarding orientation).

8.6.1   Dialogical Approaches

A central task of psychological therapists is to facilitate storytelling, that is, to create a safe space where people can narrate what has happened to them and update their story in ways that open new possibilities for future experiences. Crossley (2000) advocated for a narrative healthcare psychology and drew attention to the observation that, for people with a serious illness, "the most basic, underlying existential assumptions that people hold about themselves and the world are thrown into disarray," and that a coherent narrative is a process of making sense out of nonsense (p. 11). On this note, she considered psychotherapy to be an exercise in *story repair*. The different modes of talk-based therapy are merely different styles in which to repair or reconstruct a self-story. There is no benchmark for judging whether one talk-based method is superior to another. Suffice it to say that in sex development, facilitating story repair would require the PCP to be committed to depathologizing talk and cocreate new vocabularies about bodily diversity.

Rescripting does not have to be verbal. Caretakers can be encouraged to source socially inclusive stories to read to children or accumulate resources that contradict gendered stereotypes about bodies and bodily function. They may even be able to involve the nursery or school in these endeavors. Furthermore, many children enjoy and learn more effectively via play techniques. They can be encouraged to build their own story about bodily differences using a variety of media including collage, drawing and plasticine and elaborate on the story as they go along. Caretakers too may enjoy working with nonverbal media. In due course, with support and ideas, caretakers can guide the child toward inclusive understandings about variations in bodily appearance and function.

In "Circles and Squares" in Chapter 1, a group of caretakers with daughters with CAH intend to accept the children's potential nonnormative future identities if they must, but would prefer a heteronormative outcome if at all possible. Research suggests that across the different types of variations, heteronormativity is still the most likely outcome, although the differences between the types of variations are huge (see Chapter 11). Young people expressing different sexual preferences or gender dissatisfaction may threaten the family script. Families may struggle with their own *coming out* until they can integrate the young person's nonnormative identity into the family script. The therapeutic space can be a refuge where normative pressures on the entire household can be acknowledged. The family can be supported to move from a household of sex/gender-normative individuals to one of multiple sexualities and gender identities.

8.6.2   Dialectical Approaches

New insights are transformative, but especially so when combined with new skills. In terms of the latter, the psychology of behavior change offers practical explanations for how an individual who has learned to respond habitually in certain situations can unlearn the negative responses. Habits (e.g., staying at home to stay safe) that obstruct the client's stated goal (e.g., social confidence) are identified and modified to suit the client's purpose. Many children communicate their distress through behavior rather than words. If a child needs to build social confidence, for example, an exposure technique could start by having the child construct a hierarchy of difficulty. They can be guided to imagine or draw the least feared social situation. Cognitive therapy techniques can help individuals to challenge unhelpful viewpoints that inhibit action, leading to positive experiences.

A recognizable problem in the DSD field is genital aversion. Because the genitalia are associated with shame, anger and guilt, genital touch may automatically evoke physical recoiling, which then confirms to the individual the unpleasantness of touch. Developing skills to gradually disrupt the association is a central component in sex therapy, which I discuss in more detail in Chapter 13. On the note of genital aversion, dialectical methods can also be useful for caretakers who feel uncomfortable looking at the infant's body. The PCP can, for example, help caretakers to identify thoughts and feelings and behaviors (e.g., grimace or look away when changing diapers) and discuss how to begin to modify these experiences rather than judge them.

Cognitive behavior therapy (CBT) leans on the premise that problematic thoughts, which are associated with negative bodily states, emotions and behaviors have been learned and can be unlearned. The task of therapy is to arouse curiosity in people about their thinking styles and what may be the effects on their life goals. The client is encouraged to become aware of the effects of unhelpful thinking, such as talking themselves out of what matters to them and talking themselves into doing what they want to avoid. Changes happen when unhelpful (usually self-critical or threatening) self-talk is identified and the person is guided to brainstorm a more compassionate or balanced way of viewing the situation. The behavioral component usually involves graduating levels of exposure to avoided situations, starting with the least challenging. It may involve substituting an unhelpful habitual reaction with another. Having undergone decades of development to meet different challenges, CBT has been adapted to approach a wide range of concerns, including body image distress (Ipser et al., 2009) and trauma (Jericho et al., 2021; Lewis et al., 2020). These works may be especially pertinent to DSD services.

With a skilled provider, direct changes in behavior can happen rapidly for committed clients. These skilful changes may not follow on from the kind of story repair or discursive rescripting referenced above. However, restorying may lead to a clearer rationale for trying out the various practices that can break an unhelpful and self-perpetuating thought–feeling–behavior chain reaction.

8.6.3   Mind–Body Approaches

It is fair to say that the most significant shift in Western psychological therapies in recent years is the acknowledgment of the value of ancient religious practices originated in the East. Many of these practices are secularized and integrated into stress management interventions. The approach that has been most successfully mainstreamed is *mindfulness*. What many PCPs know as mindfulness-based interventions (MBIs) originated from the work of Jon Kabat-Zinn (2013) and a large team of mindfulness instructors at the University of Massachusetts Medical School since the late 1970s.

Mindfulness is often mistaken as a method of relaxation. Although mind–body relaxation may occur, it is incidental to rather than the goal of practice. On the contrary, learners of mindfulness are encouraged to let go of striving and grasping. Instead, they are encouraged to be attentive and curious toward all present experiences, such as moment-to-moment sensations of breathing, sound, sight, thoughts and feelings. With regular and extended practice, the learner stays with pleasant/wanted and unpleasant/unwanted experiences without losing themselves to the usual tendency to judge, compare, evaluate, interpret and reject. People learn to be with experiences just as they are and become more open to feeling the good, the bad and the ugly – the "full catastrophe" – in the here and now. A parallel instruction is to honor one's limit. For example, if a pain surges in the body during a sitting practice, the learner is encouraged to make wise choices as to whether to explore the pain, shift the posture or stop the practice, rather than to approximate some preconceived standard of sublime stillness.

The struggle with regular practice is widely acknowledged and framed nonjudgmentally as a universal tendency of the human mind to entertain itself with fantasies and imaginings that are often self-referential. The assumption is that unconditional awareness of actual experience ultimately liberates the learner from auto reactions and become more discerning on what kind of situations may require a response and what kind of response may constitute a skilful one.

Mindfulness has attracted strong evidence of physical and psychological benefits. It is increasingly extended to children and adolescents and can be practiced by families exposed to chronic stress and unique stressors associated with medical and/or social-contextual challenges (Perry-Parrish et al., 2016). There is no reason to expect the benefits to be less powerful for people impacted by sex variations, but no direct evidence exists. I have spent many years providing MBIs in large classes that included adults with variations. The emphasis of practice and de-emphasis of biographical exchange offers people with variations the intimacy of a cohesive group without any threat of exposure.

Some people (with or without variations) cannot tolerate focused attention to bodily sensations (e.g., where there is active traumatic stress). Clients who are hypervigilant of internal bodily states could try practicing with eyes open and stand up rather than lie down. These clients can also practice intentional awareness by coloring in a picture. There is no right or wrong way to be present. If the aim is to regulate autonomic responses, then a large number of other tried and tested techniques exist to suit clients who cannot tolerate mindfulness practices. The plethora of methods include slowed breathing, progressive muscle relaxation, yoga, Alexander technique, tai chi, self-hypnosis and visualization. The point is to find a helpful technique that is easily accessible (e.g., hydrotherapy may be relaxing, but it is not readily available to most people).

8.6.4   Signposting, Liaising, Triaging

Peer support is a powerful medium for shifting negative self-beliefs and mobilizing self-affirming narratives about living well with a sex variation. Over the years, however, I have met with tremendous resistance from service users about connecting with peers, although this may be changing. In "Circles and Squares," I describe the amount of personal investment that the character "Jude" has to make to attend a support group meeting. In order to be able to socialize clients to access peer support, it is important for PCPs themselves to connect with support groups, for example by providing workshops and presentations at their annual meetings and by coproducing web-based resources.

It is important to bear in mind that mental health and social care concerns are fairly common in the general population. A person with a sex variation may have grown up in a household affected by intergenerational trauma and/or substance misuse. In attributing all psychosocial difficulties to sex variations, the mental health and social care needs of many service users will remain unmet (see Malouf et al., 2010). In some situations, the level of mental health and social care needs are beyond the scope of a DSD service, even with generous psychosocial care provision. It is therefore not at all unusual for a psychosocial care plan to involve multiple agencies. I have come across numerous situations in which the sex variation is by far the lesser concern given the enormity of generic mental health and social care problems in some families.

A recent study in Italy with nonspecialist (community-based) providers has identified poor knowledge about sex variations (Prandelli & Testoni, 2021). This means the mental health and social care needs of individuals and families impacted by sex variations may not be met in the community. Generic care providers who are unfamiliar with sex variations may attribute all and sundry to the sex variation and abdicate responsibilities for pre-existing mental health problems. This is where the specialist PCP and peer worker can make an enormous difference. They can work together to educate and support community-based providers to make substantial care contributions to the client with variations.

In summary, in some instances, the most valuable contribution that an in-house PCP can provide is a detailed assessment of psychosocial needs and to situate the needs in the historical and present social, developmental and medical contexts. This considered opinion is then shared with the client. As appropriate, the assessment and formulation may also be shared with others who are making a substantial care contribution.

8.7   Evaluation

Evaluation requires a clear description of aim, rationale, baseline and meaningful pre–post differences. The aims of interpersonal work in sex development are however diverse. They may range from improving a caretaker's confidence in raising a child with genital variations, increasing an adolescent's confidence in talking about their bodily difference or helping a couple to focus on sexual pleasure rather than gender performance. These goals may not have been the original agenda of the care user. Embedded in all interpersonal work is a great deal of reframing in the interest of the client (hence my repeat emphasis in this book on being transparent about explicit frameworks).

Evaluation of remedial interventions should centralize the experience of service users, but such evaluation should not be taken at face value and deemed "objective." Recall the example scenarios in Section 8.2. Care users who accept support from a clinical social worker with the view of having their medicalized perspective verified may devalue being guided to engage with new perspectives. Therefore, PCPs who are doing ethical work could be evaluated less favorably. Furthermore, it is good practice to attribute the therapeutic gains to the client, that is, to enable the client to take ownership of what is achieved in therapy, so that they leave the process with a self-belief that they have been able to and will again problem-solve autonomously in life. In other words, the contribution of the therapist is purposefully minimized.

Hallam (2015) reminded us that decomposing a fluid interpersonal process into separate fixed components and testing how they interact, as in basic science, is unsuitable for estimating the value of psychosocial care. For interpersonal input to be remedial and enabling, all potential components (e.g., the warmth of the relationship, the techniques introduced by the therapist, the client's commitment, the theoretically and ethically informed reframing) work together in a flowing interaction with critical moment-to-moment occurrences. These components cannot operate independently of each other. In the words of the author:

> With statistical techniques, it is possible to disassociate [the process] into "main effects" but in fact we know that these effects interact in complex ways. The pie-chart strategy of examining which components predict a successful outcome could be compared to a recipe for making a cake (take 40% flour, 20% butter, 5% sugar, and a dose of raising agent). However, the perfect cake is a product of a fortuitous combination of ingredients and baking conditions. For example, the amount of raising agent and a certain oven temperature could be the catalyst to make a perfect cake of a certain kind but would not be optimal for all types of cake. (Hallam, 2015, p. 78)

At the beginning of this chapter, I suggested that the broad recommendations in DSD care documents may have limited impact without substantial translational work by psychosocial experts. A collective step is needed to refine the lofty menu of dishes in Table 8.1 and fill in the missing recipes of core activities based on theoretical and research-informed principles. Only then can evaluation be designed and implemented in ways that offer PCPs valid feedback to improve practice.

8.8 Summary

In this chapter, I adapt generic psychological processes to the DSD context. I begin by discussing *relationship to help* and highlight the kind of practitioner attributes that psychosocial service users seem to prefer. I outline an initial assessment and summarize the different types of psychotherapeutic interventions that can facilitate interpersonal work. I also pose the idea that the most important contribution that an expert PCP in the field can provide may be a robust and detailed assessment and care plan that involves close liaison with nonspecialists such as the family physician, nursery nurse and teacher. Where feasible and appropriate, the specialist PCP could collaborate with peer supporters to educate and encourage these nonspecialists to make useful care contributions. I suggest this because, much as DSD care documents aspire to lifelong care, DSD services are almost without exception located in an intensive biomedical environment designed to cure and discharge. The curative model of care may be adept at diagnosis and treatment but does not fit well with ongoing remedial input. And, given the geographical and psychological distance between where DSD services are located and where people with variations live their daily life, the community should be much more involved in future. Thoughtful facilitation of this can be a worthwhile brief of the in-house PCP working in DSD medicine.

Working Psychologically

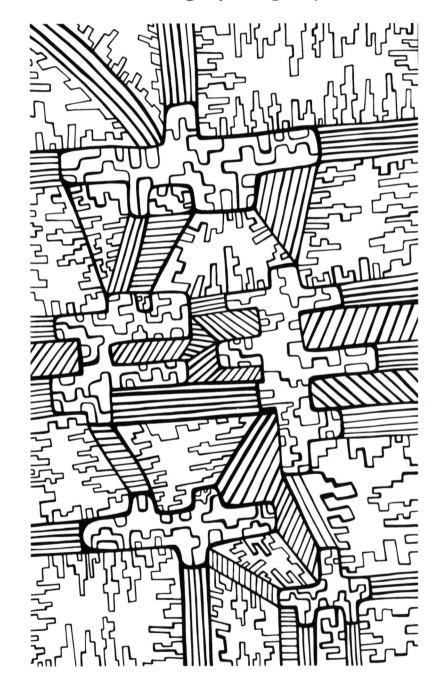

Introductory Notes

In Chapter 1, I tell a story of a meeting between several people impacted by variations in sex development. In the character "Jude," I highlight the difficulties that some people have with integrating the implacable biological facts told to them about their bodies with their fluid subjectivities. I draw attention to the labor involved in complying with gendered social scripts and the disappointment that the effort often results in. In the character "Dillon," I describe people's struggles to communicate about their variations and to interpret relationship issues that are part of everybody's lives. In the character "Karla" and her family, I draw attention to caretakers' love for their child, the dilemma that "normalizing" surgery poses to them and the thoughtful process that many caretakers engage in before they decide.

In the story, I also suggest that the positioning of psychological input in the care path can influence service users' engagement. Psychological expertise is actively mobilized by Jude, but only because all of the medical solutions have already been exhausted. Psychological expertise has much to offer Dillon, but he does not realize that this is a missing part of his care. Psychological support is devalued and resisted by Karla, because she has already made a life-changing decision for her daughter. But her devaluation is based on a mistaken view that is often perpetuated in a techno-centric biomedical culture.

All of the characters and families in the story may have acquired some psychological insight and skill to address some of their concerns. However, not everybody can tolerate thinking in depth about a painful or uncertain reality. Psychological work is therefore not a soft option, even if correctly positioned in a service. The understandable need to push away an unwanted reality can also put people off connecting with peers. In "Circles and Squares," Jude puts off the idea of attending a support group meeting for years. To finally manage it feels like a major triumph. Although peer support is a gift, people and families usually have to overcome their internal obstacles in order to receive it. Accepting peer support means coming to a realization that sex variations cannot be erased.

In the six remaining chapters of this book, I consult a much wider psychosocial literature in order to provide psychological care provider (PCPs), especially those working within differences in sex development (DSD) services, with more tools to think with and to reignite their passion for psychosocial knowledge frameworks, which can be obscured by the medical prism. Although I focus on one situation at a time, for example choosing "normalizing" interventions, all of the situations are related. Each of these six chapters ends with a practice vignette. An important note to bear in mind about the vignettes is that I do not elaborate on the therapeutic techniques that are mentioned. The techniques are generic and there are numerous resources to consult. It is also clear that I favor a consultation rather than a therapy model in DSD services. Consultation is brief and targeted. While it requires the PCP to mobilize a range of therapeutic skills, it is a different process to implementing long-term psychotherapy and is much more ecclectic. DSD clinics are generally not set up to offer a long-term therapy service, which tends to be provided in the community.

Chapter 9 is the first of the six chapters that form the "clinical area" of the book. It tackles the theme of choosing "normalizing" interventions, which concerns children and adults with variations. The chapter explores the limits of choice regarding invasive and irrevocable "normalizing" interventions in the field of sex development. It considers the role of emotion in decision-making and the complexities of obtaining informed consent. In the practice vignette, demand for surgery by a young person (with congenital adrenal hyperplasia) is a foregone conclusion – a familiar scenario in DSD services and one that places the PCP in an ambiguous position. The service user also has clear psychosocial care needs. She brings a unique suite of intersecting social circumstances that places demand on the PCP to be fluid and responsive to the dynamic and challenging context. The PCP in the vignette does not have the answers, but it is hoped that the story opens up conversation on the subject.

In Chapter 10, I suggest that there are immense possibilities for PCPs to contribute to compassionate care for caretakers following the birth of a child with variations (or before the birth, in the antenatal period). Psychosocial research and first-person accounts inform us of caretakers' brokenness. In this chapter, I suggest that PCPs work with caretakers in a grief-informed way. Grief is a language that everyone understands. It compels services to privilege psychological safety as a first care principle.

The practice vignette is built around an expectant mother in difficult circumstances with an unborn child with Turner syndrome. However, the concept of grief and the need for psychological safety is also relevant for older children and adolescents who are newly diagnosed. Indeed, processing loss is integral to adjustment, whereby taken-for-granted ideas of selfhood give way for new ways of being that are not yet known.

Chapter 11 of the book reviews potential psychological contributions in the highly charged process of assigning legal gender to a newborn with genital variations. Although a number of psychological theories exist for understanding gender development, it is the brain gender framework that has been singularly privileged in intersex and DSD medicine. Despite decades of research, it is unable to deliver the kind of certainty that health professionals and caretakers seek. PCPs have other frameworks to draw from to work ethically and pragmatically with families. In the practice vignette, I envision how a highly skilled PCP in a high-functioning DSD team could work substantially to help caretakers to cope with uncertainty and minimize the need for psychosocially motivated medical interventions. In the vignette, the psychological care path is in position before medical investigations begin. It remains highly active long after the medical and legal processes are completed. Although the vignette is built around a child diagnosed with 17β-hydroxysteroid dehydrogenase-3 deficiency, the care principles are relevant to gender assignment of children with a range of variations.

How to talk about variations in sex development is a major theme for impacted individuals and families. This is the topic of Chapter 12, in which I summarize the research literature with caretakers and with adults about the difficulties of disclosure. Considerable criticism has been levied at health professionals for failing to role model affirming communication. For sure there are gaps in health professionals' talk, but the biggest contributor to the difficulties is to do with the widespread misunderstanding about biological sex variations. PCPs are not there to put a cheerful gloss over clients' negative expressions. However, they can be part of the favorable social condition in which new meaning and narratives about bodily differences can emerge. In the practice vignette, I highlight how tentative and uncertain the process is, to facilitate decision-making to share information, when misunderstandings still abound in the wider social context.

Difficulties with communication about bodily differences are strongly implicated in relationship and sexual difficulties. These difficulties are the focus of Chapter 13. Here, I start by critiquing the framing of sex as heterosex, and heterosex as coitus in wider society. The oppressive ideas can give rise to insecurities, self-objectification and body shame for people in general and people with sex development variations in particular. Adults with variations who have been medically managed are particularly vulnerable to the effects of objectification and shame. I outline typical components of sex therapy programs but, rather than fix sexual problems, which can perpetuate people's sense of inadequacy, I suggest that PCPs support clients to process any trauma and develop a more relaxed and appreciative relationship with the body first and foremost. This work, which can draw on generic therapy knowledge and skills, can be integrated with a range of specific sex therapy techniques and resources later, to reimagine a sexual future that focuses on pleasure and closeness rather than gender performance. Although the practice vignette is built around a female couple, one of whom has partial androgen insensitivity syndrome, the care principles have applications for people with variations in a range of relationship scenarios.

In Chapter 14, I critique the research with clinic samples that has produced a problem-saturated account of the inability to have children in the traditional way. Such an account severely restricts our view of a wide range of alternative responses. I discuss the influence of pronatalist ideology on people impacted by infertility including many people with sex variations. Psychological input can help people cope with fertility treatment but, more importantly, it can guide individuals, couples and groups to explore personal meaning of nonparenthood. It can facilitate service users to grieve for what is not possible, challenge feelings of deviance and shame, reengage with a range of life goals and, perhaps most important of all, recast adult identities. Through the practice vignette built around a heterosexual couple, one of whom has a late diagnosis of Klinefelter syndrome, I tease out the difficulties of working psychologically in an aggressive fertility treatment context, where complex and layered existential issues and relational dynamics are squeezed into a pressurized treatment decision frame.

CHAPTER 9

Choosing "Normalizing" Genital Surgery

To choose an irrevocable bodily intervention for oneself in order to manage potential relational difficulties is complex to say the least. To choose a trajectory of multiple physical interventions and hospitalizations for another is exponentially more dilemmatic. While this chapter is anchored in genital surgery because it is the most talked about topic in sex development, the discussion is relevant for all forms of interventions that are steered by normative pressures, including uterine removal and transplantation, cryo-preservation and growth hormone treatment. This chapter is not a review of clinical outcomes of genital surgery, which is addressed in Chapter 4, nor is it a review of the efficacy of decision tools. Choosing "normalizing" interventions across the lifespan is so often a foregone conclusion in the field that the usefulness of decision tools may be constrained. Rather, the chapter draws from the literature on the limits of choice.

The problem of treatment "choice" is of course not unique to differences in sex development (DSD) medicine. Systemic affordance of medical technology both constructs and accommodates desires for intervention. A colleague working in an adolescent bariatric clinic laments that decisional counseling is like inviting young people to peddle backward when, from their point of view, they have already gone past the finishing line. Some young people are said to have already made up their mind with social media friends before they even meet the surgeon.

Like their medical colleagues elsewhere, DSD clinicians are committed to offer patients free choice without undue influence and experience themselves as neutral or even reluctant players in the elective treatment business (Liao et al., 2019; Roen & Hegarty, 2018). The chooser of treatment who supposedly exercises free choice is the object of analysis. The systems that shape thought, feelings and action are obscured. I suggest, however, that DSD experts are centrally involved in how clinical priorities are conceptualized, how services are configured and how options are constructed. They are deep within the system of influence on all decision-making by the consumer and not outside it. As discussed in Chapter 6, the language of pathology in DSD services confers threat, while the technology-centeredness confers hope. The distress within the system comes to be defined as medical problems in need of medical solutions. Professionals may see "normalizing" interventions as providing compassionate certainty, when it may be more ethical and productive to be honest about the uncertainties.

A rigorous and transparent process of informed consent is needed for interventions. Embedded in the principle of informed consent is the compatibility of the decision with people's values. But where do these values come from? Thus far, research suggests that there is significant variability in the thoroughness of the process of seeking informed consent in DSD services (Rolston et al., 2017). Elsewhere, colleagues and I recommended that DSD experts consider how the bioethical principles are translated into observable behaviors (Liao et al., 2018). I bring some of that discussion here. The chapter ends with a practice vignette of a young woman with congenital adrenal hyperplasia (CAH) who seeks intervention without particularly seeking to be informed, to illustrate how psychosocial input is structurally constrained.

9.1   Doing Gender

At the beginning of the Covid-19 pandemic, therapy sessions were, for many practitioners in many parts of the world, changed from in-person to remote consultation overnight. A supervisee of mine, "Ian," wanted to talk to me about "Miguel," a client of Angolan heritage who had experienced significant race-based trauma. Miguel would weep in silence and then recollect and disqualify his distress by musing that perhaps he had been somewhat "paranoid," that the perpetrators might not have been racially motivated. Ian and Miguel had never seen each other. We surmised that Miguel's hesitancy was related to his assumption that Ian was a white therapist. At the end of national lockdown, Miguel chose to continue therapy in person. He looked somewhat confused when he saw Ian. Now that Ian is seen as a person of color, Miguel is much less guarded and would sometimes end his story of social exclusion with introjections such as, "You get what I'm saying, right?"

I use the above example to show just how dependent we are on social categorization in order to know our place in relation to each other, and how confusing it is when information about a major categorization, in this case race and ethnicity, is incidentally obscured. In everyday social interaction, cues are subtly or prominently displayed or solicited to size up each other. Information about what work we do, whom we live with and where we shop, help us to tailor expectations within the complex social order, of which most of us have only limited control.

Gender is a major differentiating social category that places people in relation to each other. It is intricately embedded in politics, economics, religions, cultures and subcultures. Our sense of self and the world is so fundamentally gendered, and our relationships with each other so ordered by gender, that it is almost impossible to imagine a genderless world – who are we in such a world, how do we organize home and work lives, who are the caregivers and who is allowed to have sex with whom? Imagination is constrained by gendered linguistics and discourses that render it preposterous to imagine that gender is anything other than natural, other than how life is meant to be all along. Even when we contemplate lifeless planets and galaxies, we ascribe gender to imaginary life forms, forgetting that it is a concept constructed by a unique species on planet Earth.

At birth, the external genitalia signify whether the baby is to inhabit a female or male reality. The idea of either gender, one to either bodily sex, is not a subject of day-to-day argumentation. The nonargumentative nature of private thoughts of gender as a natural order reflects, to a large extent, a lack of public argument about it. The need to align intersex bodies to binary gender may be socially constructed, but it does not follow that such a need is not real and acutely felt. However, much as doctors, caretakers and adult service users experience their preference for interventions as freethinking, the intention to produce a certain imaginary (future) subject is decidedly powered by social structures strongly maintained by language and representation. Of course, process and outcome are not always linear. Many people who have been through various kinds of gender-affirming physical interventions go on to identify themselves as gender diverse rather than binary. Sex/gender-normalizing interventions often fail in their normative mission.

As discussed in Chapters 4 and 6, robust data on the prevalence of childhood normalizing genital surgery are unavailable, but observations based on multiple sources suggest that uptake is high for female and male assigned children (e.g., Ellens et al., 2017), despite professional protestations of a *conservative* approach (Liao et al., 2019; Roen & Hegarty, 2018) and a self-reported reduction in clitoral surgery in many DSD centers (Pasterski et al., 2010). In the most recent interview study with parents who had consented to clitoral surgery on their daughters with CAH, the need to "normalize" anatomy and psychology was so obvious that the decision was, as per previous research, experienced as rather straightforward (Alderson et al., 2022). A parent said, "I already made my mind up when I first met the surgeon when she got transferred to the hospital [where the DSD clinic is situated]." Another parent said, "So, if it was suggested that this is the next stage, we'd be like, 'Yeah, that's fine. Why should we question that?'." Significantly, over half of the parents in this study spoke of feeling unconcerned about the genital appearance of the child initially. It would seem that as the parents progressed along the medical protocol, perceptions and feelings shifted in a negative direction.

Absence of argumentation observed for many parents consenting to surgery on the child runs parallel to absence of dilemma in women with XY chromosomes consenting to surgery to create a vagina (Boyle et al., 2005). For the women in this study, surgery was felt to confer normality and entitlement to romantic love and sexual relationships. The authors suggested that the subjugation of potentially dilemmatic aspects of surgery in the medical encounter was strongly reinforced by a combination of the straightforward and authoritative presentation of surgery in a physical setting that made it difficult to discuss what surgery may not deliver: "Whenever I used to see the doctor, there would always be at least eight white coats sitting behind me, you know, scribbling down notes, and that's not really a time that you can then sit there and say, 'is it going to affect my orgasms?'" (Boyle et al., 2005, p. 578).

Considering that the women in the above study were already capable of pleasurable erotic experiences, the matter-of-factness with which they were offered the option of creating a vagina large enough to pleasure a penis suggests that absence of vaginal penetrative sex is unimaginable in heterosexual relationships. The absence of talk about pleasure as a treatment goal is also evident in surgical outcome studies, whose criteria for "success" or "normal sexual function" or "fully satisfactory intercourse" do not include enjoyment, but simply the ability to be penetrated by an erect penis without pain or discomfort. This understanding is evident in a recent study on revision surgery for a group of women whose childhood vaginoplasty had failed (Ellerkamp et al., 2021). Such narratives strongly suggest that the primary goal of surgery is to be able to meet social expectations to perform vaginal penetrative sex, that is, to do gender.

It has been more than two decades since Kessler (1998) asked a nonclinical sample of college-educated women about their opinion on clitoral and vaginal surgery for intersex. Most of the research participants stated that they would not have wanted vaginal surgery even if the condition made them uncomfortable or limited their ability to engage in coitus.

This observation is completely at odds with my clinical experience, whereby the majority of women (and not just heterosexuals) seek to modify genital appearance and increase capacity for vaginal penetration. The discrepancy may reflect population differences or the limit of vignette studies. Another explanation is that, outside the clinic, people are more able to think of different possibilities.

If people feel conflicted at all, it tends to happen *after* the intervention. Service users are often disappointed with the partial approximation to the imaginary ideal and realize that the need to talk about the variation has not disappeared. The reality of self-management to maintain the surgical result and medical follow-ups, which may have been minimized before surgery, soon materialize.

9.2   Disadvantage and Influence

The majority of DSD service users feel under normative pressures to *choose* interventions to approximate gendered esthetic and functional norms and to raise their chances of *passing as normal*, because the risks of being treated differently, which could mean being denied access to the social privileges of normalcy (real and imagined), outweigh the risks of interventions. I draw on the work of philosopher Clare Chambers (2008) to argue that factors such as *disadvantage* and *influence* may render so-called free choice questionable.

Influence on intervention uptake is rarely direct, that is, a provider rarely tells a service user "your variation needs fixing." Influence is much more likely to be indirect, for example when a provider says "the variation could be fixed, but it is a choice." Research with caretakers suggests that while they know that they do not have to choose surgery, they are rarely presented with an alternative to it (D'Alberton, 2010). Therefore, although caretakers know that they do not *have to* agree to surgery, they cannot envision how else to respond (Freda et al., 2015; Sanders et al., 2008). Until a credible alternative pathway exists, the idea of choice is disingenuous.

Even so, the influence factor alone does not render choice in this context particularly problematic. After all, people's preferences are routinely shaped by factors of availability and norms. However, where there are identifiable ways in which people are influenced to make choices that disadvantage them, that is, where the influence and disadvantage factors are combined, there are grounds for state interference (Chambers, 2008).

The disadvantages of surgery are significant. All genital surgery carries risks, causes physical pain, incurs recovery time that may mean absences from people and places, leads to scarring and involves removal of sensitive tissue from the sex anatomy or healthy tissue from other body parts such as the gut or the inside of the cheek. It may come with financial costs and status-based human cost such as guilt, shame and being devalued by self or another. Caretakers are often aware of the cost to the child and to themselves. Despite coming to an agreement with surgeons that surgery was necessary, a mother expressed her sorrow and recalled grieving for the unaltered child who had ceased to exist: "I felt sick. I felt like I'd abandoned my child or I felt like he'd died, it was horrible, really was horrible, I did honestly feel like he'd died but they hadn't given me chance to have a funeral, they just replaced him" (Sanders et al., 2008, p. 3193).

The Chicago consensus acknowledged that the purported psychological benefits of childhood genital surgery have not been evidenced and the risks of surgery have not been sufficiently acknowledged (Lee et al., 2006). In a recent study in the UK, parents of girls with CAH alluded to feminizing genitoplasty as "a big surgery" that was "eye-watering," and that which required parents to cope with the knowledge of putting their child through pain (Alderson et al., 2022). Some caretakers in the study even voiced future sexual problems as a cost: "Doctors said sensation would be slightly reduced – that's something to think about. Losing a bit of sensation – how would that affect them? That's not the only thing that matters." Despite identifiable disadvantages, there does not seem to be any other way of dealing with the child's variation. Another parent in the same study said, "Well, no, there wasn't an option. She needed it done."

What does not seem to have surfaced in research interviews with caretakers is an ethical concern of foreclosing the child's future possibilities. Lost tissue cannot be replaced should the individual choose to reassign gender and opt for reconstructive surgery later. We also know that surgery is not a one-off fix but part of an ongoing trajectory involving further clinic visits, examinations and hospitalizations. From a developmental perspective, hospitalization, treatment regimens, invasion of personal space, pain and discomfort, absences from school, parental anxiety and evasive responses can impact upon socialization. Financial hardship may result if one parent has to give up work. Siblings have expressed to me their experience of being "farmed out" to other caretakers from time to time without understanding the reason. The capacity of childhood surgery to reduce adult anxiety is mixed (Ellens et al., 2017). And, as already discussed, surgery does not always deliver the intention to produce sex/gender-normative subjects (Schweizer et al., 2014).

Choosing under societal pressure in ways that put people at a disadvantage is dependent on a social context in which interventions are normalized and healthy bodies are pathologized. Influence and disadvantage, according to Chambers (2008), renders choice a *normative transformer*, that is, the idea of choice transforms an otherwise unjust practice or situation into a just and acceptable one.

The pressure brought on by "choice" is palpable in a mother's reference to the unbearable weight of decision-making over limb extension surgery for her child: "When it came to surgical fixes," she said, "all you can be sure of is doubt" (Abelow Hedley, 2006, p. 48). Decision-making relating to elective and nonlife-saving medical interventions is emblematic of dilemmatic decision-making in conditions of uncertainty and subject to influence of complex psychosocial factors. The aforementioned mother further described how, in the end, caretakers may still have questions and doubts but have no more capacity to go over the grounds again. They simply cave in: "Nothing is clear or irrefutable. It is just that at some point you get exhausted by statistics, possibilities, and probabilities and decide just to act and that is when the internal arguments end . . . and you go for it . . . whatever it is you have decided on" (Abelow Hedley, 2006, p. 48).

In an article about the 2006 BBC Radio 4 series *Am I Normal*, the author of the article posed a rhetorical question (Parry, 2006): If medical tests show that you are not normal, is that a reason to medicate and treat or a reason to celebrate your individuality? Dr. Linda Voss, a psychological expert in growth studies, was quoted saying that shortness only became a disease when a treatment became available. The show's presenter suggested that it is usually "doctors with charts" who get to define normal but that "they constantly change their minds." Voss and her colleagues had observed that the threshold for normal stature was raised with the availability of growth hormone. In their longitudinal research on the psychosocial disadvantages of short stature in healthy children, Sandberg and Voss (2002) concluded that shorter children wanted to be taller and reported more experiences of bullying than their taller peers, but that neither of these variables had a measurable effect on school performance or self-esteem. They concluded, "[studies] have demonstrated that the psychological adaptation of individuals who are shorter than average is largely indistinguishable from others, whether in childhood, adolescence or adulthood" (p. 455). The resilience of the children in the growth studies resonated with that of young people with exstrophy diagnoses in a study published around the same time (Wilson et al., 2004). The participants in the exstrophy study also reported being bullied. However, they also described a range of coping strategies and identified positive aspects of their situation. The authors observed that "maturity, self-sufficiency and independence came early" for the young people who had to cope with unexpected circumstances (p. 610).

9.3   Psychological Barriers to Informed Consent

While the provision of balanced information is pivotal, it is by no means the only requirement in informed consent. Care providers must be certain that the patient has a sufficient understanding of their medical problem and the treatment proposed and is able to weigh up the risks and benefits of all available options including no or delayed treatment (Tamar-Mattis et al., 2014). In situations where a caretaker provides consent, respect for the child's rights requires decision-makers to consider the child's open future and best interests in the long term. There are, however, psychological barriers in upholding these broad principles in practice, even with strong professional intentions (Liao et al., 2018).

Emotional arousal can impair understanding and alter computation of probability and value. Under pressure, the typical care user may rely on cognitive heuristics such as magnification and minimization to selectively attend to what has or has not been said (Liao et al., 2018). Emotional arousal does not just affect care users. Care providers are human too. They are vulnerable in emotionally charged transactions and feel under pressure to fix the problem. To avoid upsetting the patient further by belaboring on what the patient does not want to hear, the clinician may gloss over risk information, the demand on self-management after surgery and the impact of ongoing medical reviews.

Throughout this book, I cite research to suggest that many caretakers and adults service users feel that genital surgery does not require a decision at all, that it just has to be done. However, even if service users do not wish to be informed in detail, it is a requirement, as a starting point, that the provider is informed about both the scientific and the ethical debates, as Morland (2009) contended:

> Were doctors to trust patients entirely about treatment decisions, they would squander their medical training. There is no reason at all why an intersex layperson – unfamiliar with the thousands of research papers published on intersex treatment – should be asked to judge whether they have been provided with enough information to assess fully the risks of genital surgery. But there is a good reason why a doctor can and should: because they are a doctor. (p. 204)

I suggest that if the provider were to familiarize themselves with the scientific and ethical debates of "normalizing" treatment, a different kind of conversation with service users would emerge. In that conversation, absence of questions is not misconstrued as clarity of mind, and any mismatch in expectations between provider and user is thoroughly addressed.

A series of guided, open conversations that enable the decision to emerge over time is preferable to a single consultation (Karkazis et al., 2010). Rather than information giving, which connotes a one-way process, doctor–patient interaction is best considered as an information exchange. It is incumbent on the provider to prompt expressions and check meaning. Any information about the intervention should be tailored to the patient or surrogate's level of health literacy and language capacity. In practice, this is not always straightforward. A degree of pragmatism is required, and I explore this in the practice vignette in Section 9.4. Explanations using a variety of media and the use of recordings may help. What is especially helpful for the service user is a conversation with other people with variations who have elected to have the intervention in question and those who have not.

If the intervention is conducted in infancy or early childhood, the treating clinician is obliged to disclose to the caretaker to what age their young patients have been followed up, and what is known and unknown about further treatments, lifetime complication rates and patient reported outcomes. As well as talking and listening, it is crucial to also check understanding. Research suggests that caretakers rarely have their understanding checked when choosing genital surgery for the child (Sanders et al., 2008), which leaves many caretakers opting into interventions without being aware of the debates. To check understanding, a closed question such as "Do you understand?" will shut down conversation. Open questions such as "What would you like me to expand on?" are more likely to open up discussion.

A decision support tool is currently being developed to improve the process of decision-making in childhood interventions (Sandberg et al., 2019). It remains to be seen whether such a tool improves the quality of the exchanges between DSD experts and caretakers and, if so, whether such a tool is routinely and consistently utilized. Suffice it to say that if surgery were allowed to be a foregone conclusion, such a tool is unlikely to be acceptable to the decision-maker.

If surgery is delayed, respect for the older child's developing autonomy means explaining the complex information in such terms that can be understood and respecting their disagreement with treatment where appropriate. Older children who can understand the basic aspects of an intervention can provide assent (informed agreement). By the age of 14 years, many children have the cognitive ability (if not the legal capacity) to make medical decisions (American Academy of Pediatrics, 1995).

The process of obtaining informed consent can be described in terms of the discrete behaviors required of each party with the recognition that the

Table 9.1. *Example guide for informed consent*

Guidance for professionals to support informed consent to elective interventions	Guidance for patients and surrogates giving informed consent to elective interventions
• Consider whether this decision is appropriate for a surrogate, or if it should be made by the patient at a later time	• Decline to sign a written consent after a single discussion
• Decline a written consent after a single discussion or if there is any doubt about the patient or surrogate's understanding or freedom to choose	• Decline to sign a written consent if you are not comfortable with the recommendation or any aspect of your interaction with the treatment team
• Provide the patient or surrogate with guidance on informed decision-making (see right-hand column)	• Prepare your questions in advance if at all possible
• Find out what the patient or surrogate already knows about the intervention and ask how they think and feel about it	• Include another family member or close other to help you listen to the information if possible
• Ask what additional information they seek	• Take notes or audio record the information (people typically remember about 30% of what doctors say)
• Give information about the intervention, a segment at a time, for example:	• Update the treating clinician about what you know so far and your thoughts and feelings about the information you already have
– Information about the problem that treatment is targeting	• Ask direct question
– Information about the procedure	• Listen to the answers
– Information about known physical and psychological benefits and risks	• Tell the clinician what is not clear
– Information about unknown physical and psychological benefits and risks	• Repeat the information in your own words to check that you have understood what is meant
– Information about post-treatment demands including self-management, follow-on investigations, examinations, monitoring, additional procedures	• Ask the treating clinician about his or her experience in giving the treatment
• Check understanding after each information segment; if unsure, ask the patient or surrogate to repeat the information in their own words	• If at all possible discuss what is known and not known about the physical and psychological benefits and risks of treatment now and later
• Encourage the patient or surrogate to express their thoughts and feelings after each information segment, picking up cues that might have meaning for decision-making including that of no treatment or postponement of treatment, especially for a minor	• Ask what happens afterwards, such as how often will you need to come back to the clinic and for how long, how much will it cost and what is likely to happen at those clinic visits
• Discuss the observations with the multidisciplinary team and give due consideration to postponement to enable a	• Ask what will you/the child be required to do to manage the impact of the treatment afterwards, and what happens if you cannot manage
	• Discuss the information with people who are helpful to your situation before making up your mind, such as people who have decided for or against the treatment

Table 9.1. (*cont.*)

Guidance for professionals to support informed consent to elective interventions	Guidance for patients and surrogates giving informed consent to elective interventions
child to participate in the decision at a later time; minute the discussion and action points • Feed back to the patient or surrogate the team's reflections • Create time for the patient to process the implications of the information you have presented • Offer or encourage second opinion if appropriate	• Ask further questions until you are satisfied • Seek second opinion for major decisions, or if you are not comfortable with the recommendation • If you have doubt after signing the consent form and before treatment commences, communicate this clearly with the team

behaviors exhibited by one party would influence the perceptions and expressions of the other and vice versa. For example, the enthusiastic presentation of an intervention by the treating physician may inhibit further questions from the patient. Alternatively, a plea for treatment on the part of the patient is likely to inhibit clear communication of the controversies relating to the intervention. Table 9.1 is an example behavioral checklist to introduce more consistency to a process that is prone to erroneous mutual assumptions and mismatched understandings (see Liao et al., 2018).

9.4 Practice Vignette

Hetty is 16 years old and self-identifies as female. She lives with her father and stepmother and four younger half siblings. They are a loving family that is part of a close-knit traveling community. Hetty has salt-losing CAH (see Chapter 2). She has had two feminizing genitoplasties at age 18 months and 9 years. The family stopped taking Hetty to the specialist DSD clinic a few years ago. It is far away and expensive to get to. They have a good relationship with the local endocrinologist who seems well able to provide care. This physician has now referred Hetty back to the DSD clinic for a gynecological review and more genital surgery.

Hetty attends with her stepmother Mrs. B who tells the gynecologist that Hetty is getting married next year and needs "more tidying up at the front." On examination, the gynecologist feels that a small operation to open the entrance to the vagina (introitoplasty) followed by dilation would be required for sexual intercourse. However, the clitoris, though "prominent," does not require further surgery. Mrs. B is not satisfied with this opinion. She feels that Hetty looks different to her other daughters. She worries that Hetty's future husband "might get suspicious." She is angry at having to come back for another appointment to discuss surgery.

The DSD team, on the other hand, is concerned how little Hetty seems to know about her diagnosis and medical history. It is difficult to have a direct conversation with Hetty with Mrs. B present. The team psychological care provider (PCP) "Eva" subsequently telephones to ask the referring doctor to explain to Mr. and Mrs. B that a conversation between the DSD team and Hetty is necessary before agreeing on any surgical treatment. This only results in Hetty missing the next appointment and apparently seeking an opinion elsewhere. Five months later, she comes back to clinic, this time with her father Mr. B. Below is a summary of the psychological involvement in the overall care process.

9.4.1   Assessment

After a tense beginning, whereby Mr. B expresses no small measure of exasperation with the clinic, he agrees for the gynecologist "Dr. Mills" to meet with Hetty alone. Dr. Mills has to examine Hetty before advising her about more genital surgery. But before that, Dr. Mills needs to meet with Hetty alone to check her understanding about CAH and the medical process.

Eva uses the time to speak with Mr. B alone. She stays as closely to Mr. B's language as possible and draws on her core counseling skills in active listening and verbal following:

EVA: What do you call Hetty's medical condition at home?

MR. B: We say it's her illness. She needs medicine. She's fine.

EVA: Who is aware of her illness?

MR. B: Everyone. She's our miracle baby. She was sick. But look at her now.

EVA: I can see she's doing beautifully. What's been the most challenging thing about the illness?

MR. B: She's a girl. I don't want anyone to think anything else.

EVA: It's important that everyone knows Hetty's a girl. Is there anything else about the illness that has troubled you or your loved ones?

MR. B: My ex-wife [Hetty's birth mother] couldn't handle the medication . . . . She ran away, you know, had an affair . . . . My now wife [Hetty's stepmother] is confident with drugs and all that, maybe because she wasn't spooked by how Hetty used to look before the surgery. It was all very confusing when she was born.

EVA: I see you've all been through a lot . . .

MR. B: It's all behind us now. No point looking back.

EVA: No point looking back. Maybe we can talk about what you all look forward to?

MR. B: She'll be great.

EVA: What a wonderful fatherly endorsement! Tell me what you admire the most in your daughter?

MR. B: She's happy, doesn't let things get to her. She's been looking after the young ones full-time. She's just so capable.

EVA: Full-time? Hetty doesn't have school any more?

MR. B: Nope. She left at 14, the kids were horrible to her . . . . One girl in particular called her "backward" . . . . If Hetty's backward, I think we might have noticed. She hates doing sums that's all. She's great with the animals, more an outdoor girl . . . . She's just different.

EVA: She's good at many things, but school was hard and the kids were horrible and you had to take her out of school. Did anyone help find another school for Hetty?

MR. B: Send her to another school? And have her beaten up again? She had stitches behind her left ear you know. All our kids get bullied at school. People don't like our community, they don't know us, they're scared of us . . . . Still, we've got each other.

Clearly there are additional concerns about Hetty's well-being to consider, not just her CAH. Meanwhile, Hetty is being informed in her meeting with Dr. Mills that her clitoris is within the "normal" range and that more surgery is not recommended. The introitus, however, has shrunk and the scarring means that it is not stretchy enough for dilation without "a small procedure to free the scar."

As the gynecologist leaves the room, Eva steps in to spend some time with Hetty. She sees that Hetty is quiet and makes limited eye contact. Asked how she feels about the physical examination and conversation with Dr. Mills, Hetty passes to Eva the diagram of her genitals drawn for her by Dr. Mills. Hetty expresses her disappointment of being denied further clitoral surgery. Eva asks Hetty about the wedding plans. Hetty smiles and turns toward Eva instantly. She talks happily about having met Vano [her future husband] and his family a few times and that he doesn't mind her illness, though he "doesn't know everything."

Eva asks Hetty whom she talks to if she gets upset or feels unsure about anything. She is interested in hearing how Hetty now feels about what had happened at school, being separated from her birth mother, her big responsibilities at home and so on. Hetty seems to be holding some difficult feelings around her birth mother, but she is more worried about her father's health. She says that she has an aunt to confide in.

The two health professionals now meet with father and daughter together. Eva sets up the four-way consultation as follows:

Thank you Hetty, thank you Mr. B. It has been very helpful to listen to you both. Dr. Mills and I would now like to talk to each other about what we have understood about your situation. Would it be ok for the two of you to listen as we speak? At the end of our discussion, I will ask what may have struck you about our conversation, and whether you wish to add to our understanding or have any questions for either of us?

Here, Eva draws on a family therapy technique to position the family as listeners. Her intention is for Hetty and her father to be present to the professional opinions on Hetty's care needs. Eva and Dr. Mills reflect on Hetty's many capabilities, the strength of the family relationships, how timely the meeting is because it enables them to form an ongoing working relationship with Hetty who is now an adult. The two professionals also reflect on the dilemma of having Hetty undergo more interventions that carry risks. They also emphasize their own need to be convinced that Hetty is making her own decisions.

Afterwards, father and daughter are invited to comment on the conversation, correct any misunderstanding and ask questions. As the waiting time for surgery is 4–6 months, it is agreed that Hetty is provided with bespoke psychosocial input outlined below. It is explained to both father and daughter that the psychosocial program is important to help Hetty to make up her own mind about surgery and for her long-term well-being. Mr. B agrees to encourage Hetty to attend appointments. Additional assessment information can be found in Table 9.2.

9.4.2   Formulation

Eva's "best guess" of Hetty's situation is figuratively represented in Figure 9.1. The insistence on (more) genital surgery makes sense within the Power Threat Meaning Framework (Johnstone & Boyle, 2018). Within the wider culture, the female genitalia are constructed as smooth, flat and without protrusion. The capacity for coitus, pregnancy and motherhood is central to the shared understanding of female sexuality and identity. Having a protruding clitoris and being unavailable for coitus carries meanings of shame and inferiority and threatens social sanction.

Marginalized by gender, ethnicity, class and education, Hetty's social disadvantages require Eva to think in intersectional terms. Intersectionality is a concept that takes account of simultaneously belonging to multiple intertwined social categories such as gender, race and class and examines how power acts on the individual who belongs in each of the intersecting categories. For Hetty, who is disempowered on multiple counts, the

Table 9.2. *Summary of initial assessment with Hetty*

Inquiry domains	Summary of content
Goal of assessment – Information gathering for formulation and care planning as appropriate	– Find out more about understandings of CAH – Find out about the expectations of intervention – Identify potential to avoid unnecessary interventions – Identify psychological care needs for best possible long-term whole-person outcome
Relationship to help – Who is referring who for what reason – Who are in the system – Relationship with specialist services and community providers – Patterns of engagement with services	– Re-referral by trusted family doctor – Strong faith in medical doctors to "normalize" body – Belief that the current team is there to "put everything right" so future partner will not notice any bodily difference – Psychology is for "mad people" ("I am not mad, I don't need psychology") – Good relationship with same family doctor since childhood
General health and psychological well-being – Current – Past	– Well-controlled CAH – No other health problem – No mental health history in family – Physically active lifestyle – "I'm happy" / "I don't let things get to me" – Query re. sufficient healing from bullying and trauma at school?
Personal strengths and needs – Psychosocial skills (e.g., communication, emotion regulation) – Family relationships (e.g., closeness and distances) – Peer relationships – Capacity for independence – Education, work, creativity, interests – Hopes and fears	– Capable of independent living – Capable of responsibility for younger siblings – No current means of financial independence – Calm, quiet, introverted, well liked – Skilled in internet access – Left school early; limited literacy – Main interests – animal husbandry; camping – Aspires to stable married life with children – Dream: "Have my own pony" – Fear: "My dad's cancer coming back"
Understanding of variation and treatment past/present – Factual knowledge – Understanding of immediate and long-term MDT care plan – Knowledge of respective roles of providers involved	– Knows name of diagnosis but no other detail – Knows how to take medication – Does not know rationale for regular medical reviews at specialist clinic – Expects surgery to make any difference invisible – Does not know risks of surgery – Does not know names of surgeons and how to get in touch in case of concerns

Table 9.2. (*cont.*)

Inquiry domains	Summary of content
	– Does not know role of nurse and psychologist before and after surgery
Emotional responses to variation and treatment past/present – Emotional reactions – Immediate and future concerns	– "I'm used to it" (living with CAH and taking medication) – Worries that future husband may think she's not a "full woman" because her genitals are "a little boy-like" – Concerned about not being able to "have sex and have babies like a normal woman" – Query re. how true is assumption of future husband's inability to accept CAH?
Social and cultural aspects – Family relationships – Community support – Access to confiding relationships – Cultural and religious attitudes relating to diversity – Knowledge of education and support resources; and capacity to navigate	– Supportive extended family – Supportive closed rural community – Confiding conversations with aunt and two best friends – Does not warm to professional support services ("strangers") – No interest in support groups – "Not religious" – Does not want to question heteronormative and gender stereotypes – The family doctor is aware of the situation and supportive
Gender and sexuality – Sex/gender identity – Attitudes, preferences – Sexual experiences – Current relationship	– "I only like boys" – Engaged to a young man – Denies any previous history of solo or partnered sexual experiences – Limited sex education – poor understanding of sex anatomy

traveling community that offers a sense of belonging and inclusion and the healthcare system are two of the few power resources that she can access. She mobilizes her right to interventions to respond to the meaning-based threat of her genital variation and, by passing as "normal," she can withhold information about her variation. This enables her to survive and access a purposeful life.

Surgery is meant to remove the threat and protect Hetty's access to social inclusion. But Eva can see from the formulation that a vaginoplasty does not address any of the negative elements in Hetty's life. She also understands from research that vaginal construction itself will not deliver the best psychological and sexual outcome for Hetty. However, Eva is also

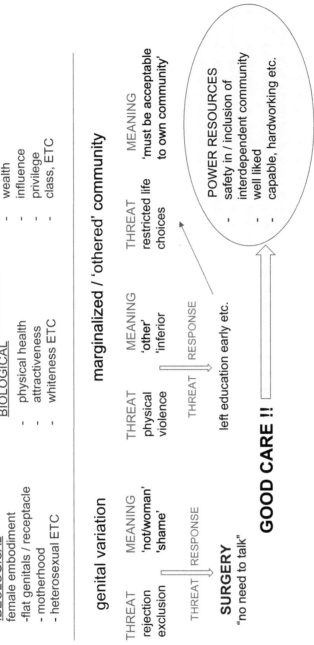

Figure 9.1   Formulation chart for Hetty. A colour version of this figure can be found in the plate section.

aware that Hetty's reasoning is not at all unusual. In a consecutive audit of 50 girls aged between 12 and 20 years seen at a specialist DSD clinic over a six-month period, the care users were most often referred to the clinic for urological or gynecological reasons (accounting for 70% of indications for referral) and least often for psychological reasons (accounting for 14% of indications for referral). On reviewing their diagnoses, history of interventions and ongoing care needs, the service providers agreed that 46% of the individuals required ongoing psychological input to address the various problems such as anxiety, low mood and social isolation (Liao et al., 2010).

Like many of the girls and women in the above study, there are gaps in Hetty's psychological care that vaginal construction will not be able to fill. However, Hetty has the right to choose surgery. Guided by her formulation, Eva considers Hetty's overall care needs and how she and the team might become a resource for Hetty. Vaginal construction could be understood as one component of a comprehensive care plan. The other components of the care plan are to provide her with some education about CAH so that she can navigate her own care in future, help her to make sense of her body using the least pathologizing language, support her to make a more informed decision about disclosure and monitor her overall well-being.

9.4.3   Dialectical Consultation

The components of the care program, all of which require creative use of a range of media, are outlined as follows:

1. Psychoeducation of CAH: This involves checking understanding, filling in knowledge gaps, trying out different vocabularies, and discussing possible disclosure. Eva also creates a poster of the DSD service with names and photographs of different clinicians, to encourage Hetty to navigate her own care in future.

2. Surgery: This involves ensuring that the client can repeat back the information on procedure, risks, limitations and postintervention requirements (knowledge, skills and feelings about dilation to prevent narrowing of the introitus, access to privacy, etc.). The dilation booklet by the UK support group dsdfamilies is used as an aid to explain to Hetty about postsurgical dilation. The nurse demonstrates to Hetty with a hand-held mirror the techniques, with pauses for Hetty to practice simple exercises to relax her body, until Hetty can do this herself.

3. Psychosexual counseling: This aims to increase knowledge of sex anatomy and responses, diversity in sexual preferences, factors that

can affect sexual pleasure (e.g., communication, quality of relation-ship, mood, stress, energy, etc.), sexual health and birth control. Eva makes use of Joani Blank's *Femalia*, Jamie McCarthy's "Great Wall of Vagina" sculpture and the Labia Library put together by an Australian group to illustrate female genital diversity. A key moment in the process is when Hetty giggles and gasps at the wide range of vulval appearances in these works. Though she cannot stop herself laughing, she sees that every vulva is unique. She giggles again when Eva talks to her about pleasure and shows her a book with a range of sexual positions. Hetty is surprised to be told that erotica has been around for thousands of years and exists in almost all cultures.

4.   Overall well-being: This provides opportunities to process the effects of difficult past experiences (e.g., fractured attachment with birth mother, bullying at school) and gives voice to any general psycholog-ical concerns in current life (e.g., worry about father's health).

Eva engages Hetty in a cognitive therapy–informed conversation (Hays & Iwamasa, 2006) to explore the all-or-nothing thinking about disclosure (e.g., "He mustn't never know I've had any surgery") and catastrophic self-talk (e.g., "If he finds out, he'll run a mile"). This work, however, is interrupted by a number of missed appointments. With Hetty's agreement over the telephone, Eva writes to the family doctor whom Hetty is most likely to consult in case of any difficulty. The report outlines the care plan and where the nurse and PCP have got to so far.

9.5   Reflexivity

In the West, people have been systemically maneuvered to imagine them-selves as self-determining choosers, when choice is already structurally predetermined, by and large. For many service users, preferences and options are often a foregone response to the threat of breaking the cultural code, yet uptake of interventions is often constructed as a free choice. The PCP's role is not to push clients into a moral dilemma. The responsibility is double-edged, to acknowledge care users' deep wish for normalcy *and* make influence and disadvantage legible to encourage argumentation. We do this work while remaining sensitive to the fact that people's capacity to resist social norms is constituted in (unequal access to) social, economic and interpersonal power. In many circumstances, though by no means all, we can become a power resource that the client can access.

CHAPTER 10

Caretakers' Grief and Growth

The birth of a child demands some adaptation from every member of the household. Caretakers of a neonate with variations face many additional challenges. What can professional and peer supporters do to encourage the kind of "positive psychological adaptation and well-being" (Sandberg et al., 2017, p. 280) that is so talked about? We know from first-person accounts that service users' silence, passivity and compliance is often mistaken by health professionals as coping, when it may be a manifestation of the opposite.

Research in caretakers' emotional reactions is summarized in Section 10.1. Research suggests that caretakers may 1) not receive enough information about the child's condition, 2) receive too much information or find the information too fast paced and unusable, 3) be upset by excessive professional interests in their child's genitals, 4) flounder on how to approach practical problem such as talking to the family about what is happening, 5) lack confidence in their ability to take care of their child, 6) have too little psychological care or do not understand how psychological expertise can make a difference, 7) want to meet someone with similar experiences and 8) dread what other people may think.

Strong support for caretakers is important in its own right, but it will also have the biggest impact on children living well with their bodily difference. Citing a mother with two daughters diagnosed with congenital adrenal hyperplasia (CAH), Magritte (2012), herself a mother of a child with a variation, passed on the following advice to other worrying parents: "I believe that there are two key factors in helping [children] to come to terms with their condition. One is that their parents accept and are comfortable with the physical effects of their condition and the other is that the emphasis of their condition is not placed on these obvious physical effects" (p. 573).

In Section 10.2, I suggest that healthcare is grief-informed in the neonatal period. Much like caretakers whose child is born with a chronic illness or disability, caretakers with a child with variations grieve for the idealized child that they have longed for. Grief is a typical response to loss.

It is a universal language that every clinician can relate to – personally and professionally. Grief-informed interaction can help the entire system to respect the turmoil and bleakness, however transitory, of the caretakers' internal world and help them to mourn for and let go of the imagined child.

Being grief-aware in healthcare is not based on the premise that intersex variation is inherently a tragedy. Rather, it encourages differences in sex development (DSD) providers to give caretakers time to prepare for new life experiences. Giving false hope can be an obstacle in the caretakers' emotional journey. Based on the literature briefly summarized in this chapter, I suggest three care principles in the early days: 1) safeness/containment, 2) emotionally competent communication and 3) peer support.

I end with a practice vignette that explores grief work with an expectant mother by drawing ideas from the Power Threat Meaning Framework (PTMF) (Johnstone & Boyle, 2018) outlined in Chapter 7 as well as basic therapeutic principles that are familiar to most psychological care providers (PCPs).

10.1 Research with Caretakers

In his 2004 paper, pediatric endocrinologist Gary Warne described an unpublished interview study carried out in the mid-1980s by two social workers in Australia, Elizabeth Loughlin and Margaret Sahhar. They asked a group of parents whose children were born with *ambiguous genitalia* what they found most difficult to cope with. The parents described the strong emotions they were feeling at the time and needing help from an experienced social worker or psychologist whose role it was to assist them to "understand and work through their intense emotions" (Warne, 2004, p. 100).

A subsequent publication by a group of Dutch medical specialists reported on parental reactions based on interviews with 18 mothers and 15 fathers with a child with androgen insensitivity syndrome (AIS) (Slijper et al., 2000). Feelings of shock, sadness, guilt and shame at the time of the child's diagnosis were rated as absent or present retrospectively by the interviewer. The same emotions were also rated in the same way at the time of the study. The methods were crude, cumbersome and unclear in some places, but the account resonated with clinical observations, if predictably, that the majority of mothers and fathers had experienced all of the emotions. Grief, according to this study, was more commonly recorded for fathers, while guilt was more commonly recorded for mothers due, the authors surmised, possibly to having been a genetic carrier.

Guilt and other strong emotions were likewise observed in an unpublished qualitative study involving 20 parents with daughters with AIS around the same time in the UK (Le Maréchal, 2001). Guilt was expressed in the following excerpts:

> Well you do feel guilty because ... you want to ... you would give them your right arm, your left arm, your everything and you've ended up giving them AIS [laughs]. So there is that, and, of course, I've made [daughter] a carrier. (p. 82)

> I think my first reaction was, you know, sort of "Get rid of it" type thing almost. It was ... it was really that, you know, that I'd had this feeling that I'd ... the way it was presented to us was that we'd created this "creature" ... and it was that ... I mean I was quite shocked at my reaction to it, you know ... "just don't want it" type thing. (p. 81)

Gough et al. (2008) emphasized the impact of the shock engendered by the uncertain sex status of a child. The authors argued for more commitment in specialist services to develop a nuanced and in-depth understanding of the complexity of sex and gender in society. This understanding is said to be foundational to decision-making relating to the child's sex characteristics.

Discordance between XY karyotype and female embodiment was reported to be one of the most psychologically challenging aspects of the diagnosis of AIS in the aforementioned Dutch study (Slijper et al., 2000). Parents whose daughters had partial AIS (i.e., involving some genital *masculinization*) were additionally noted to find it hard to cope with perceived cross-gender behavior in their child later. Many of the parents found infertility to be a difficult aspect of AIS and wondered about their child's eligibility for pair bonding without fertility. Parents by and large chose not to share their concerns with other people because they did not know how to, because they feared stigmatization of the child and themselves and because of concern about the child's privacy. Many hesitated to confide in close family members at any level.

Caretakers who are denied opportunities to process their concerns in confiding relationships would have to hold the information and reactions within themselves. Unsurprisingly, 28% in the Dutch sample reported that AIS had had a negative impact on their relationship with their partner, and 40% of the mothers indicated a lack of support from their partner in coping with AIS (Slijper et al., 2000). In a US study, a mother of two daughters with variations said:

No one wanted to talk about the gender issues, how my daughter wouldn't play with their dolls. Both girls are gay. No one wanted to talk about that. The father didn't want to deal with the gender issues at all, and his family thought that we had turned two little boys into girls. We divorced in 1976. (Feder, 2002, p. 297)

In the UK study, a parent said that, as a couple, they would have wanted more children but would not take the risk of having a child with AIS again (Le Maréchal, 2001). Twenty years later, in a study with caretakers with girls with CAH, a parent said something similar: "If [daughter with a variation] was my first baby, she'd be the last" (Alderson et al., 2022).

As little as one-third of the Dutch sample reported having received psychological support (Slijper et al., 2000). The depth, type and quality of the support was not recorded. Chivers et al. (2017) interviewed eight mothers about their experience of support. The four master themes identified were 1) the various stages in the child's development when the mothers most needed support, 2) the importance of developing an understanding of the child's condition, 3) the lack of acknowledgment of the emotional needs of parents and 4) the importance of having close and trusted networks. The study also concluded that the relationship between the extent of the child's variability and the scale of parental distress was not a linear one. While all of the participants prioritized privacy about the child's variation, a minority felt that their guardedness had negatively affected how much support was available to them.

10.2   Understanding Grief

Grieving has important biological, cognitive, emotional, behavioral and spiritual dimensions. It is the most fundamental and universal of human experiences, and also the most unpopular. Here, I draw from research with caretakers of children born with disabilities to argue for emotion-focused care within a grief model (e.g., Solnit & Stark, 1961/2017) in sex development services. Such a model provides DSD services with a language for knowing and talking with and about families. It protects the child and family from undue preoccupation with technological fixes. It gives meaning to patient-centeredness.

Based on the expectant parents' own experience of being a child, the role models that they wish to emulate and, of course, cultural ideals subscribed to, parents have expectations of the unborn child, who is usually perfect. These expectations are thought to be adaptive, because they motivate expectant parents to prepare to make sacrifices and to invest in raising the child in alignment to their values and expectations. The high hopes are brutally crushed when a child is diagnosed with a chronic illness or disability, which may be in utero, at birth or later. A mother with a child with disability spoke movingly about her grief:

> The news that your baby is damaged is devastating to any parent. Devastating is actually putting it very lightly. It rocks the world of the parents. All the dreams, hopes and desires come crashing down. The process of grieving begins. Yes, it is grieving. You grieve for what could have been, what should have been and why it isn't what should have been. The parent grieves for the loss of the perfect child, the imagined child. (Anonymous, 2018)

10.2.1   Processing Loss

Many caretakers with a child with an illness or disability express guilt that they may have unwittingly done something to cause the problem. Despite clear medical causes, a wide range of other causes may run through their mind, ranging from exposure to X-rays and dental amalgam to living too close to a power line. Caretakers may feel rejected by the world and disappointed with how life has turned out. They may direct anger toward themselves or accept their fate as punishment for past sins. These strong feelings can prevent them from talking with each other or with family and friends about how they feel.

In an extensive qualitative study involving caretakers of children and young people with an appearance-affecting condition or injury and their healthcare professionals, a mother said: "I'd done something wrong, my body had failed my little girl" (Thornton et al., 2021, p. 422). The caretakers spoke candidly about feeling repulsed by their child's appearance and feeling guilty and disloyal for the feeling of aversion. They spoke of feeling broken, of not knowing how to approach the situation.

Acknowledgment of fantasies of what might have been is considered by most therapists to be a necessary step in becoming less involved with what is lost. This is an assumption shared by psychoanalytic and cognitive theories of grief resolution. The bereaved need to turn toward rather than block internal thoughts and feelings. Engagement with their pain and sorrow can help people to extricate themselves from what is irrevocably lost. Failure to express the highly charged emotions is assumed to put individuals at risk of delayed and complicated grief. These assumptions underpin grief work.

Suffice it to say that there are social differences in the experience of loss. In some cultures, the idea of *working through* loss may be considered unhealthy or detrimental to the future (Stroebe & Schut, 1999). Many caretakers may not want to talk about loss. They may not want to talk at all. They may hold different and perhaps contradictory beliefs about acknowledging and expressing their feelings. Thus the broad principle of supporting caretakers to process feelings of loss requires sensitive (and sensible) translation when working with people from diverse backgrounds.

Furthermore, the psychological labor of mourning does not bring restitution, in the sense of someone returning to their previous existence. In other words, a caretaker of a child with a variation cannot return to their prevariation existence and must learn to relate to themselves and the world differently. The emphasis is important here. Health professionals are not there to put pressure on caretakers to love their child but to support them to embark on a journey of discovery, along which they grow new perspectives on difference and diversity.

Grief is often described as a journey associated with intrapersonal growth, relationship deepening and emergence of different roles and identities. Within this formulation, grieving has the potential to facilitate adaptation, signified by existential transformation and enhanced family functioning (Doka, 2017). This idea has strong support in disability studies as well as psychosocial research in childhood illness. The personal transformation is reflected in the moving words of a mother adjusting to her child's disabilities:

> When you are a parent busy adjusting to the loss of the idealized child and raising the one you do have, it takes time to come to terms with a couple of facts. First, flaws are an essential part of real, normal human lives. Second, the pursuit of some imagined, flawless life obscures the real parental work, which is to raise a resilient child who values her self. (Abelow Hedley, 2006, p. 43)

Contrary to the popular notion of the stages of grief, some cognitive scientists understand grief as a nonlinear process. Central to their idea of *dual processing* (Stroebe & Schut, 1999) is the dynamic phenomenon of *oscillation* between loss-orientation (lamenting and yearning, focusing on what might have been) and restoration-orientation (social reintegration, doing what needs to be done). What this means is that at times the caretaker is gripped by guilt, shame and fear and, at other times, they are distracted or seek relief by concentrating on other aspects of life. They engage in a back-and-forth process that could feel confusing for them. It is not uncommon to hear someone say, "I thought I was getting better but I seem to be back to square one." Caretakers can be reassured that these fluctuations are to be expected, and that they can hold different and even contradictory feelings about their situation in the same moment. For example, they may yearn for the dream child yet also experience deep love and protectiveness toward the real child.

Sheehan and Guerin (2018) identified a shift toward restoration-oriented coping when parents begin to envision a future with their child with an intellectual disability and reflect on what they have learnt in the process. The dual processing model makes an assumption that the ability to cope with feelings of grief depends upon the capacity of parents for oscillation between processing the meaning of loss and moving forward, despite a high care load and stress, such as required by some disabilities or by changes in the family, like the parental dyad breaking up.

However, disability studies suggest that the caretakers' sorrow could become chronic, so much so that the term chronic sorrow has been coined to describe the experience of loss by parents whose children suffer from chronic disease (Coughlin & Sethares, 2017). In an early study, Pianta et al. (1996) assessed the resolution of the loss or threat associated with learning of the child's disability or chronic illness. While all of the mothers in the study had received similar levels of input concerning their child's condition, half of them remained unresolved about the diagnosis. Furthermore, the researchers identified a strong link between the parents' resolution and the quality of their child's attachment to them and stated that the unresolved parents had not yet integrated the experience of the diagnosis within their views of themselves and their relationships. The degree of resolution was not related to the severity of the child's incapacity or developmental age. They concluded that a mother's capacity to grieve the loss of the child of her imagination was related not only to her own but also to parent–child adjustment.

A recent study in Spain involved 16 parents of adults with intellectual disability (Fernández-Ávalos et al., 2021). The study identified five themes in the parents' reflections of their experiences: receiving the diagnosis, emotional bonds with the child, experience of loss and feelings in response to the diagnosis, recurrent grief and coping strategies. In the emotional bonds theme, parents talked about not knowing whether the disability was a tragedy or a blessing. They also expressed overprotecting the child more than the rest of the family and not feeling able to leave the child to anyone else's care despite offers of help. These resonate strongly with what caretakers of children with sex variations say. Despite ongoing challenges, which may include a stable sense of sadness and ongoing search for meaning, virtually all participants in the Spanish study reported that their children provided positive elements in their lives. In line with previous research, many of the caretakers in the study stated that no one could bring them the love they received from their child every day, that the pleasure of being with their child was incomparable, that their priorities had changed and that they had been helped to become stronger with a keener sense of what should and should not matter in life.

10.2.2 Adaptation

Western psychology understands the perinatal and postnatal periods to be critical for the formation of reciprocal attachment, sometimes to the point of minimizing the realities of many parents in diverse circumstances and those from diverse communities. The perfectionism can result in a premature push for caretakers to have positive feelings toward the child. Reciprocal attachment is much more variable than how it is described uncritically in popular childcare manuals. I discuss ideas about attachment and bonding in this section as they often come up in DSD publications but suggest that these concepts are applied flexibly. Parents who do not live up to cultural ideals may need reassurance by the PCP not to panic.

Research with caretakers of children with genital variations suggests that some caretakers judge themselves by the popular ideology of bonding (Sanders et al., 2008). Some of them negatively compare their experience of bonding with the child with variations to their previous experiences of bonding with their other children. Preoccupation with the child's bodily difference will add to the distress, as a research participant reflected:

> I never ever felt maternal with P, I never felt like I'd had a baby, I felt like I'd woke up and she was 7 months old after she'd had the operation because then she was a girl. The first six months of her life it was like you were, it's like looking after somebody else's child cos you can't form a bond a proper bond with a baby that people are just fiddling with constantly... (Sanders et al., 2008, p. 3191)

The concepts of attachment and bonding are interchangeable in popular culture, but they are not equivalent. Attachment refers to the infant's connection to their caregiver. Bonding, on the other hand, refers to the connection of the caregiver with the infant (Kinsey & Hupcey, 2013). A large-scale concept analysis (Goulet et al., 1998) identified three core elements in reciprocal attachment (attachment and bonding). *Proximity* refers to the physical contact between infant and caregivers. *Reciprocity* refers to the extent to which the infant's behavior elicits appropriate responses from the caregivers. *Commitment* refers to the caregivers' ability to centralize the infant's needs and integrate this new responsibility into their overall identity. Despite more empirical studies in recent years, scientific evidence for these concepts is thin, not least because they (and their temporal relationships) are difficult to operationalize.

The idea of reciprocal attachment resonates strongly with the idea of adaptation. Barnett et al. (2003) defined adaptation as "an ongoing process whereby parents are able to sensitively read and respond to their child's signals in a manner conducive to healthy development" (p. 184). On the basis of their review of numerous studies that have documented the unique emotional and physical demands of raising a child with additional needs, the authors concluded that working with caretakers on their understanding and feelings is still the most effective strategy for promoting adaptation.

However, adaptation should also reference the well-being of caretakers and, where they exist, siblings. Thus far there has been no research that involves siblings of children with variations. Care of siblings is rarely considered in DSD publications, yet research shows that sickness and hospitalization of one sibling can have a significant impact on behavioral and emotional distress in the others. A meta-analysis of 50 published studies from 1976 to 2000, representing over 2 500 siblings of children with chronic illness, offers a useful perspective (Sharpe & Rossiter, 2002). While no alarming blanket effect was identified across clinical contexts, not least because myriad factors are involved, the reviewers identified sufficient risk to the well-being of siblings to recommend high-quality research to explore the effectiveness of psychoeducational interventions for siblings.

Based on what we can learn from disability studies, it is worth asking how care protocols in sex development services could be restructured to facilitate adaptation rather than chronic sorrow, as exemplified in this quote from a caretaker: "We love him because of his differences, not in spite of them. And we are grateful to have the opportunity to accompany him on his journey, wherever it might take him" (Anonymous Parents, 2021, p. 167). A take-home message for PCPs is that they can lean on their scientific credibility to leave caretakers in no doubt that a range of factors can affect interactions with the newborn in the early months, that not all caretakers bond with the child immediately or smoothly and that this need not have significant long-term consequences. Caretaker–child attachment is much more variable than what popular discourses suggest. Parents who judge themselves against cultural ideals need compassion and reassurance to let go of self-blame.

10.3   Service Principles for Grief and Growth

Based on the literature summarized above, psychologically informed care means respecting the caretakers' internal world and reflecting on how the team can interact with them so that they feel held and cradled by the system, so that they can in turn hold and cradle the child. I suggest that DSD teams operate under the principles of safeness, emotionally competent communication, and facilitating peer support.

10.3.1   Safeness/Containment

Parents who give birth to a child with variations may experience themselves as having messed up. They may feel threatened by the risk of being shamed and excluded at the very time when they feel most in need of inclusion. Caretakers need signals of safeness in order to down regulate mind–body arousal and to rest, self-soothe, recover, explore what is new and integrate new learning. The simple message "not your fault" can be a helpful starting point and may need to be repeated in different ways. Rather than retreat into the self, overt expression of sadness and anger may be preferable. Early on, PCPs can describe the pattern of emotional vicissitudes that is to be expected, including the process of oscillation described above, and confidently cite published narratives of caretakers who have overcome similar challenges.

It is important to structure care so that caretakers achieve early success, experience control and feel rewarded. Just like caretakers of newborns with disabilities, caretakers of children with variations are often denied the rituals and rights of passage integral to the early period. The simple act of birth announcement can be fraught with difficulties. In order to resist invisibility and self-abnegation, early on, caretakers may be encouraged to resist any sense of nonentitlement by showing off the baby, talk about the baby's interesting personality and look after themselves in ways that only proud parents would.

Caretakers differ markedly in their capacity to negotiate dynamic relationships with complex social systems of hospitals, schools, friendship networks and community-based services. Those who have experienced childhood trauma or ruptured relationships in their own upbringing may struggle the most in coming to terms with the additional cognitive, emotional and practical challenges posed by sex variations. Working collaboratively with caretakers who manage less well and appear to be retreating into their own world or are in discord with each other can be challenging for the DSD team.

Holding in mind parental and child needs in complex healthcare systems, Kazak et al. (2002, p. 135) described a family consultation model for PCPs in pediatric settings. They named three major tasks that families face every day and may need help with. I have adapted their recommendations within a grief-informed ethos and suggest that the PCP in DSD services 1) enables caretakers to express their strong emotions and at the same time teach skills to moderate arousal, 2) cultivates a trusting relationship with caretakers and encourages them to be proactive over what happens to the child and 3) helps the team to identify points of tension and conflict within the family and between the family and the healthcare system.

Health professionals suffer greatly when they do not have answers and cannot fix the problem. Kazak et al. (2002) suggested parallel engagement with the medical system. In DSD services, the PCP can work with the team to 1) express how they feel (for example about uncertainty) and regulate anxiety and/or excitement, 2) trust each other and the family in the face of uncertainties and 3) be alive to conflicted and dilemmatic experiences (which are often not verbalized) among themselves, within the family and between team and family. If the PCP is not in a position to help family and team in that way, by the time a referral is made to the PCP, it can be surmised that at least one of the three sets of tasks (for family and/or team) has gone awry (Kazak et al., 2002).

10.3.2   Emotionally Competent Communication

In the most recent UK care guidance document for newly diagnosed people and loved ones, the family with a child with genital variations must access a specialist DSD service as soon as possible (Ahmed et al., 2021). The reason is not because the baby is literally a medical emergency or that genital variation is some kind of human disaster. Rather, professionals unfamiliar with genital variations are more than likely to talk to caretakers in ways that can shock them even more. But, how psychologically literate are DSD professionals when they communicate with families? What switches on the threat system of caretakers may not always be obvious to clinicians. For example, a new parent said, "I was exhausted and bewildered. The doctors had lost me at the first hurdle: the introductions. I did not understand their expertise, nor how they were going to 'evaluate' my child, and so I could not begin to understand what was the matter with my child" (Magritte, 2012, p. 572).

Caretakers should be left in no doubt as to who is responsible for the oversight of the entire care process. A pediatric endocrinologist usually assumes overall responsibility and coordinates contributions from other team members. It is a tacit requirement that this physician makes a point to familiarize everyone with each other's roles, responsibilities and timing, to socialize families to engage with the whole team productively and to encourage every team member to verbalize the potential emotional impact of what they are planning to do.

Being emotionally competent can mean as little as conducting ordinary conversations about the infant, such as showing an interest in their feeding and sleeping habits. It means emitting confidence that the caretakers are well capable of being good parents, that the child is capable of flourishing and that lots of people can help to make this happen. In other words, services need to create an environment in which the dominant focus is on the baby's immense possibilities rather than their genetic defect, as suggested by a caretaker speaking from experience: "And I needed someone to empower me, to tell me that even if I didn't understand much of this yet – my/our parenting would play a really important part in my child's well-being, and that they would help me and give me strategies to be the best possible mum" (Magritte, 2012, p. 573).

In a study with parents of children diagnosed with CAH in the neonatal period, however, the participants talked about their inability to digest unmanageably dense medical information (Boyse et al., 2014). They reported looking online to help them make better sense of the information. Sadly, a recent analysis suggests that online information is poor both in terms of quality and quantity (Ernst et al., 2019). Parental confusion and anxiety on account of a biogenetic language and the pace at which information is delivered is identified in other studies (Sanders et al., 2012). Parents may avoid asking for clarification and repetition because it may sound like a criticism of the physician's poor explanation (Freda et al., 2015). In the case of discussing test results concerning older children with variations, some parents reported that they did not want to ask questions in front of the listening child who could be left feeling anxious (Sanders et al., 2017).

Audio and written records of early discussions are a helpful suggestion (Ahmed et al., 2021), but only if every health professional is well versed in a socially inclusive language. It is also important to recognize that when caretakers express confusion or a lack of understanding, they may be struggling with a crisis of meaning, or a fear of not managing the challenges ahead. Rather than burden them with more biology lessons, care staff can try to get behind the confusion first, for example, by asking, "What does the information mean to you so far?"

10.3.3   Facilitating Connections with Peers

Peer support is recognized as a core care component in all DSD documents (Ahmed et al., 2021; Cools et al., 2018; Lee et al., 2016). It is different from but can dovetail with professional psychological input beautifully. It is characterized by nonhierarchical interaction, positive role-modeling, mutual learning, identity-based support and a sense of belonging. Peer support offers people new to the scene the kind of "know-how" and "can-do" that comes from lived experience (Magritte, 2012). These benefits are irreplaceable and cannot be substituted by professional input (Baratz et al., 2014). In the words of Melissa Cull and Margaret Simmonds (2010), two peer support leaders in the UK in the 1990s and 2000s: "A support group is often referred to as a second family; somewhere a person can go in order to talk with and listen to others, air concerns and worries, share break-throughs and experiences, good and bad" (pp. 310–311).

Research shows that confiding in another can enable the person to feel more able to cope with the secret, which in turn predicts higher levels of psychological well-being (Slepian & Moulton-Tetlock, 2019). Feeling more able to cope can change how preoccupied people are with the secret. The reluctance to share information about the child's variation with others and feeling separated from one's social reference group represents a major loss to caretakers. Peer support provides caretakers with opportunities to confide in one another.

Even so, peer support involves social risks and emotional costs. Service users speak of a continuous trade-off between talking and not talking about their variation. They explain that the diagnosis only exists when they think and talk about it. Engaging with peer support and indeed psychological care brings the variation into the foreground. In Chapter 1, the character "Jude" has had to make multiple attempts to attend a support group meeting, despite encouragement from her PCP. When she finally succeeds, she experiences it as a major triumph. This is a common observation in my years of practice in the field.

Indeed, an early study with caretakers of children with AIS found the caretakers to be ambivalent about peer support (Le Maréchal, 2001). However, a later CAH study suggested that the majority of parents felt that support groups were important (Lundberg et al., 2017). When caretakers can clearly benefit from connecting with peers yet reject the idea, it may be because the peer community is not yet accepted as a reference group. Alternatively, rejection of peer support and indeed psychological care more generally may reflect distancing or denial of the reality of the variation because engaging with the reality is too overwhelming. Therefore, although information about peer support should be made available without exception, service users must be allowed to decide for themselves in terms of timing.

10.4 Practice Vignette

"Oxana" and "Bill" meet during their career break in the USA. They fall in love and travel for several weeks together. At the end of their long sojourn, she returns to England where she works, and he returns to South Africa where he lives. There is a mutual strong wish to continue the relationship, though it is not obvious how.

Upon returning home, Oxana discovers that she is pregnant. She had chemotherapy in her teens and was told that she would not be able to conceive. Bill and his family are just as shocked. Under the circumstances, Bill and his family feel strongly that it would be irresponsible to continue the pregnancy. At age 36 years and with her medical history, Oxana sees the pregnancy as her only chance to have a child. She continues with the pregnancy and tells Bill that there is no expectation for him to be involved. He is unhappy and silent.

Because of her social circumstances, Oxana sees the community midwife and family doctor regularly. She attends all her antenatal appointments alone and in tears. At a weekly maternity safeguarding meeting, the midwife expresses his concern that Oxana "has no maternal feelings" and is at risk of "PND" (postnatal depression). He asks PCP "Izmini" for input. Between the time of the midwifery referral and the psychological assessment, the fetus is diagnosed with Turner syndrome (TS).

10.4.1 Assessment

At the first appointment, the PCP introduces herself as Izmi and tries to put Oxana at ease. However, Oxana is so distraught that she struggles to breathe. Izmi intervenes several times to ask Oxana to look around and name what she sees, to prevent her from dissociating. What upsets Oxana the most is the fact that Bill has not been in contact for weeks. She is conflicted – she feels guilty toward Bill because he will soon be a father because of her unilateral decision. And, although she tells him he does not *have* to be involved, she has allowed herself to hope that somehow they would become a family. She now dreads telling Bill that the baby is diagnosed with TS. She repeats to Izmi: "this baby will have only me" and "she will need me all her life." Izmi meets with Oxana for a further appointment, to consider antenatal and postnatal psychological care needs. The information gathered is summarized in Table 10.1.

Table 10.1. *Summary of initial assessment with Oxana*

Inquiry domains	Summary of content
Goal of assessment – Information gathering for formulation and care planning as appropriate	– Referred by midwife concerned about unplanned pregnancy, low mood, "lack of maternal feelings" and "risk of postnatal depression" – Assessment of needs for antenatal and postnatal psychosocial support
Relationship to help – Who is referring who for what reason – Who are in the system – Relationship with specialist services and community providers – Patterns of engagement with services	– Diligent attender; values all professional contact – Attached to "Eva"; is disappointed to hear she will be directed to another service for postnatal support when the baby is born – Family doctor aware of situation, is monitoring mood, has prescribed antidepressants, which Oxana wants to stop when breastfeeding
General health and psychological well-being – Current – Past	– Currently physically well – Upset by baby's father's disinterest in her and the unborn child – Cancer successfully treated at age 16 years, considered cured – Extensive bereavement counseling at college when older sister died in car crash ("It was helpful"), no other mental health history
Personal strengths and needs – Psychosocial skills (e.g., communication, emotion regulation) – Family relationships (e.g., closeness and distances) – Peer relationships – Capacity for independence – Education, work, creativity, interests – Hopes and fears	– Has lived independent and autonomous life and traveled widely – Well liked at work – calm disposition, unassuming, gets tasks done – Does not find work fulfilling; does not know what she would like to do instead – "not ambitious" – Small friendship group – mainly women, similar age, full-time work, see each other some weekends – "I don't have hobbies"; "I'm a quiet person with a quiet life" – Close family but they are all in Mexico – Best hope: "Bill changes his mind . . . and we are a little family . . . I don't mind where I live"

Table 10.1. (*cont.*)

Inquiry domains	Summary of content
	– Worst fear: "Bringing up a disabled child by myself, I don't know how I am going to do that"
Understanding of unborn child's variation – Factual knowledge – Understanding of immediate and long-term MDT care plan – Knowledge of respective roles of providers involved	– TS is "a life of being in and out of the doctor's office – heart, kidney, diabetes, growth hormone, school problems, hands and feet, childhood menopause. . ." – Understands baby will stay in neonatal unit for assessment – Understands there is a community team for children with additional needs – Understands family doctor will help her access everything available
Emotional responses to child's variation – Emotional reactions – Immediate and future concerns	– "Still in shock" about TS – Worries about telling baby's father about TS – Not ready to process care plan – "too real" "still in a fog" – Will go home to Mexico for parental leave but "can't think what happens after that" – "May be I have to move back to Mexico permanently, but I moved away to be independent" (family used to be "'overprotective" because of her cancer and because of sister's tragic death)
Social and cultural aspects – Family relationships – Community support – Access to confiding relationships – Cultural and religious attitudes relating to diversity – Knowledge of education and support resources; and capacity to navigate	– Mother and father have offered practical help with the baby though in Mexico – Lifelong friends from school in Mexico have all offered help – Self-identifies as a Buddhist – committed, belongs to sangha, "comforting" "my spiritual compass" – Knows about TS support resources; open to peer support but not ready yet
Relationship to diversity – Exposure/experience – Attitudes/preferences in relation to child's future	– Accepting of diversity, but had assumed she would have a "normal" baby who would grow up and go to college and travel around like her – TS would have been fine, if she could co-parent with Bill, but not by herself – Sadness around losses in life exacerbates catastrophic thinking about future

While her marketing job pays enough to enable her to be financially independent, Oxana will not be able to afford childcare. Friends and family are excited and can give substantial practical help but they live in Mexico. They have no means to finance childcare. Oxana has a few friends near where she lives, but they work full-time and cannot offer practical help. Furthermore, Oxana will soon have to move out of the apartment currently shared with three people, because it is not a suitable environment for the baby.

With some prompting, Oxana talks about her childhood cancer to the extent that she can remember. As she tells her story, she realizes that, although she does not usually think about the cancer, at the back of her mind, she has always prepared herself that she could have cancer again later in life. She now ruminates what would happen to the child if she were to die.

Asked what she understands about TS, Oxana references worst-case scenarios, even though she has been made aware that TS is a spectrum condition. Izmi explains to the fetal and neonatal doctors that the information about TS, however balanced, has led Oxana to lose herself in terrifying information on the Internet. The medical experts agree not to overfocus on TS until Oxana has more emotional capacity.

10.4.2 Formulation

Izmi draws ideas from the PTMF and other resources for a meta view of the situation. Her "best guess" about the layers of influences on Oxana's current grief and potential for growth is summarized in the formulation chart in Figure 10.1.

Izmi reflects on the shared ideology of children as perfect and happy. This construction creates a psychological space between actual and imaginary children. Children who fall outside the perfect/happy imaginary can be a source of ongoing threat for caretakers. How caretakers respond to that threat is variable and context-dependent. To Oxana, TS will end all hope of Bill agreeing to co-parent with her. The emotional pain of his rejection loops in catastrophic thinking about the future. The child with TS is constructed as not perfect/therefore incapable. She becomes preoccupied with many what-ifs (e.g., what if I die of cancer later). She misses her late sister acutely and yearns for the imagined support. Overnight, her dream becomes a nightmare.

Although Oxana and Bill had an equal role in conception, they have different choices relating to the pregnancy. Even though she had never desired to be a mother, the pervasive idealization of motherhood made it

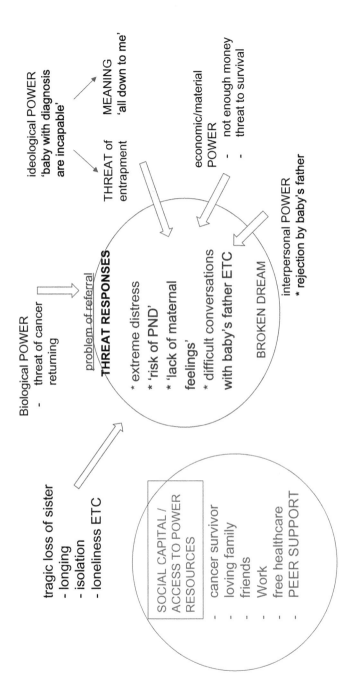

Figure 10.1 Formulation chart for Oxana. A colour version of this figure can be found in the plate section.

"natural" for Oxana to grab the (potentially only) opportunity to have a baby. She exercises her legal and biological power and continues with the pregnancy. Her expectation to change Bill's mind reflects an unawareness of his disempowerment. Bill is less culturally primed to accept fatherhood but he is catapulted into fatherhood nevertheless. Now that the choice is made, however, he holds a disproportionate amount of interpersonal power within the dyad, to choose how much to participate or withhold support. Oxana's distress at Bill's apparent disinterest is also shaped by her lack of material power to provide for her child.

Oxana's low mood and "lack of maternal feelings" is at odds with cultural representations of the blooming expectant mother. Valorization of motherhood successfully obscures a mountain of evidence attesting to the negative impact of motherhood on maternal mental health. A different formulation of postnatal depression focuses on the changes that all mothers face, which include losses in terms of financial independence, career advancement, social status and connections, intellectual stimulation and personal identity, not to mention physical vitality and access to leisure and self-care (see, e.g., Nicholson, 2011). While there is undeniable joy, the paradoxical experiences that are often felt postnatally are generally overlooked. With a broken dream, Oxana is feeling the threat of the losses early. Although her low mood is entirely understandable, it is "unnatural" for an expectant mother and is being medically managed (with safeguarding measures in place).

Oxana's strengths are obscured by her intense negative emotions. She forgets that she has survived cancer and the tragic death of a sibling. She minimizes the fact that she has actively chosen to leave behind the protectiveness of family and community to forge an independent life abroad. Her family and community in Mexico are committed to helping her to raise her child. The workplace has agreed to offer maximum flexibility. She is part of a Buddhist sangha, even though she has not actively engaged with it in recent months. There are many community resources that are free to her. She can look forward to forging new and supportive friendships in future. Peer support for TS is thriving.

The antenatal staff want Oxana to be proactive and start discussing care planning for the baby. They are concerned about the impact of PND on the child and want to effect a change in mood as soon as possible. However, Oxana does not have the emotional capacity at the moment. Izmi is confident that by listening to Oxana's losses and creating an atmosphere of emotional safety and containment, Oxana will have the best chance of regaining her composure and becoming agentic again to do what she needs to do.

10.4.3 Dialogical Consultation

Oxana is now 25 weeks pregnant. This allows time for around 10 weekly counseling episodes – if the baby were to arrive around the due date. Izmi's intention is to build rapport and help Oxana to mourn for what is not to be and look to the future. Meanwhile she praises her antenatal colleagues for the sense of safety that they have provided for Oxana. She shares Figure 10.1 at a weekly maternity safeguarding meeting and explains the psychological care plan. She draws attention to ideological constructions of attachment and bonding in popular culture and encourages her colleagues to keep an open mind. She further explains that she will identify opportunities and timing to introduce the idea of peer support and asks that her colleagues join with her to encourage Oxana in due course.

Izmi first focuses on building a nonthreatening relationship by asking open questions and listening actively, using prompts to draw out the richness and depth of Oxana's current and past life experiences. She uses silences to ensure that the conversation is spacious, reflective and unhurried. To address the highly charged physical and mental states observed in the assessment phase, Izmi draws on mindfulness practices to help Oxana regain some of her physical composure when they meet.

Oxana feels attached to Izmi almost right away. She confides in Izmi about the broken dreams in her life. Drawing on mind–body awareness further, and in the interest of encouraging processing, Izmi would sometimes ask her client, "Where in the body are you feeling this deep sadness?" and "What is the shape and color of this pain, where is it now?" The intention here is to help the client to turn toward difficult experiences rather than block them. Sometimes, when Oxana becomes too distressed, Izmi would inquire, "What would you like to do to take care of yourself right now?"

In time, when Bill comes up in conversation, Izmi would arouse more flexible thinking by asking, "What do you think Bill would want us to know about his experience?" Oxana begins to see that perhaps Bill has needed more time to process the shock of his impending fatherhood. This new awareness paves the way for her to connect with Bill differently over the phone. He is now aware that the baby is diagnosed with TS.

A major component of the therapeutic work relates to the impending birth, the postnatal period and a more balanced understanding about TS. Izmi asks what Oxana knows about TS. What comes back is: "heart trouble, short-stature, menopause, diabetes, shield shape breast, growth hormone, infertility, hearing and balance. . ." About halfway through the grief work, Oxana is ready to speak on the telephone with a peer support worker diagnosed with TS who then introduces her to a father who is raising a child with TS. The conversations are transformative. Izmi takes the opportunity to explore the way in which society positions children as either perfect or incapable/unlovable and distorts the reality of many children who are lovable, loved and thriving despite their physical and/or psychosocial challenges.

As Oxana becomes less involved with the dream baby and dream family, she meets with neonatal and pediatric experts to discuss care planning. She begins to shop for clothing and equipment for the baby and look in earnest for a place to move to. She makes friends in antenatal classes and learn about all the free facilities that are open to new parents. And, she is also expecting Bill, who is taking a month's leave between jobs, to be at the birth and to help in the postnatal period.

When Izmi gets to meet Bill, in anticipation of his unease, she says to him, "This may come as a surprise to you, but I have always thought of myself as your psychologist too. Your welfare has been an important part of all our conversations in this room. Everyone in this situation is valuable and deserves the best attention." She facilitates the conversation with the future co-parents around the following questions:

What does normal mean in your world?
Looking back, what and how were you taught these ideas?
Looking ahead, what ideas do you want to commit to?
What is your dream for your child?
Who can join with you to be part of this beautiful vision?

Izmi shares part of the formulation chart with the couple to place their dilemma in context. She invites them to name their strengths and resources. The co-parents agree on the name Elinor. Izmi is curious about how people in Mexico and South Africa celebrate new life. She asks who in their respective communities will sign up to Team Elinor.

Boundaries and limits are integral to all therapies, and ending is part of the experience. However, ending can be especially difficult for people with attachment issues or who have suffered major losses. Oxana has benefited from secure attachment in early life but has subsequently endured a serious illness and the tragic loss of her only sibling. Izmi invites and guides the client to design the final session with her in the interest of mutual reflections and learning.

10.5 Reflexivity

The concept of loss is not based on the premise that variations in sex development are a tragedy. Rather, grief is a language that all care providers can understand. It reframes the caretakers' experiences and demedicalizes their needs. It defines patient-centered care and operationalizes the concept of growth and adaptation. It commands emotionally competent interactions with families.

Grief is understood not as a linear process but one that oscillates and, with skillful professional and peer input, if all goes well, eventually eases the caretakers out of their emotional entanglement with the imaginary child and the pre-DSD self. It is only then that space is freed up to question "normal" – a task that is vital for everyone impacted by variations but one that can be obstructed by hasty promises of fixing.

CHAPTER II

Assigning Legal Gender

Each culture prescribes standards of appearance, comportment and behavior for boys, girls, men and women. Gender differences are therefore observable in almost all cultures in any given period, though the quality and quantity of the differences are clearly malleable by time and place. Gendered socialization is not usually consciously orchestrated. People tend to experience themselves as acting naturally, as a matter of course.

The designation of a newborn as female or male organizes how s/he is interacted with. When a baby's genitals do not signify either gender, which world should the baby inhabit? Gender assignment has been said to be one of the most stressful processes for caretakers (Magritte, 2012). No amount of blood tests and pelvic imaging can overcome the arbitrariness of fitting a nonbinary body into a binary gender. Changes in the law have been made in a number of countries to try to accommodate the considerable struggles of assigning a binary gender to a child with variations. In a world that fails to acknowledge the heterogeneity of bodies and identities, these changes are unlikely to remove the uncertainties that surround caretakers, who feel as if they are gambling with their child's future. In this chapter I examine the knowledge bases that psychological care providers (PCPs) in differences in sex development (DSD) medicine may bring and contribute to the process of legal gender assignment and discuss how to work pragmatically.

According to the World Health Organization (2021), the term gender describes characteristics of females and males that are socially constructed, that is, an individual's subject position and social roles (which, by definition, are contingent and negotiated). Sex, on the other hand, refers to biological characteristics, that is, chromosomes, hormones, the reproductive system and urogenital anatomy. However, medical publications continue to refer to sex and gender interchangeably, reflecting how they are represented in popular culture and echoing the point made by Chase (1998) that, if physical female sex is understood to be congruent with female gender, and physical male sex with male gender, is sex not gender all along (p. 208)?

The Chicago consensus recommends that psychologists contribute to the process of gender assignment. What kind of knowledge do psychologists bring to the process? A number of psychological theories exist about gender development, including psychoanalytic and social and cognitive theories. However, it is brain organization theory that has dominated research in intersex and DSD medicine. Masculine attributes are understood to be hardwired by exposure of the brain to androgens during fetal development. Chromosomal females exposed to fetal androgens and subsequently assigned to feminine socialization are considered "natural experiments" (Berenbaum & Meyer-Bahlburg, 2015, p. 362). Therefore, psychological research used to mostly target girls and women with congenital adrenal hyperplasia (CAH). The definition of masculine is seductively simple, that is, preference for stereotypic boy play (e.g., wanting to play devil rather than witch at Halloween) and occupation (e.g., wanting to be a truck driver rather than a nurse), being sexually attracted to females and having a male core gender identity.

If it is unsound to reduce the complexity of gender to a culture-free hormonal manifestation, does dismantling of gender offer solutions for intersex? The scholar/activist Emi Koyama's (2003) frustration in how intersex is mobilized by nonintersex experts to verify their own political standpoint is evident in the following words: "Intersex people are reduced to their peculiar organs, then are further diminished into a pure theoretical device, the exhibit A in the case against essentialism and for social constructionism. In other words, people's bodies were used to support abstract social theories, rather than social theories being used to support people" (p. 1). Here, Koyama exposed how intersex people could be stuck between biomedical scientists who see their bodies as a route to learn about "normal" development and gender scholars who see the same bodies as a strategy to disrupt the gender binary to serve nonbinary communities. The iterations by Chase (2003) that intersex struggles are a problem of stigma and trauma, not gender, were a call for activists and their allies to prioritize changes to how patients, especially children, are treated.

The goal of gender assignment is to advise caretakers on a legal gender that minimizes interventions and to ease them toward bringing up a child with a nonbinary body as a laudable way out of their grief. For the PCP involved, this means proceeding pragmatically to 1) build a warm and robust alliance with the whole family from the beginning (see Chapter 8), 2) familiarize with relevant literatures (medical, psychosocial and lived experience) to work with the whole system on choosing the best legal gender that minimizes invasive interventions and developmental interference, 3) prepare caretakers to build and maintain relationships with the community as they reenter their social world and 4) collaborate with peer workers where possible to conceptualize and deliver a bespoke and clearly punctuated program of compassionate and supportive mentoring for family and community. These tasks, which are explored in the practice vignette in Section 11.3, are far from well supported by traditional psychological research in intersex/DSD.

11.1   Brain Gender

The main role of the sex chromosomes is to determine whether the bipotential gonads differentiate into testes or ovaries. Brain organization theorists posit that after gonadal differentiation, the ensuing prenatal and perinatal hormone milieu shape development of certain brain regions and produce permanent changes and enduring behavioral patterns. During puberty, hormonal surges activate brain circuits already in place and extend them from the central to the peripheral nervous system. These mechanisms are said to be foundational for gendered attributes.

Laboratory experimentation with animals is integral to research in brain organization. Experimental manipulations such as hormonal injections or lesions along hypothesized neuroendocrine pathways of rodents enable researchers to assess corresponding variations in reproductive markers (e.g., sperm production in males, lactation in females) and mating behavior (e.g., intromission in males, lordosis in females). The extent to which animal data can be extrapolated to humans remains a moot point in the behavioral sciences. Human sexuality is clearly not just a question of copulation. Every autoerotic and partnered sexual act involves a complex interplay of thoughts, emotions, behaviors, sensations and physiological activations and feedback. More than that, subjective interpretations are framed by language and discourses. There is a fundamental problem of conflating the elusive and dynamic quality of human eroticism and the mechanics of reproduction.

However, brain organization theory does not just rely on animal research. An important aspect of the investigation paradigm is observations of humans combined with psychometric testing. Experiments are set up so that boys and girls choose between various toys and play activities, playmates, imaginary future occupations and so on. Children, caretakers and teachers may be asked questions about the child's gendered preferences. An engaging and accessible account of this fascinating body of work can be found in Melissa Hines' (2004) volume, *Brain Gender*. Research has demonstrated that boys as young as three years old show a preference for stereotypic masculine toys and games. By kindergarten age, boys are observed to be less likely to show a preference for feminine toys than girls to show a preference for masculine toys. With increasing age, boys and girls make increasingly more gender-stereotyped choices, with boys consistently making more of them than girls. Researchers are careful to point out that within-gender variability can be as wide as between-gender variability. Therefore, it is difficult to define "normal" ranges of either gender. On the whole, the predictive power of brain organization theory is strongest in relation to mating behaviors of animals and weakest in relation to adult gender identity.

11.1.1   Research in Intersex

Brain gender as a field of study marks psychology's longest relationship with intersex medicine. In a review published by the pediatric clinical psychologist David Sandberg and coworkers (Stout et al., 2010), the authors identified 98 original research studies published between 1955 and 2009 that examined psychosocial endpoints in intersex. The research team reported that the majority of studies (68%) investigated endpoints related to psychosexual differentiation. They explained: "The preponderance of studies (76%) examined a direct relationship (i.e., inferring causality) between prenatal androgen exposure and psychological outcomes" (p. 1). The authors criticized the imbalance between academic brain gender research and psychosocial research in clinical settings. They expressed a clear wish for their review to stimulate new research to address the many complexities in the lives of impacted children, adolescents, adults and families.

Brain gender research has focused upon chromosomal and social females with CAH. Investigators of gender outcomes have concentrated their effort on three key areas: 1) juvenile play patterns (usually involving direct observation and/or interviews with caretakers), 2) adult erotic interests (usually involving direct questioning and psychometric tests) and 3) core gender identity (usually involving direct questioning and psychometric tests).

Girls with classical CAH have consistently been reported to show increased preferences for "boy toys," boy playmates and rough and tumble play style and fewer female-typical preferences (Hines, 2004). And yet, a study also showed that, while masculine gender identity scores were higher for girls with CAH compared to their sisters, they were lower than those of healthy "tomboys" without CAH (Berenbaum & Bailey, 2003). Researchers acknowledge the extensive evidence that children are rewarded for gender-appropriate behaviors and learn the rules from a young age as to which behaviors lead to social approval.

The majority of women with CAH are said to identify as heterosexual. As a group, however, they are also more likely to report bisexual and homosexual erotic interests compared to their sisters, demographically matched controls and the general population (Hines, 2004). Attraction to females is said to correlate moderately with degree of prenatal androgen exposure (Berenbaum & Meyer-Bahlburg, 2015), which is inferred from the degree of genital masculinization. By contrast, 46,XY individuals raised as female with very low prenatal exposure to effective androgens, as is characteristic of complete androgen insensitivity syndrome (AIS) or complete gonadal dysgenesis, are typically attracted to males.

Brain organization research in core gender identity is inconclusive. It is generally thought that the majority of female-assigned individuals with CAH and other variations remain female-identified, even in the presence of "highly masculinized" behavior (see Berenbaum & Meyer-Bahlburg, 2015). Taken as a whole, the current understanding is that, compared to the general population, adolescents and adults with DSD diagnoses other than Klinefelter syndrome and Turner syndrome are more likely to express gender dissatisfaction and change gender (Kreukels et al., 2018). Prevalence of gender transition is said to vary as a function of diagnostic and treatment factors (Berenbaum & Meyer-Bahlburg, 2015). Brain gender research, which has spanned many decades, remains limited in its capacity to confidently inform gender assignment of newborns.

A recent publication that aimed to provide guidance on gender assignment acknowledged the uncertainties surrounding gender identity outcomes of children with variations (Bangalore Krishna et al., 2020). The authors criticized the literature that gives percentages of gender transition without any attempt to account for the multiple factors that could impact upon such an outcome. The criticism is fair, when so much research has yielded so little help for DSD clinicians with responsibilities to counsel families in real time. Implied in the criticism, however, is that better science in future will afford clinicians more confidence and certainty. However, gender is a social construction. The fluidity in gendered subjectivities and expressions afforded by an evolving society may always trump biological predictions.

Brain gender affords a comfortable fit with biomedicine, which also conceptualizes gender as normally either feminine or masculine and congruent with biological sex characteristics. Feminist scientists have scrutinized the vast body of psychoneuroendocrine research, which is critiqued for being complicit with patriarchy and heterosexism and for its methodological weaknesses. A notable reexamination of brain gender research is in *Brain Storm*, a major monograph by Rebecca Jordan-Young (2011), who concludes that psychoneuroendocrine research is characterized by widely variable and conflicting results, limited effect sizes and overconclusions and who argues for a better science that does not begin with heteronormative presuppositions.

11.1.2   Needs for Theoretical Development

In a recent commentary, Hines (2020) maintained that early testosterone exposure has some effects on gendered behavior but acknowledged that the influence can only be understood by taking account of the socialization context. After some seven decades of research, knowledge of how early testosterone exposure interacts with postnatal socialization "is currently incomplete" (p. 89). A new generation of neuroscientists/sexologists increasingly emphasize the growing understanding of social modulation of hormonal effects.

Research in the "reverse relationship" between socialization and biology, that is, study of the "profound social influences on testosterone" (van Anders et al., 2015, p. 13805) represents a paradigm shift. In a non-DSD context, scientists have known for some time that poverty-modulated social experiences can exert profound neurobiological effects on humans. Without being saddled by linear causality, more may be learned about a potential gender to testosterone pathway of influence as well as vice versa. Studies have also moved beyond a pure androgen focus to include research in peptide hormones such as vasopressin, oxytocin and cortisol. Van Anders (2013) called for integration of research in several domains that have been gaining grounds including adult–infant interactions and adult sexual desire, behavior and partnering. The idea is to work on "seemingly orthogonal perspectives to allow for transformative approaches to an empirically-supported social phenomenology of testosterone" (p. 198).

Away from the hormonal focus, a growing body of social psychology research by Susan Egan and David Perry (2001) and their coworkers offer a useful framework for making sense of children's cognitive understanding and social experiences of gender and how such experiences affect adjustment. Based on work with school-age children in the general population, the researchers proposed that gender identity is understood as having multiple dimensions. In their 2001 formulation, five components were proposed and hypothesized to follow different developmental trajectories, serve different psychological functions and relate to adjustment in different ways. The first dimension is *membership knowledge*, which means knowing one's membership in a gender category. Secondly, the dimension *intergroup bias* refers to the belief that one's own gender is superior to the other. The third dimension, *felt pressure for gender differentiation*, refers to perceived pressure to conform to gender stereotypes. Fourthly, *gender contentedness* refers to satisfaction with one's gender. Lastly, the dimension *felt gender typicality* refers to perceived similarity to others of one's gender. Two of the five components, felt pressure and felt typicality, were found to relate reliably to aspects of adjustment in middle childhood, but in opposite directions. Felt typicality was associated with positive outcomes (especially high self-esteem) and felt pressure is consistently linked to maladjustment (Egan & Perry, 2001).

An example of this interesting field of inquiry is a nuanced study based on a large (if mainly white) sample that examined perceived maternal support, a factor in child adjustment, as a moderator of gender identity dimensions (Menon et al., 2017). Perceived maternal nonsupport was shown to magnify ill effects of felt pressure and sometimes nullify benefits of felt typicality. The authors concluded that the relationship between gender identity development and psychological adjustment required simultaneous consideration of the family context. Where children did not perceive maternal support within and beyond the home, gender-related pressures can operate in a relatively harmful or aberrant way. Research to identify intersex children's felt typicality and felt pressure as well as environmental moderators may offer useful insights to PCPs working in sex development and related services in future.

11.2 Gender Uncertainties in Context

Gender assignment is, to some caretakers of children with variations, akin to hedging a bet that will result in a win or a loss. It is worth placing the dilemma in the evolving social context, whereby no one can tell whether a child born today will choose to remain in the same gender in future and, if they do, what their sexual preferences may be.

Recent statistics suggest that young people, at least in the West, are increasingly endorsing minority sex and gender preferences. Citing recent literature, Stewart et al. (2019) reported that approximately 15% of adolescents in the USA identify as lesbian, gay, bisexual, queer, pansexual and bicurious. They conducted a general population study to examine fluidity in adolescent girls' and boys' self-labeled identities and romantic attractions over time, and to examine what extent these variables coincided with sexual behavior. They reported that 26% of girls and 11% of boys reported fluidity in identity, and 31% of girls and 10% of boys reported fluidity in romantic attractions and a high prevalence of same-gender sexual behavior.

Aside from adult sexual preferences, if we were to consider children's gender satisfaction per se, gender services for children and youth in several countries have seen a sharp increase in referral in the past decade (Butler et al., 2018). Among preadolescent school-age children who are referred, the natal sex ratio appears to be evenly split. Among adolescents, there is a preponderance of children with female natal sex being referred but especially in Finland. In the UK, children and young people from minority ethnic communities are thus far underrepresented at gender services (compared to referral patterns to child mental health services and population statistics). The reasons for the overall increase and sociodemographic differences therein are unknown.

It has been suggested that destigmatization of gender identity diversity facilitated by social media combined with service availability have coalesced to give rise to more gender questioning (Kaltiala et al., 2020). A Dutch study identified an association between gender identity dissatisfaction with gendered bodily characteristics and felt gender identity incongruence in children (Verveen et al., 2021). One interpretation of this finding is that pressure on sexed appearance is potentially implicated in gender dissatisfaction. The increasing support for nonbinary gender identity options in the USA is reflected in the option of nonbinary identity in 15 states (see Ernst et al., 2020). However, although an increasing number of youths describe themselves as nonbinary and gender-queer, many do not proceed to change their legal gender and/or undergo physical interventions.

11.2.1 *Working with Limitations*

In the past, production of a future heteronormative subject was the goal of gender assignment. Even today, young people impacted by sex variations feel under pressure to conform to cultural norms for body and identity and struggle with healthcare services that fail to challenge the oppressive norms (Steers et al., 2020). There is, however, mounting pressure for gender assignment of newborns to be seen as the beginning of an ongoing care plan that ends with flourishing children, teens and adults who are socially engaged, whatever their gender and sexuality.

In order to prepare caretakers that a sizable minority of children will become uncomfortable or dissatisfied with whatever gender assigned, Lee et al. (2016) suggested that the legal gender in childhood is best considered a probable adult gender identity. To advise families in this way will require an inclusive way of knowing and talking about sex and gender. DSD experts are in a powerful position to lead by example on inclusive knowing and talking, not least because families' reluctance to share information outside the clinic renders them almost solely reliant on DSD experts for guidance.

Bangalore Krishna et al. (2020) offered guidance for four challenging gender assignment scenarios: late onset 46,XX CAH being raised as male, 46,XY ovotesticular DSD diagnosed at birth, 46,XY partial AIS diagnosed at birth and 46,XY 5αR2D diagnosed at birth. While the guidance is almost exclusively anchored on a biological perspective, for example with a strong focus on DSD etiology, testosterone level at birth, androgen receptor gene, potential virilization, need for a gonadectomy and so on, there is clearly a strong intention to individualize the approach and provide the most humane possible care.

Although medical experts infer from their technological expertise a tacit authority to advise caretakers of the best legal gender for their child, a study by Timmermans et al. (2019) suggests that many caretakers already have a firm opinion about the child's gender when they present themselves to a DSD clinic. The authors of the study suggested that medical experts' primary involvement in gender assignment was to put a distinct biomedical spin on the ontology of gender. Importantly, the study showed that clinicians are more comfortable about considering the possibility of future gender dysphoria and reassignment than the social stigma of genital variations. This observation chimes with my reading of the aforementioned case studies by Bangalore Krishna et al., whereby surgical and hormonal options are firmly in place, but narratives about children growing up with genital differences and adults living with genital differences are scant.

Gender assignment typically takes place when parents are still grieving for the longed-for imaginary child (see Chapter 10). In threat mode, and in the absence of any professional input for addressing the stigma of genital variations, many caretakers can be expected to want to salvage a degree of the familiar imaginary. Medical personnel who assert a leadership position in the gender assignment process yet do not acquire the skills to talk about genital variability as a livable social reality will perpetuate the conflation of gender assignment and genital "normalization."

Despite references to a multidisciplinary approach, education and counseling relating to gender assignment are largely framed in terms of helping caretakers to understand the biology rather than to question "normal." What does questioning "normal" look like? In Timmermans et al.'s analysis of audio recordings of real-life consultations, a father asked if his daughter would have a normal sex life in future. The pediatric endocrinologist was quick to reassure the father with the offer of treatment options in future. By contrast, the gynecologist reframed the father's inquiry as a complex question that needed unpicking. She explained to the father that many women with a different sex anatomy enjoy sex and many women with a so-called normal anatomy do not. She went on to say that growing up feeling loved and supported and able to accept oneself was the route to happy and healthy adult relationships.

For the PCP involved in gender assignment, it is clear from the discussion so far that the task is not to speculate what toys the child will prefer, who will turn them on sexually later and what gender will they inhabit in life, but what decisions will minimize controversial interventions and what kind of ongoing support does the family need. Warm and compassionate connections with caretakers at the very beginning of their medical journey can pave the way for a robust alliance, whereby caretakers are encouraged, even challenged, to think about the child's variation in different frames. As seasoned therapists, the PCPs would have the skills to empathize with caretakers' fear but also the confidence to moderate their shame-based predictions about genital variations.

11.3 Practice Vignette

A baby girl is born at a local hospital late into the evening. The mother "Lilly" is asleep. She had wanted a natural birth, but labor did not progress and she had to be induced. "Dympna," a trainee midwife, is on night duty. She changes the baby's diaper. Under the spotlight, Dympna wonders if the baby may not have some genital swelling. She creates an alert in the electronic notes. The next day, a neonatologist examines the baby. He asks Lilly about the conception and pregnancy, rereads the notes several times and asks another colleague to help. After 2–3 hours, the neonatologist tells the parents that the baby may not be a girl and could be "intersex." Lilly suddenly feels very awake. Her partner "Ralf" falls silent. The baby is transported to a tertiary hospital some distance away. The parents have to stay at a hotel nearby; they ask Ralf's father to stay on to take care of their older child "Ben." Lilly and Ralf are confused but hopeful. They have been told by maternity staff that the "big hospital with all the latest equipment and experts will clear everything up soon."

The expert DSD team is assembled at the tertiary hospital. The excitement is palpable. The pediatric endocrinologist "Professor Waseem" and pediatric urologist "Professor Maranto" agree that the baby's external genital appearance maps onto Prader 2 staging. But they are far more concerned with how the baby has developed physically, what are the internal structures and what the hormone assays can say about gonadal function. The baby has to undergo many tests, not all of which can be done right away. Results are not instant and, in any case, the tests could come back with very little information or information that contradicts other features. The baby has to stay in hospital for a few more days. Lilly and Ralf are worried about how Ralf's father will manage at home because he is not very mobile. Friends and neighbors offer to assist and ask about the sex of the baby. At one point, Ralf says to someone that the baby could be a boy or a girl. Lilly is furious with him but cannot come up with an alternative response herself.

Professor Waseem, who leads the DSD team, pleads with her colleagues not to second-guess the diagnosis, because the supposition could subtly steer communication with the family in unhelpful ways. But, already, there are whispers about what intervention options are available should the parents go with a boy or a girl. However, the clinical lead's cautious tone opens space for in-house PCP "Masako" to articulate a psychosocial perspective: "Whatever the test results," she explains, "gender identity won't be on the table." She continues, "the tests can help us to advise the parents on the best legal gender that minimizes unnecessary interventions. But we don't actually know anything about the family, like, their values and life experiences, and what they will find difficult. I am guessing that they want us to appreciate what they are like as a family and how they are feeling right now."

Here, Masako's intention is to remind the team of the risk of an overreliance on technology to deliver the answers. She also tries to expand the professional focus and to place the team's relationship with the family at the heart of the focus. The team agrees with Masako's proposal and she and the nurse specialist "Aditi" meet with the parents right away and stay in close touch with them. These early meetings with the parents pave the way for Masako and Aditi to do substantial work with the entire family in the months to come.

11.3.1   Joining with the Family from the Beginning

Masako congratulates Lilly and Ralf warmly and asks the usual questions that people ask about newborns – how are they feeding and sleeping, who do they look like in the family and how is breastfeeding going. She also asks the parents about their experience of the birth, how well they are recuperating and how much parental leave they will have. She is interested in the strengths of this family and curious about who are in the baby's "village." She asks who will be there to welcome and champion the new member of the community.

Masako returns on the same day with a poster of the team with photographs and contact details of all the relevant team members. She explains everyone's role in a simple language and, with Professor Maranto's agreement, she emphasizes his contribution as an expert in anatomy and deemphasizes his role as a surgeon. At the back of the poster, there are several stock phrases drawn from *Clinical Guidelines* developed by Consortium on the Management of Disorders of Sex Development (2006a) and *First Days* produced by dsdfamilies (2018a) to enable the parents to politely limit conversations with people in their social network about the child:

> The doctors have some questions about how our baby has grown. It's complicated to talk about. We will be in touch soon.

> I'm not sure how to explain it to you yet and hope to have some good news soon. Thanks for taking Ben to school and picking him up.

> The baby is adorable. We're impatient to send out a birth announcement too. Because of a genetic variation, which is not uncommon, the hospital needs a bit more time to figure out whether Baby is going to feel more like a boy or a girl. We appreciate your support and will introduce you to our little one soon.

> Our baby's doing well. The pelvic organs may have developed a little differently. Doctors have to do a few more checks to make sure that our baby stays healthy. We will get in touch soon with more news.

Lilly and Ralf infer from Masako's ease that their situation must be very familiar to her and her colleagues and therefore more common than they have imagined. They enjoy their first good night's sleep since before Lilly's first contraction.

11.3.2   Working with the System

The baby is diagnosed with a deficiency in 17beta-hydroxysteroid dehy-drogenase-3 (17βHSD3), which is one of several enzymes that regulate hormonal activity at the prereceptor level. A deficiency in this enzyme affects how testosterone is processed and actioned. A baby with a diagnosis of 17βHSD3 deficiency has 46,XY chromosomes. However, the testes do not produce enough testosterone and tend to stay in the abdomen, at least for a time. At puberty, the testes become more active and, with more testosterone released, the young person develops male-typical secondary sex characteristics.

At the preassignment team meeting, viewpoints and research papers are passionately exchanged. "If the parents decide to raise the baby as a boy," a clinician says, "then DHT cream should be the first port of call (for stimulating the external genitalia)." Another clinician feels certain that this would not make any difference and that the parents are likely to choose masculinizing genital surgery for the boy. "If the testes can be preserved until puberty," this clinician explains, "they will produce testosterone to enable the boy to virilize spontaneously." Other team members feel that the baby can do better as a girl. "The clitoris is only mildly enlarged, so it doesn't need any surgery." Another clinician points out that the retained testes may migrate and the baby will have hernia later. Still another team member suggests that, at puberty, if the girl should feel more male, she can naturally virilize. "Yes, indeed," echoes another, "if she is happy to stay female, puberty blockers will buy her time, and we can have help with breast development, and vaginoplasty, and gonadectomy." A researcher raises the question of the advantage of early gonadectomy because the gonads can now be preserved for future fertility. "What fertility?" asked a colleague. "This kid has no fertility, whom are we doing that for?" Aditi points out that the parents are still grieving. "Talk of fertility is a bit like putting a fake carrot in front of them," she suggests, "isn't that a little bit cruel?" The team agrees that, at the moment, gonadectomy is only confidently recommended for Swyer syndrome. Therefore, they should not confuse the parents in the current scenario.

Masako worries how anyone could digest such complex information, which is framed entirely biomedically, with no acknowledgment that all of the interventions that have come up in discussion are psychosocially motivated rather than medically indicated. Refocusing her mind on the care principle on emotional safety (see Chapter 10), she asks the group quizzically, "Which of us need to be physically present to advise the parents on the best legal gender?" Before anyone can answer, Professor Waseem quickly suggests that as a minimum, she, Professor Maranto and Masako will be present. Masako holds Professor Maranto in high esteem but ponders on what it would mean for the parents to meet with a surgeon so soon.

At the meeting, all three clinicians congratulate the parents again for their healthy baby. While Lilly and Ralf express a sense of gratitude that their baby has no immediate health concerns, they are both in tears. Lilly says, with some irony, "When that doctor in our local hospital said 'intersex,' it was monstrously cruel at the time. Turns out he was right after all!" The medical specialists in the room criticize the word empathically. Masako takes a risk here before the conversation about intersex is shut down:

MASAKO: Intersex?
RALF: That's the word that seared my mind.
MASAKO: Just curious, with hindsight, is there another word that could have been used?
LILLY: Maybe not, as it happened.
MASAKO: Are there situations in which you can imagine the word intersex being less searing?
RALF: Maybe if I've heard it before, and I've met nice people associated with it.

Professor Waseem makes use of a range of support group resources and her own drawings to explain about regular sex development and the many ways in which it can vary. She then explains how the reproductive and urogenital systems grow where there is a deficiency in the 17βHSD3 enzyme. She pauses frequently to enable the parents to ask questions and emphasizes that there will be many more opportunities to hear this information again. Before going further, however, she makes several points and invites Lilly and Ralf to "think of them often." She reminds them that 1) they have a child who is as capable as any other child; 2) the biggest factor is love; 3) every week, hundreds of parents all over the world are receiving a similar kind of news; and 4) reaching out to other families can make a big difference.

All three clinicians stay with the language "assigning a legal gender" so that this is understood as a social process rather than a reflection of the baby's biological destiny. Masako explains to the parents that assigning legal gender has always been a social process for everyone. Having spoken with them many times by this stage, she is able to emphasize to Lilly and Ralf that in the current climate of gender fluidity, exploration and uncertainty among many young people, it is advisable that every parent stays flexible and open about how their child may want to live their life in future.

A third segment of the conversation concerns what happens next. Professor Waseem looks to Professor Maranto to lead on this part of the conversation. Masako preempts the conversation with, "This is where some professionals in the field are debating whether there should be any more medical steps for a while, and whether the next step isn't just about working out a support program to help you enjoy your lovely baby and regroup as a family with as little intrusion as possible." Professor Maranto expresses his agreement and begins with a statement that any surgical option is "not actually needed for the baby's physical health" and that no decision will be made today or even soon. He introduces the broad concept of surgery without going into details and talk about "various known and unknown risks." He also prefixes his sentences with "some parents may," "not all parents would," "other parents think" and so on.

Before they leave hospital, Lilly and Ralf have already decided to raise their baby as a girl. They reject gender-neutral names and call her Carrie because, Ralf says, "if Carrie should transition later, it would be easier if we get used to an entirely different name then." Masako seizes the teaching moment with further clarification:

> I am impressed how flexible and open you are. Your children are lucky to have you as their parents. But remember, just because Carrie has XY chromosomes and has grown slightly differently inside doesn't mean that she will transition. Many girls and women in a same situation are happy being female. It's just a question of not being too fixated about the future.

11.3.3 Continuity of Care

A major agenda after gender assignment is to facilitate caretakers' reengagement with the wider community, and it is the role of the PCP to inquire into the anticipated challenges in the immediate days and weeks. Asking "what are you worried about" is less helpful than questions about the family's daily schedule and upcoming tasks, such as: "What will you do when you arrive home? What happens tomorrow, and the rest of the week?" The PCP can also make suggestions, such as "How about switching off the world for a day or two for some family downtime?"

Masako draws up a tentative psychosocial care program for the couple to take home. The care plan involves finding out how the child and family are doing psychologically, talking through the diagnostic information again, reflecting on what the information means, consulting relevant peer resources together to find the best language and preparing for degrees of disclosure in different social contexts.

Three months later, the couple goes back to see Professor Maranto to find out more about surgical options for Carrie. Professor Maranto asks the couple to think about the information with Masako before they meet again to talk about it. When conversing with couples and families, Masako tends to mobilize *circular questioning* techniques (e.g., Penn, 1982), to elicit similarities and differences in sense making within the system. The intention here is not to get to the bottom of people's reasoning but to understand how they relate to each other's ideas and language (see also Section 14.4 in Chapter 14). The conversation with the couple begins as follows:

MASAKO: What did you find most useful about your conversation with Professor Maranto this week?

RALF: Oh, we haven't decided, but it's a relief to know there are options.

MASAKO: Having options is a relief. [Turns toward Lilly] What are your thoughts about the options?

LILLY: A lot of parents like to have their daughters looking more normal.

MASAKO: [Turns towards Ralf] More normal?

RALF: Yeah, after the surgery, the clitoris is like a normal girl. Hopefully, no one will notice any difference when Carrie starts nursery. Lilly is going back to work. We worry about nursery staff freaking out. Lilly can't stop thinking that the staff will gather around our baby and laugh.

MASAKO: How upsetting! Let's talk about those worries soon. [Turns toward Lilly] How does your expectation of surgery compare to Ralf's?

LILLY: [Looks at Ralf] Ahh, I didn't hear the word normal. I think the professor said "less noticeable," whatever that means. He also said, he said that, that there could be this altered sensation and and and . . . and this makes surgery controversial. But we kind of knew that already.

MASAKO: [Turns to Ralf] How do you understand what Lilly's just said about "controversial"?

RALF: Lilly is referring to people on the Internet who call all clitoris surgery FGM. That's ridiculous. We're not sending our daughter to the bush. This doctor has done dozens of clitoris, clitoral, clitoral surgeries. He even gets invited to operate abroad. He's a safe pair of hands.

MASAKO: Professor Maranto is indeed a famous surgeon, and a terrific doctor. What else do you need from him to help you decide?

RALF: The point is that Lilly is not so confident about the gender assignment. Carrie is already a big strong girl at three months. Should she have been a boy?

MASAKO: [Turns to Lilly] Ralf thinks you have some doubt that Carrie may be happier as a girl?

LILLY: I'm wondering if we're giving her the best chance to be happy as a girl, and whether having her looking more girl-like can help, can help her more . . .

MASAKO: More girl-like can help . . . [Turns to Ralf] What are your thoughts about what Lilly's just said?

RALF: I don't know. My sister was a big and strong baby, and I was not. Maybe Carrie needs us to make more room for her uniqueness. Maybe whatever we do, at the back of our mind, we will always have doubt. That's not great . . .

Masako empathizes with the couple and does not gloss over their reality. She suggests, however, that coping with the biology is usually more of a challenge for the caretakers than for the child. She proposes a four-way conversation with Professor Maranto to think together about the surgical trade-off in more detail, such as how many likely operations altogether and what are the known and potential physical and emotional complications, follow-up requirements and adult surgical options if Carrie were to have different ideas later. Masako suggests that she and Professor Maranto primarily listen to the family's goals, values, day-to-day concerns and anticipated challenges ahead before advising them. Lilly and Ralf's part of the agreement before the meeting is to have spoken with peer caretakers of children with a range of variations who are satisfied and dissatisfied up to a point about their child's genital surgery for a balanced view.

The conversation also preempts some psychoeducational input around adjustment. Masako is able to explain to the couple that in the process of adjustment, mental preoccupation with the situation is to be expected. Furthermore, people often oscillate between feeling better and feeling worse (see Chapter 10): "When your mood is up, you are confident that you have made the right decision. When it's down, you start to doubt lots of things." Masako also reminds Lilly and Ralf that they are experienced parents. However, she suggests that they take their self-care more seriously, as this is foundational for the welfare of the whole family. She also explains that risk-taking is integral to adjustment and growth, and that finding a reputable nursery and assessing their competence in meeting children's additional needs is a valuable opportunity to practice such risk-taking.

As an awareness-raising exercise, Masako creates a scenario whereby Lilly and Ralf imagine themselves as Carrie's potential adoptive parents. She asks them to note down what they would do to prepare to adopt Carrie and to discuss their ideas with each other. This exercise highlights to the couple that there are several advantages that adoptive parents have over biological parents. First of all, Lilly says that she would feel no guilt toward Carrie, that is, she would not be asking whether she should have started on folic acid before conception. Secondly, in choosing Carrie, they would have read all about 17βHSD3D and similar variations. They would also have spoken to other caretakers of children with variations and received lots of encouragement from them. Lastly, they would take upon themselves to educate people around them and would only accept as friends those who are prepared to love Carrie with them.

The exercise led to a conversation about the impact of the shock, the mourning of the imaginary perfect baby, the guilt toward Carrie and the effects of the lack of preparation, knowledge and support. Lilly and Ralf realize that as Carrie's biological parents, they carry strong and mixed emotions that are unresolved. Masako places the couple's distress in a grief-informed understanding (see Chapter 10). As Lilly acknowledges her psychological struggles and stops judging herself, she asks for help to find a therapist who can help her to process her loss and separate her needs from her child's.

In the months that follow, Masako meets with Lilly and Ralf regularly. Between these episodes, Aditi keeps in touch with the couple via brief telephone contacts. Between them, Masako and Aditi manage to source a broad range of play materials that embrace diversity. They use the resources to devise play opportunities that also involve Carrie's older brother Ben. They are able to demonstrate to the parents how readily children ease into nonstereotypic ideas and enjoy moving between sameness and differentness.

11.4 Reflexivity

Assigning legal gender is a highly charged process. The PCP has multiple roles that require multiple skills. Although their role is not to speculate about the gendered brain or deconstruct binarism, they are nevertheless required to be familiar with the different knowledge frameworks for understanding gender so as to be able to think about the topic with people holding different perspectives.

Most caretakers aspire to raise happy and confident children, but what does this mean? With a PCP who has a strong grasp of children's psychosocial development and family systems, DSD teams do not have to rely on psychological guesswork when advising caretakers on the implications of interventions. However, socializing caretakers and teams into psychological thinking requires advanced interpersonal skills. Where care users' wellbeing is at risk of being jeopardized, often inadvertently in a complex system, the PCP must have the authority and a willingness to take risks to engage colleagues in difficult conversations in the interests of child and family.

A DSD service that takes seriously the idea of a nonsurgical care path will need to recruit a PCP with a broad skill set, centralize their presence in the process of gender assignment and provide them with resources to follow up families from the very beginning and in the months to come. A robust psychosocial care path staffed by an expert practitioner may minimize interventions that do not address biomedical concerns and center the rights of the child to an open future as far as possible.

CHAPTER 12

Disclosure

Talking about variations in sex development in the social sphere is a monumental step that is typically avoided. Although suppression of significant information may feel burdensome, most psychological care providers (PCPs) working in this field will have come across people who seem to live happy and productive lives with minimal disclosure of their variations (even in intimate relationships). However, a recent questionnaire study with adult clinic attendees diagnosed with Turner syndrome, Klinefelter syndrome, congenital adrenal hyperplasia (CAH) and XY conditions suggests that openness about their condition is associated with better mental health (van de Grift, 2021). The analysis is based on a usable response rate of 25%, which vastly limits generalizability. Nevertheless, the finding should encourage PCPs to probe into the possibility of self-disclosure, at least when working with adults.

Presentation of oneself in a positive light is a social process involving verbal and nonverbal behaviors to construct preferred meanings and preserve relationships. Therefore, disclosure of sex variations in the social sphere is never a simple case of regurgitating biological information about the bodily variation. The huge effort that has been made to plumb complex biology into care users may actually emphasize their difference and, it has been said, secure the position of doctors as arbiters of knowledge about their bodies (Holmes, 2009, p. 4). By contrast, resources developed by intersex-identified adults only give limited air time to biological facts, if they are even mentioned. The Interface Project (interfaceproject.org), for example, comprises more than a dozen short videos of individuals who role model dignity and pride as they tell their story that ends with the motto "No Body Is Shameful." *YOUth&I* (youthandi.org), an Australian publication of individual stories of intersex youth involving artwork and poetry, is another example of open celebration of diversity and difference.

Facilitating self-disclosure is the subject matter of the current chapter, which summarizes what caretakers (Section 12.1) and adults (Section 12.2) say about it first of all. The summary is followed by a conversation about ways of knowing and talking about sex variations that have been put forward by people with lived experience (Section 12.3). The practice vignette (Section 12.4) provides an example of how motivational and behavioral techniques may be mobilized to help a service user to prepare to share information about genital variation with peers.

12.1 Research with Caretakers

Being told that their baby is not typically female or male is profoundly disorientating for caretakers (Gough et al., 2008). The information, however well communicated, cuts deep into the minds of caretakers with lasting effects. One of the earliest studies with parents of children with androgen insensitivity syndrome (AIS) said, "I'll have to be honest with you – at the moment we parents are lost. That's the fact" (Le Maréchal, 2001, p. 105). In the past, caretakers were advised not to reveal the intersex diagnosis on their own accord to the child (Karkazis, 2008). Today, they are told that it is their responsibility to talk to the child (Lee et al., 2006) – in an appropriate and timely manner. This is easier said than done. Caretakers tacitly accept this brief, but they struggle to carry it out. They feel that they lack skills and confidence for the task and report an absence of professional guidance on how to approach it (Lundberg et al., 2017; Sanders et al., 2011, 2012). In a CAH study, a parent recalled being told by health professionals to be open and shame free and build their daughter's self-esteem (Lundberg et al., 2017). The parent responded to the tall order with "so what do we do?" (p. 526).

Research shows that many caretakers actively avoid talking about the child's variation within the family and their social network (Karkazis, 2008; Le Maréchal, 2001; Sandberg et al., 2017; Sanders et al., 2011, 2012; Slijper et al., 2000). Some parents report feeling conflicted out of a concern for the child's right to decide for themselves as to who should know about their variation (Lundberg et al., 2017):

> [W]e had to learn techniques of conversation which we weren't expecting, because we're quite open people. ... [I]t was in my mind, "Why are we being like this, why don't we be open about it?" But I didn't want to be devil's advocate for my daughter really, 'cause it's not, it wasn't for me, it was for her and her future. (p. 524)

In a relatively large study for this field, 27% of parents indicated that they were unwilling to share information about their child's diagnosis with relatives, and 20% indicated they were not willing to share information with close friends (Sandberg et al., 2017). Even when parents managed to talk about their child's condition within their immediate social network, they would labor over how much information to meter out and to whom. An example strategy of partial disclosure is, for example, to reference CAH as "adrenal deficiency" for which the child needs medication to stay healthy (Lundberg et al., 2017).

Caretakers have to consider what the child may do with the information. They could tell the child to keep the information private, but this may imply shame. Other caretakers are concerned that disclosure may trigger a gender identity crisis in the child. Some find it stressful to have to be continuously guarded about the child's condition (Crissman et al., 2011). The UK peer support charity dsdfamilies recommends talking to children from the preverbal stage. Their *Top Tips for Talking* booklet (dsdfamilies, 2018b) is an attempt to help each family to explore the space between privacy and secrecy.

Carroll et al. (2020) carried out a substantial qualitative study involving female children with CAH due to 21-hydroxylase deficiency as well as their caretakers in the USA. The study provided evidence that caretakers do actually talk to younger and older children about CAH. In terms of the children's reactions, many of them said that CAH was out of sight and out of mind ("It's like I just have this condition that will always be with me . . . sometimes I think about it, and sometimes I don't") until they had to take medications or were socially restricted by the treatment in some way (p. 675). The children recalled having early conversations with caregivers, even if they tended not to remember the content or specific words. Some caregivers described being "matter-of-fact" about communication (p. 676). The authors could not identify a common language among caretakers to describe CAH to children. Caretakers mainly felt that they had not done a very good job. The researchers asked about potential improvement to care. The children expressed not wanting CAH to be made into a big deal. The researchers suggested that health professionals expand the focus of CAH beyond the sex development aspect. Indeed, sex and gender as a theme did not emerge as a key concern in either the USA (Carroll et al., 2020) or a recent European study (Lundberg et al., 2017).

PCPs have an important role to enable caretakers to communicate with the child. However, a study involving parents of girls with AIS suggested that caretakers were divided about the benefits of counseling (Le Maréchal, 2001). Some caretakers identified clear needs to speak in confidence to a professional and expressed their frustration at the lack of availability. Others felt that it was too challenging and uncomfortable to confront their situation in the early days, especially with a stranger. Whatever the feelings about counseling at the time of diagnosis, the majority of parents expressed a specific need for help with disclosure when their child was older.

Slijper et al. (2000) asserted that girls with AIS (and perhaps other XY conditions also) were informed in the following three broad steps: 1) early education about the biological and psychological aspects of "normal" sexual development so that they have a baseline from which to be able to understand the ways in which their own body differs, 2) from around the age of 11 (i.e., before hormone replacement therapy commences) all information about AIS should be given with the exception of the XY karyotype and 3) from age 16 to 17 years, disclosure of karyotype should be completed (although this may need to become earlier as children are more able to gain access to such information though the Internet). The idea of educating children about "normal" first and then about how they deviate as "other" is considered out of date. Furthermore, the deferring of disclosing karyotype to late teens has also become questionable.

With reference to AIS, Warne (1997, cited in Le Maréchal, 2001) suggested that between 6 and 11 years, most children only needed practical explanations for their clinic visits. It is generally assumed that reasoning capacity is sufficiently developed by age 12 years, so that discussion about the complex nature of AIS would be more possible. The author also suggested that since children learn about chromosomes at school in their mid-teens, girls with AIS should be fully informed about their diagnosis before this time.

The idea of staged disclosure makes sense and has broad support. However, it is rarely backed up by the kind of micro skills that caretakers need to do the job. Disclosure is often understood to be a biology lesson carried out in stages, but what parents struggle the most with is how to help their child to find meaning and manage the sense of threat posed by sex variations.

Interesting parallels can be drawn from disclosure to children about their HIV status, because talk about HIV is also taboo, and families live in fear of stigmatization of the child and the family. As for DSD, research has identified a significant proportion of caretakers who either practice complete concealment or actively deceive the child. A systematic review identified 14 studies that discussed the impact of disclosure on HIV-infected children (Vreeman et al., 2013). Similar reasons, such as parental guilt, shame and fear and a desire to protect the child from social rejection and mental health problems were the reasons for nondisclosure.

Lamentably, none of the studies in the review evaluated the children and families pre and post disclosure, when it is this very evidence that can help caretakers to decide how and when to share information with the child.

Drawing on multiple literatures and clinical experiences in sex development services, the reasons for total or partial concealment of information from children include a fear of causing 1) negative self-evaluation and/or poor mental health in the child, 2) the child to become uncertain about their gender and sexuality, 3) information sharing with peers that can lead to painful social consequences for the child and the family and 4) blame of or estrangement from the caretakers and/or the rest of the family. Supporting caretakers to share information with their child would mean exploring all of these fears and preparing them for strategic and constructive risk-taking.

12.2   Research with Adults

In a study involving eight women's experience of complete AIS (CAIS) (see Chapter 2), fear of devaluation was the overarching theme in the women's talk (Alderson et al., 2004). References to AIS as "an unfortunate twist of nature" (p. 87) and other similar metaphors were not uncommon. Although nearly all of the women had experienced positive responses from others to instances of AIS disclosure, it remained the biggest psychological challenge of living with AIS. Likewise, in a study with women with Mayer-Rokitansky-Küster-Hauser syndrome (MRKHS) (see Chapter 2), negative meanings such as being repellent to potential partners abounded (Guntram & Zeiler, 2016). Fear of rejection was a key observation, even though actual rejection had not happened to any of the research participants.

Women with CAIS have spoken about altering what they consider to be the most unpalatable sound bites. For example, they have spoken of referring to ovaries rather than testes. Just like parents of children with variations, the women reported using partial disclosure as a risk reduction strategy, for example: "[Friend] knows I can't have children and she knows I haven't got a womb and I think she knows I take hormones as well so I don't quite know whether she would need to know any more than that really" (Alderson et al., 2004, p. 88).

While it is easy not to disclose in many situations, nondisclosure is difficult in situations involving physical intimacy. Disclosure to new partners is felt to be high risk even for people who have had positive experiences of disclosing to previous partners (Liao, 2003). Having to talk about the variation is often cited as a reason for not seeking relationships. Fearful of leaking information unintentionally, care users have reported terminating social interaction well before it became sexual. In a study involving eight men with mixed diagnoses associated with prepubertal hypogonadism, informant "Joe" summed up this kind of fear:

> Being capable of having sex. Was a lot of it. And yeah because you think that if you've got small genitals sort of thing you can't. One you think you can't and don't even think of yourself in that position ... basically, you think "oh they're gonna find out and that will be it." You lose all confidence, any shred of confidence that you had is shattered. (Chadwick et al., 2005, p. 538)

If talking to potential partners is difficult, over half of the research participants in Alderson et al. (2004) reported difficulties in talking openly even within the immediate family, and even where other siblings were diagnosed with AIS, for lack of discursive tools. Guntram and Zeiler (2016) reported that one of the barriers to disclosing about MRKHS is the anticipated "poor you" response. The women talked about not wanting to be an object of pity and being positioned as inferior relative to their peers.

In order to gain insight into patterns of disclosure in clinic samples, I devised a questionnaire with response categories extracted from therapeutic conversations, for a study that achieved an exceptionally high participation rate from attendees at a single center with mixed diagnoses (Liao et al., 2010). Mothers were identified as the most likely people with whom the adult service users had shared almost/all information (74%), followed by partners (71%) and ex-partners (34%). A significant minority had not confided in stable partners about some aspects of their variation (29%) and an even higher proportion (37%) had shared nothing or next to nothing with siblings with the same diagnosis. I asked clinic attendees to think about the person who knew the most about their condition and which of the component aspects had they disclosed to this person. The most frequently disclosed aspect was primary amenorrhea where applicable (91%) and the least frequently disclosed aspect was having had genital surgery where applicable (71%).

More recent research suggests significant variability in how impacted adults manage the information. In a qualitative study, some young people have described highly controlled decisions about what aspects of their variation to share with whom, while others have reported positive experiences of high-risk approaches, such as doing a school project relating to their medical condition (Sanders et al., 2015). Some of the adults in the study explained that they had been much more guarded about sharing information in early adolescence but that as they moved toward adulthood, they had learnt to self-disclose with greater confidence.

Sharing secrets is said to be "a crucial element of friendships in adolescence" and withholding information is said to be a potential barrier to the benefits of social support, self-acceptance and coping (Ernst et al., 2016, p. 158). This assumption makes sense to me too. However, in the absence of strong research evidence, the idea of overriding benefits of openness remains an assumption. Disclosure per se did not uniformly lead to a reduction in social isolation for women with CAIS (Alderson et al., 2004). Likewise, disclosure did not achieve the cathartic effects imagined by women with MRKHS (Guntram & Zeiler, 2016). However, there are other reasons to self-disclose.

In the research participants' talk, Ernst et al. (2016) identified two reasons for wishing to disclose to romantic partners about MRKHS: 1) a responsibility to be open and honest in the context of a potential long-term relationship and 2) to enable the partner to choose not to remain in a relationship where there was no possibility of conceiving biological children together. The women reported not wanting to become too attached to a partner in case the relationship was to discontinue. This resonates with my practice experience. Many care users have alluded to the difficulty in determining the appropriate timing for disclosure (Liao, 2003).

Some adults have expressed to me that they are preoccupied with thoughts of disclosure even in the absence of any call to talk about their variation. For example, a research participant said that even if surgery could remove all the anatomical signs and there was no pressure to disclose, they have been "found out" by themselves, so to speak: "Like I said, people say they would – people wouldn't know, but I mean, I know . . . and to me that's, that's enough. . . . That is a stumbling block" (Boyle et al., 2005, p. 580).

Despite an increasing amount of resources developed by advocacy groups in recent years, the UK support group dsdfamilies concluded from its survey in 2018 that the vast majority of families, young people and adults actively conceal the reality of sex variations. An article talked about *fetishizing* intersex as a new phenomenon that is making it less safe for people with variations to share information with others (Cadet & Feldman, 2012). This may have special implications for information sharing with strangers online. Successful mainstreaming of online dating means that many people self-introduce to one another virtually. While it is possible to choose intersex as a gender category, the majority of dating app users would not understand what that means. Some people may even carry mythological constructions of intersex bodies. In general, online disclosure of private and intimate information to strangers is ill-advised. Sharing information about bodily differences is best understood as integral to a mutual and trusting relationship. Therefore, until there is evidence to suggest otherwise, online disclosure of sex variations is best avoided at present.

In "Circles and Squares" in Chapter 1, the character "Dillon" first shares nothing with one girlfriend and then everything all at once with another. In the majority of situations, neither of these approaches is optimal. Psychosocial research into disclosure rarely reports about the techniques that have led to positive experiences that people can draw on. In Section 12.3, I draw attention to some of the suggestions provided by advocacy groups to demedicalize communications but also highlight an ongoing tension between a biological and a psychosocial focus in communication about sex variations.

12.3 Contested Knowing and Talking

Biological explanations are important. However, when service users say they do not know how to talk to their child or friends, they may also be expressing a lack of usable vocabularies and positive meanings. In one of the earliest published first-person accounts, a woman with CAIS said that being asked what made a person female had been the most impactful intervention for her (Anonymous, 1994). This resonates strongly with my experience of talking with adolescents and adults about a range of variations. Disclosure is a process of negotiation of meaning. The dialogue would have to involve questioning socially constructed sex and gender norms. Below I first provide a published example (Liao & Simmonds, 2013) to evidence the need for accurate medical information. This, however, needs to be balanced with the kind of knowing and talking produced by advocacy groups, which I draw attention to afterward.

In 2012, the then AISSG-UK received an inquiry from a woman who self-identified as female and had inherited partial AIS (PAIS) (see Chapter 2) from her father alongside two sisters who had biological children including a son with PAIS. The AISSG-UK explained to the inquirer that AIS, if inherited, is usually passed on by the mother, and that affected people do not have ovaries or uterus and cannot conceive. The inquirer replied: "My dad has the PAIS. As it is his X that is affected, he passed on his bad X [to all three daughters]." The inquirer went on to state: "We all have 50% good X and 50% bad X" and that the three sisters all had "internal and external female organs" but had "definitely got PAIS" with a one in two chance of passing this on to their offspring (Liao & Simmonds, 2013, p. 57).

Confusion such as the above may have inspired the kind of painstaking educational effort by advocacy groups, as exemplified in *The Story of Sex Development* (see Figures 2.1a and 2.1b in Chapter 2) developed by dsdfamilies (2019). The booklet seeks to explain and demystify variations in sex development in order to help impacted people to become effective care users. While it is important to break down the complex biology for laypersons, it is equally important to translate the biological to the relational. It is this translation that many service users find difficult.

Intersex-identified adults have an important reassuring message for caretakers, that is, they did feel negatively about their variations initially but these feelings generally became more positive over time (Davis & Feder, 2015; Simmonds, 2004). Far from viewing disclosure to children as a threat and a dreaded obligation, care providers can help users to reframe disclosure as an opportunity to overcome their worst fears and learn together with the child about difference and diversity. Disclosure can be an opportunity to nurture the child to:

1. make sense of bodily variations and changes
2. voice concerns and ask questions
3. develop a curiosity about diversity of body and embodiment
4. grow skills to moderate rather than catastrophize reactions
5. understand the reasons for hospital appointments
6. develop mutually trusting and respectful relationships in healthcare transactions
7. expect care providers to keep them informed and treat them with dignity and respect.

The *Handbook for Parents* (Consortium on the Management of Intersex Disorders, 2006b) makes discussion about genital variations relevant to the developmental context of the child. The ballpark suggestions are:

1. Always let children know that they are loved and accepted just as they are.
2. Have answers ready for questions that may come up. For example, when a toddler asks why his penis is different from his father's, a possible response could be a version of: "Just like people's faces look different, everyone's parts look a little bit different, too. Pee-pees can come in many shapes and sizes. Yours turned out different from daddy's, so it looks different from his."

3. Help the child to voice feelings, and talk to them about how to respond to teasing generally, that is, before any specific issue of their genital variations arise. For example, caretakers can talk to the child who is unhappy because their toy has been snatched away or when a friend would not play with them.

4. Early on, opportunistically educate the child about average bodies and body parts but also many exceptions.

5. It is recommended that by preschool, some conversation about bodies and bodily differences should have taken place, because some children will have become quite interested in their genitals. School-age children expressing a wish to look the same as other boys and girls could be invited to make a list of questions for the next visit to the doctor's and find out what the options are later. Adolescents may be distressed about their bodies and experience a deep wish to be the same as their peers. It is important for caretakers to demonstrate their acceptance of this and offer the young people an opportunity to talk to a psychosocial professional if it is too difficult to have an embarrassing talk about their sexuality within the family.

6. Speak the truth. For example, when a child asks why they are different, if the caretaker is unsure, say something like: "Lots of times nobody knows why our bodies develop how they do." If it is a genetic condition, the caretaker could say something like: "Just like some of your toys come with instructions . . . every person comes with a set of instructions called genes ... . You came with your own set of instructions . . ."

Additionally, dsdfamilies (2018b) suggests that we use a relativizing language, as in "many people but not all have," "some girls can," "not all boys do," and so on. They also provide strategies if caretakers are caught by a surprise question and suggest responses such as: "I'm not sure how to explain that, let me ask someone who knows." The *Handbook for Parents* recommends that caretakers explain to close family and friends that the child is different yet unique and lovable like any other child:

> By honestly telling your friends and family about your child's DSD, you begin to "normalize" the issue so that it's not a horrible family secret or a tragic mystery. When your child is old enough to begin to understand the information about his DSD, chances are he will have heard from you about the DSD since he was born. Your child will also know he can talk to certain other loved ones about having a DSD, since you will have paved the way for open talk. (Consortium on the Management of Intersex Disorders, 2006b)

Perhaps the most strategic input from PCPs here is to help caretakers and adults to question, from the very beginning, the norms and values that are giving rise to communication difficulties. Rather than advising caretakers on how to "talk to" children, it may be more manageable to think of the task as "socializing" and "orientating" young children toward a world of diversity from the word go.

There are many everyday opportunities to role model how to subtly challenge cultural ideals without turning the challenge into a big militant act. It is possible to introduce children to books where heroes are not all white, male and nondisabled. Furthermore, the entire family could question gender-based stereotypes by starting to apply the word family to a range of configurations including those that are childfree or with same-gender parents. Every day, there are numerous occasions for adults to casually demonstrate self-acceptance of their own bodily imperfections – there is no need to preach to a child. For example, every time a skincare advertisement comes up, there is a chance to say, "I wish I had nicer skin, but I have so many exciting dreams to focus on." This may lead to a conversation about other "cool stuff" to focus on in life.

Social comparison is what all human beings do, but it is possible to practice a shoulder-shrugging "no big deal" response to negative social comparisons with, for example, "too bad I can't please everybody." Little by little, children take on the family culture. If the family embeds heteronormativity as preferred or natural, then talking about bodily sex differences will be a lot harder than it needs to be.

Clinic visits are superb opportunities for caretakers to show the child how to command respect for their body. In the face of multiple spectators, a caretaker could remark, "wow, so many people today, what's the excitement?" When another physical examination is proposed, the caretaker could pose a question politely: "May I ask what it is for?" They could check with an older child, "how do you feel about it?" and "hey, isn't it your turn to ask the doctors to explain?"

12.4 Practice Vignette

Kereem is nearly 16 years old and identifies as male. He was born in the USA. His parents Mr. and Mrs. H divorced when he was 6 years old. Mr. H soon remarried and moved to another town. Mrs. H and the children later moved to England where her extended family has resettled having emigrated from Turkey.

Shortly after birth, Kereem was diagnosed with 5α-reductase deficiency type II (5αR2D, see Chapter 2). A doctor had already told the parents that they had a baby girl. When the karyotype testing came back as XY, Mr. H was furious with the hospital for the "mistake." The baby was to be registered as a boy. The parents severed their relationship with the clinic and told relatives that the baby was born premature and unwell, and that an inexperienced trainee doctor had made a mistake about the child's sex.

Kereem had three episodes of genital surgery between 1 and 5 years at a different hospital. A fourth episode was proposed, but Mrs. H hesitated. When the family moved to England, Kereem attended a specialist DSD clinic, where he had further surgical "repairs" at age 9 and 11 years. After that, Mrs. H stopped taking Kereem to the clinic. She was back in full-time teaching and had no time to spare. She also felt very let down by the clinic that had chastised her for not explaining 5αR2D to Kereem. Her thought was, "I am not a doctor, how would I begin to explain such a complicated thing to anyone? Surely that's the doctor's job." Because Kereem seemed to be developing well, Mrs. H gained confidence and ignored the appointment letters.

Kereem is currently preparing for his national exams and expecting excellent results. He plans on going wild camping with his best friend "Mish" this summer, to mark the end of their exams and to celebrate their 16th birthday jointly. Mrs. H is deeply concerned about the young men's lack of experience. Privately, she worries about toileting facilities for Kereem. She asked to be fast-tracked back to the pediatric DSD clinic. At the medical review, the doctors are urgently concerned that Mrs. H has not spoken to Kereem about his diagnosis. Mother and son are asked to meet with PCP "Alex," who is warned that Mrs. H is "chaotic and difficult" and does not engage well with the service.

12.4.1 Assessment

Kereem and Mrs. H attend the first meeting with Alex together. Mrs. H looks very tense. She apologizes for raising her voice at the receptionist. She starts to list her objections to the camping trip right away. Alex promises to listen to her concerns soon, but begins the conversation by asking each of the participants "what's working well in your life at the moment?" He then asks about safety and limits of the conversation and what is the most important topic to discuss. They agree that the purpose in this instance is to orient Kereem to his care and prepare him to navigate the care system in future.

Mrs. H. recalls telling Kereem when he was a little boy that he has a small problem with his pee-pee and that he must always pee in private and not show his "private parts" to anyone. She has told the schools that Kereem has a lung condition that makes him prone to pneumonia, so that he must avoid showering at school and have warm baths at home instead. Kereem tells Alex that he is among the handful of "body-shy" boys in class. He thinks his peers consider him a "geek." Everyone including the teachers go to Kereem for technical advice.

In the middle of the conversation, Mrs. H is shocked to hear that Kereem had self-diagnosed himself on the Internet. As the conversation turns to the camping trip, Kereem reveals that he plans on talking to Mish about his condition. Mrs. H nearly falls off her chair. She starts to talk over Kereem and expresses many worries. She insists that "private matters should always stay private." Alex intercepts by empathizing with Mrs. H about her worries:

ALEX: Worrying is an important way to protect the people we love. The flip side is that sometimes worrying can also upset the people we love. For example, they do not feel trusted . . .

MRS. H: But I trust him all the time! He has a lot of freedom! You know, once you tell someone, you can't take it back. At some point, it will be used against you . . .

ALEX: Used against you?

MRS. H: [Wells up in tears] You know, it's all on me, if either of my children falls apart, everything is down to me . . . . No one else is interested. I'm all they have . . .

ALEX: I can see it has been very hard on you to shoulder all the responsibilities of parenting your children . . . . Who's aware of how you're feeling?

Mrs. H feels aggrieved that the children's father has flatly refused to co-parent, though he keeps in touch with them at a social level and provides adequate financial support. She considers herself a burden to her extended family who have given her so much help over the years. As a divorced woman and lone mother, she sees herself as the "odd one out" in the Turkish community. Yet she also feels excluded by "English people." Alex is interested to hear Mrs. H talk more about her experiences of unfairness and how they might have affected her sense of threat and the need to worry for herself and her children.

At this point, Kereem reveals that he was bullied when he first started school in the USA, not for his variation but for being bilingual and therefore different from other children. Alex asks Kereem how he survived the bullying. Kereem explains that he stopped speaking Turkish. Mrs. H has never heard her son articulate his difficult life experiences so candidly before and sees a new maturity in him.

At the end of the appointment, Alex asks Mrs. H if she would like to invite her daughter Esra to join in the next family conversation. When this is declined, Alex asks Mrs. H if she would like some support just for herself. This too is declined. Mrs. H expresses that it is time for Kereem to have some counseling and make his own choices in future.

Alex would like to help Kereem to think more broadly about his life experience, such as how it might have been for him to be uprooted in childhood and how he feels about his relationship with his father. But Kereem only wants "a few strategies" from Alex: "What's the best way to bring up the subject? How do people react?" Alex understands from Kereem that, at least for now, his role is confined to helping Kereem to identify and overcome the obstacles to his stated wish to confide in his best friends about his bodily difference. However, Alex needs more clarity from Kereem:

ALEX: You say you want some strategies for speaking with your friends. So far, how do you talk to yourself about it? What words do *you* use with yourself?

KEREEM: I think of myself as having a hormone imbalance. It's called 5-alpha something. I was born with it – something to do with my genes. I'm kind of a normal boy, very healthy, but shy in groups, and I will have problems with sex, unfortunately.

ALEX: That's a lot to process. Let's think together about some of that later. For now, tell me, who do you think should know that you are a normal and healthy guy? Who should know that you see a doctor for a health condition, like lots of people do too? Who needs to be made aware of the genes or hormones? And who should know about the 5-alpha something?

The above exchange enables Alex to introduce the idea that, first of all, meanings are negotiable and, secondly, communication is not all-or-nothing. It also enables him to learn more about Kereem's social network. Kereem explains that he has a "sort of girlfriend," that they have been "quite physical" and that one day he would have to talk to her about his genital variation. Thus he wants to "practice" with one or two friends whose support he will need.

The information from the assessment meetings is organized in Table 12.1. Alex formulates his understanding as in Figure 12.1 and shares his thoughts with Kereem.

12.4.2   *Formulation*

The formulation, or best guess, as informed by the Power Threat Meaning Framework (PTMF) (Johnstone & Boyle, 2018), is diagrammatically

Table 12.1. *Summary of initial assessment with Kereem*

Inquiry domains	Summary of content
Goal of assessment – Information gathering for formulation and care planning as appropriate	– Kereem is becoming independent. He feels the need to talk about his condition with friends but does not know how. – His mother has different ideas – she wants the clinic to help Kereem understand his condition but keep it private.
Relationship to help – Who is referring who for what reason – Who are in the system – Relationship with specialist services and community providers – Patterns of engagement with services	– Rereferral to specialist service triggered by Kereem's mother Mrs. H. – Family doctor very aware of situation and is supportive. – The current specialist clinic has not engaged the mother well. The clinic has not anticipated the mother's need for support. The mother has not been able to voice her dissatisfaction.
Understanding of variation and treatment past/present – Factual knowledge – Understanding of immediate and long-term MDT care plan – Knowledge of respective roles of providers involved	– Has read about 5αR2D on internet and understands the biogenetics but has not spoken about it with doctors or family. – Does not remember much or understand about previous operations – what was he like to start with, what was done, how has it improved function and appearance, what else can doctor do. – Does not know about long-term health needs and role of clinicians. – Mentions some "leakage" which is being assessed by a urologist.
Emotional responses to variation and treatment past/present – Emotional reactions – Immediate and future concerns	– Cannot remember early reactions, is now guessing that perhaps he has been upset at different points about his penis being different but "iIt wasn't on my mind the whole time." – Is fairly satisfied with overall physique and secondary sexual characteristics – "it helps coz I think I'm fit" – wants to join the gym and build muscle. – Has started dating first time and wants to explore genital sex but is worried about talking to girlfriend about the variation.
General health and psychological well-being	– Describes physical health as very good.

Table 12.1. *(cont.)*

Inquiry domains	Summary of content
– Current – Past	– No other health concern.
Personal strengths and needs – Psychosocial skills (e.g., communication, emotion regulation) – Family relationships (e.g., closeness and distances) – Peer relationships – Capacity for independence – Education, work, creativity, interests – Hopes and fears	– Highly academic and ambitious. – Optimistic about future education, career and financial independence. – Has lots of interests. – Is close to an elder sister Esra. – Has a good relationship with mother but describes her as a worrier. – Has a date. – Has two confiding male friends. – Responsive to ideas if they are logical and they "work." – Claims to have a calm disposition.
Social and cultural aspects – Family relationships – Community support – Access to confiding relationships – Cultural and religious attitudes relating to diversity – Knowledge of education and support resources; and capacity to navigate	– Good contact with extended family – aunts, uncles and cousins on mother's side but "we don't talk about personal things." – Having lived in different places, the family feels "rootless." – They are beheld as a Turkish family but the Turkish community think they are a bit "eccentric." – Fractured relationship with father and uncertainties around relationships with stepmother and half siblings. – "Technically Muslim; but we are not religious." – Appears to be semireceptive to the idea of peer support – is able to navigate if wished to.
Gender and sexuality – Sex/gender identity – Attitudes, preferences – Sexual experiences – Current relationship	– "I feel male; I'm not intersex" but does not object to the term. – Self-identifies as heterosexual. – Has been "physically intimate" with date; has not engaged in genital sex and wants to.

represented in Figure 12.1. The formulation takes account of ideological constructions of bodies as either female or male. Genital variations are confusing to hospital staff and caretakers and break a fundamental cultural

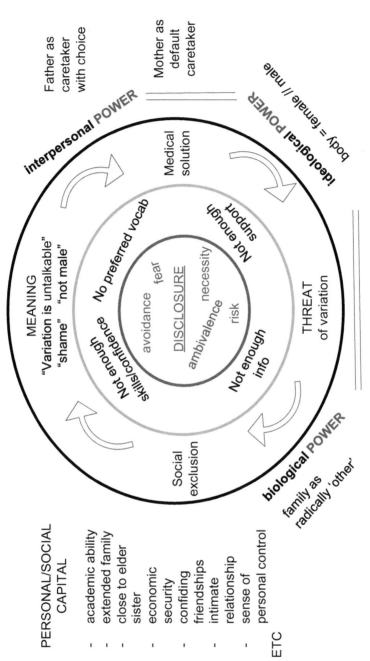

Figure 12.1   Formulation chart for Kereem. A colour version of this figure can be found in the plate section.

code, which can threaten the core human need for social inclusion. Many families may have chosen to stay safe by remaining silent and invisible. For the H family, however, additional dimensions of power are operating negatively to produce the current tense situation.

Alex places the difficulties of disclosure from mother to son in a wider context and also takes account of the ruptured family relationships and cultural displacement of the H family. The parental divorce displaces Mrs. H socially from one community, while her ethnicity displaces her from another. Alex is also struck by what seems like a tacit, social acceptance that it is down to Mrs. H, as mother, to raise her children, when it is optional for Mr. H, as father, to choose how much he is involved. Alex understands Mrs. H's helplessness as a manifestation of the gender and ethnicity-based inequalities acting on her life rather than as her personal ineptitude.

Mrs. H is understood to have survived the threat of genital variations, a threat accentuated by her precarious reliance on her extended family, by avoidance. Because the DSD clinic put pressure on her to face the difficulties, she avoids them too. Her survival strategy has served to maintain her fear, leave her unsupported and delay what is inevitable.

Still, as a survival strategy, avoidance has worked for a time. However, Kereem is growing up. His need for knowledge and skills has precipitated a crisis for his mother. Adolescence is a time of rapid physical and psychosocial transformation (Suris et al., 2004). Kereem is preoccupied with his own ideas as to how he wants to live his life. One of his current preoccupations is to be genitally intimate with his date. This requires him to prepare her to anticipate his bodily difference. He is not debilitated by shame but feels unskilled and lacks confidence in approaching the task. There are many reasons why Kereem should feel underskilled and underconfident. First of all, negative meanings of variations are generously supplied but positive meanings are limited and have to be negotiated. Secondly, in order to educate others, he needs to educate himself first. The healthcare system expects his mother to keep him informed. Mrs. H contests the brief in her mind but, like many disempowered people, is inarticulate, which leads to her being judged by the DSD service as being noncompliant. The souring of the relationship between the patient's mother and the DSD service is a manifestation of systemic factors rather than individual fault.

Alex recognizes that the H family, while disempowered in some ways, has access to power in others. They are an educated family. Mr. H, though not available emotionally, does at least support the children materially. Mrs. H is clearly a very capable person. Mother and children live in relative harmony in a safe area. The extended family is available to help. Kereem is a brilliant scholar with a bright future. He is close to his sister. He enjoys confiding relationships (and clearly has a sense of adventure). While he does not yet understand his genital variation well, he has escaped some of the more negative meanings, and he is motivated to take control and make the best of his life.

Having made sense of the referral and the information gathered in the assessment, Alex is left feeling concerned about Mrs. H's unattended sorrow but, as Mrs. H declines psychological support for herself, Alex accepts that for now, his brief is to help Kereem to 1) meet with a medical expert to go over his diagnosis and treatment history; 2) explore the meaning of the information and, in relation to that, develop skills to talk to people about his variation in ways that serve him well; and 3) codesign a plan for Kereem to transfer out of the children's hospital to an adult care environment that is more suited to meet his ongoing adult care needs.

12.4.3   Dialectical Consultation

Alex is interested in what Kereem makes of his meeting with the doctors, what were the high and low points, how he feels about the vocabularies, whether there were any surprises, and so on. Informed by the literature, he probes to elicit any difficult memories about his care, such as being hospitalized for surgery, and being examined. These aspects can have a significant bearing on how Kereem makes sense of his variation. Thus far, however, Kereem is rather matter-of-fact about it all.

Alex tells Kereem that he is in the process of designing "The Delta Program" to prepare people to communicate about sex development variations. Kereem agrees to try out some of the "strategies" in the program. He is encouraged to think aloud the hopes and fears about disclosure. Their exchanges drift toward a motivational interviewing style (see Arkowitz et al., 2015). Alex summarizes Kereem's responses in the form of an "ambivalence grid" in Table 12.2. He especially draws out the *change talk* (talk that promotes movement toward a stated goal) from Kereem, such as "I'm bored with arguing with myself, might as well give it a go." Alex is equally interested in working on the roadblocks with Kereem (Table 12.2, box B) especially the internal roadblocks in the form of catastrophic thinking. He invites Kereem to estimate the likelihood of the worst scenarios and consider what he could do to cope if they should arise. Below is a truncated version of their dialogue:

Table 12.2. *"Ambivalence grid" on self-disclosure by Kereem*

A. Good things about talking	B. Less good things about talking
Not having to think about it anymore, it's done.	Some people ask too many questions; I haven't even figured everything out yet.
Relieved; feel free; nothing to hide.	What if they wish I hadn't said anything?
Having someone to talk to about my worries.	They may feel awkward and move away from me.
Having someone advise me on how to talk to my date.	They may tell other people – not to hurt me just to offload.
Trusting people back; be more genuine.	Being an object of someone's pity.
Being accepted for what I am.	Angry if I get the wrong reactions.
	Becoming suspicious – what do they ***really*** think???
C. Good things about not talking	**D. Less good things about not talking**
Relieved.	Feel guilty; I know quite a lot about my friends' private stuff and I don't trust them with mine.
Safe.	
No effort; carry on.	
Family feel better, less worried – maybe??	The stress can build up and I start arguing with myself.
	Might blurt it all out accidentally, that's even worse.

KEREEM: What if my friend just walks away.

ALEX: Walk away? How likely is that?

KEREEM: I've seen him walk away in the middle of a conversation, when people are still talking.

ALEX: Tell me more?

KEREEM: Mish, you know, he doesn't do details. When a conversation drags on, he sometimes goes off to a corner to play with his phone.

ALEX: Important to stay brief then. But suppose he does lose interest and walk away, what would you do?

KEREEM: That's what I'm asking you.

ALEX: Think back on a social occasion when you felt challenged but stayed calm, how did you achieve that?

Kereem does not say much in therapy. He prefers to be given tasks to do. He follows up on Alex's suggestion to look up the YOUth and I Project (youthandi.org). Having consulted these resources, Alex asks Kereem how confident he now feels about talking about his variation on a 1 to 10 scale, with 1 reflecting the minimum and 10 maximum. To his surprise, Kereem rates his confidence as only 5 out of 10. Alex inquires:

ALEX: What makes you a "5" on the scale at the moment?

KEREEM: The stuff you told me to watch, I've got a few ideas . . . . But I'm not intersex, I'm not cool like that . . .

ALEX: Let's come back to intersex later . . . . If seeing confident people makes your confidence go down, what needs to happen for your confidence to go up, say to 6, or even 7?

KEREEM: . . . My sister. She's the blunt instrument of the family. If she thinks it's a bad idea, I probably shouldn't try. If she thinks I should go ahead and talk to Mish, I know she's right . . .

ALEX: What if you were to rehearse with your sister, or me?

KEREEM: You mean like a role-play? I hated that at school . . .

ALEX: And what will make your confidence go down, like down to 4, even 3?

KEREEM: Nothing . . . I suppose if my mother and my sister were to gang up on me and tell me to keep everything a secret. But then I shouldn't let that affect me . . .

ALEX: But it could affect you, so we should give time to that . . .

The above dialogue leads to a discussion to recruit Esra to join the "team." Kereem's homework is to look up the Interface Project (interfaceproject.org) with Esra. He is surprised to learn later that Esra knows quite a lot about his condition already. Esra confronts Mrs. H for "hiding everything from Kereem." Mother and daughter have a heated argument. At Esra's insistence, the whole family watches Interface together. After a few of the video clips, the three of them compare notes about their most and least favorite clip. They all smile at the simple message "no body is shameful."

Rehearsals are opportunities to experience challenges in a safe environment in which to practice coping strategies. Prior to that, inspired by the idea of expressive writing (Pennebaker & Smyth, 2016), Alex invites Kereem to hand scribe everything that he can think of about his variation without looking up any information, underline the words that he prefers and strike out the words that he dislikes. When Alex and Kereem meet for the final time, they rehearse by swapping roles and seats and asking each other awkward questions that could come up. They note down all the potential reactions that they can think of, even jaw-dropping ones. Kereem has to think about an action or coping thought to respond to every possibility. At the end of the rehearsals, Kereem thinks he might say the following to Mish on day 2 of the camping trip:

You might have been wondering why I disappear behind the bushes to pee. It's kind of a long story, which I'll make super short. I was born with big hair, big eyes, big cheeks and a small penis with the pee hole closer to the base than at the tip. Turns out I had a rare biology with a big long name.

Anyway the doctors did some operations to straighten me out, but I still can't pee like other guys. There are many men with this kind of pee issue. It's a big deal, even though I haven't been obsessing about it. I'm ok about it, and I'm not. It depends. I'm interested in what you think, and what questions you may have, coz I might need your help later, on how I can talk to my girlfriend about it.

12.5   Reflexivity

How to talk about variations is a major theme for people with lived experience. Considerable criticism has been levied at health professionals for failing to role model affirming communication about sex variations. While there are gaps in health professionals' talk, there are other factors that underpin care users' struggles to talk about sex variations. No matter how well the information is communicated to patients or parents – and I personally have witnessed exemplary professional communication – talking about sex development variations is fraught with difficulties, because of the widespread ignorance in society.

It is important to empathize with clients' negative thoughts and feelings rather than supplant them with positive and affirming narratives prematurely. Under favorable social conditions, including those created by a skilled PCP, self-affirmation and acceptance is something that people may come to in their own time.

CHAPTER 13

Sexual Intimacy

Sexual experience is neither natural nor inevitable. Consider what counts as sex, with whom one should have sex, what is deemed a normal amount of sex, who is sexually desirable and deserving, and so on. Think about the many views on these questions and how they may have shifted over time. Then ask how the ideas behind the answers may have been transmitted, for example, through conversations at school and in the home, or through advertisement, books, movies, television series, pornography, music, social media platforms or video games.

Sexual interest, disinterest, pleasure, pain, satisfaction and disappointment vary throughout the lifetime. The variability is subject to changes in personal circumstances including health, well-being, stress, aging and relationship quality. In a sexual relationship, each partner may be affected differentially by these variables and make sense of experience in prevailing cultural mores. Rather than relativize experiences, people are strongly taught to judge their experience in absolute terms against cultural scripts, which are often contradictory. For example, there is an increasing expectation for older people to be sexually active, yet older bodies are also held to be unattractive and therefore undeserving of sexual attention (and perhaps all the more in need of appearance- and function-enhancing products). Different social groups are subjected to different messages. No one is spared.

People of all ages may ask for help because they feel that they are falling short in specific ways. A range of dedicated professional services exists to provide assessment and treatment of sexual difficulties in the general population. The services range from surgical and pharmacological to psychological and relational. Currently there is limited knowledge as to what type of intervention works best, for whom, for what and how.

This chapter discusses some of the sexual difficulties of adults with variations. To prepare to work psychosexually with individuals and couples, it is important to hold in mind the prevailing discourses about what counts as "sex" and how these discourses work with medicalization to produce sexual failings and compress the complexity, fluidity and elusiveness of sexual preferences and experiences into a treatment frame. The chapter ends with an overview of core sex therapy techniques, some of which are explored in the practice vignette in Section 13.5.

13.1   Sexual Difficulties

A *New York Times* article reported that while many people with variations feel too ashamed of their bodies to date and seek partners, others talk of a rich and stimulating sex life (Angier, 1996). The author quoted a 32-year-old pre-medical student, whose ambiguous genitals were never surgically modified and who was raised as a girl, as saying, "I'm a heterosexual in the truest sense of the word" (p. 2). Many clients have spoken to me about positive sexual experiences. I have met some of their dates and partners who attended clinic with them. I begin this section with these observations for important reasons. Narratives of actual sexual experiences – positive and negative – of people with variations are underresearched. Although sexual difficulties are common, they are certainly not the whole story. Future research could take a different angle. Rather than being preoccupied with sexual *dysfunction* and problem-saturated accounts, research could seek to be more informed about most and least pleasurable fantasies and experiences and how people with variations with a range of identities make sense of their preferences.

Sex research in the era of intersex medicine focused almost exclusively on women with congenital adrenal hyperplasia (CAH) and is of variable quality. Taken together, the studies are suggestive of delayed sexual debut, sexual anxiety and inexperience, sexual pain, impaired genital sensitivity, problem with orgasm and reduced rates of erotic interest and stable partnership. While most participants in the studies had undergone childhood feminizing genitoplasty, it is important to bear in mind that women with CAH who have not undergone surgery also report sexual difficulties though not with orgasm (e.g., Minto et al., 2003a). Women with variations other than CAH who are without a history of childhood surgery also report psychosexual concerns (e.g., Boyle et al., 2005; Minto et al., 2003b).

Due to the high demand for vaginal construction by women with Mayer-Rokitansky-Küster-Hauser syndrome (MRKHS) and the need to develop nonsurgical approaches, a number of studies have focused on sexual experience associated with MRKHS. In a UK study, currently sexually active women with MRKHS reported reduced sexual desire, arousal, lubrication, orgasm and satisfaction and increased sexual pain

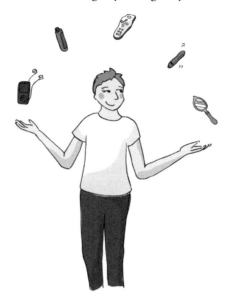

Figure 13.1   Making it fun (*Top Ten Tips for Dilation*). Printed with permission from
dsdfamilies.org. A colour version of this figure can be found in the plate section.

(Liao et al., 2011). A contemporary Dutch study identified more lubrication difficulties among women who had had vaginal surgery compared to
nonsurgical dilation (Callens et al., 2012). In general, despite vaginal
construction, women with MRKHS self-report more sexual distress and
functional difficulties, reduced sexual esteem and poorer genital self-image
compared to non-MRKHS controls (Weijenborg et al., 2019). The
amount of difficulties despite anatomically successful vaginal construction
suggests that whichever method of construction is deployed, the care
pathway is undersupported by psychosexual expertise.

It has been a while since I drew on therapeutic principles relating to
motivation, behavior change and sex therapy to reduce surgical risks with a
program that combined psychosexual education and counseling with self-
managed dilation (Liao et al., 2006). Aspects of the program are embedded
in *Top Tips for Dilation* published by an advocacy group (dsdfamilies.org,
n.d.). Figure 13.1, for example, suggests that dilators are substituted by sex
toys to refocus on sexual exploration and pleasure. Psychologically
informed first-line dilation has enabled a good proportion of women to
avoid surgery (e.g., Dear et al., 2019). Sadly, many services still carry out
complex surgery as the first port of call for MRKHS, leaving the women to
work on their emotional difficulties afterward (Shao et al., 2022).

As for XY conditions, a German review examined sexual quality of life relating to XY variations identified 21 studies published between 1974 and 2007 (Schönbucher et al., 2010). Sexual function and satisfaction was reported to be problematic, though the authors warned that any conclusion is hampered by poor methodological quality across the studies.

In a subsequent study, all 14 men, the majority of whom had had 1–6 genital operations, reported experiencing erection and orgasm (van der Zwan et al., 2013). However, half of them reported ejaculatory concerns and not every man was able to experience penetrative sex. The men reported decreased sexual desire and activities and being less satisfied with genital appearance compared to controls, although their overall body image satisfaction was similar to controls. Male gender assignment is on the increase, and more studies with men with variations can be expected in future.

Meanwhile, a recent questionnaire study involving adults with a range of differences in sex development (DSD) diagnoses, gender identities and sexual preferences resonated with previous findings of a range of sexual difficulties, with greater sensitivity problems associated with childhood genital surgery (Kreukels et al., 2019). Overall, people with variations are less sexually active compared to the general population and less satisfied with their sexual lives. Differences from general population estimates include delayed sexual debut, lower rates of pair bonding and more problems with sexual function. Thus far, with a few exceptions, almost all of the research has failed to examine the ways in which the sexual difficulties are shaped by the social context.

13.2 Ideological Constructions of "Sex"

Many people with genital variations seek surgery to approximate cultural constructions of "normal" sex. Such constructions lay the ground for pathologization of differences and imperfections. In recent decades, critical reformulations that emphasize context and fluidity have shifted understanding, but the cultural shifts are matched by an escalation of medicalization powered by the corporate thrust of the pharmaceutical industry (Gavey, 2011).

13.2.1 Coital Imperative

In an article with the intriguing title "Would you say you 'had sex' if. . .?," Sanders and Reinisch (1999) reported their research with a large, randomly selected and stratified sample of undergraduates in the USA. They observed that only penile-vaginal intercourse was considered as having "had sex" for almost everyone. Fifty-nine percent expressed that oral-genital contact did not count as having "had sex." The US report was swiftly followed by a UK study that asked an opportunistic sample of university students which behaviors constituted "having sex" (Pitts & Rahman, 2001). The majority of respondents regarded having sex as involving penetration. Only one-third of respondents regarded oral-genital contact as having sex. The study provided broad support for the conflation of sex with one body penetrating another.

The cultural indoctrination of sex as involving genital penetration is embedded in and reinforced by psychiatric classification of sexual *dysfunction*, critique of which is captured in the following words: "Full *genital performance during heterosexual intercourse is the essence of sexual functioning*, which excludes and demotes nongenital possibilities for pleasure and expression. Involvement or noninvolvement of the nongenital body parts becomes incidental, of interest only as it impacts on genital responses identified in the nosology" (Tiefer, 1995, p. 53, emphasis original).

People in the general population may enjoy nonpenetrative sexual activities (more), but these activities are constructed as "foreplay" rather than "full sex." In a small study with an opportunistic sample of heterosexual women, the participants reported a lack of sexual desire but positioned themselves as wanting to want sex (Hayfield & Clarke, 2012). They predictably expected penis-in-vagina intercourse to be an inherent part of (hetero)sex, and some of the women had engaged in unwanted but consensual sex to satisfy imaginary male needs.

The coital imperative (McPhillips et al., 2001) is integral to a nexus of discourses relating to lifelong, monogamous, heterosexual coupledom and reproduction. It is an extremely resilient ideology. Even though the digital age opens possibilities to disrupt constructions of gendered bodies and sexual practices, normativity is identifiable in digital sexual encounters. A study of teledildonics, a form of digitally mediated sexual interaction that permits nonheterosexual exploration, suggested that the penetrative act remains a reassuring presupposition in the sexual scripts (Faustino, 2018). Essentialist assumptions in a denaturalized environment prompted the author to say that remote-controlled sex toys offer new extensions to the coital imperative: "Teledildonics sex appears as digital intercourse, rebooting an old script by new means" (p. 255). The author further concluded that "in spite of structurally disrupting the reproductive model of sex, teledildonics promotes its strongest corollary" (p. 243).

On one hand, ongoing resistance offers hope for a level of reworking of sexual norms. On the other hand, history suggests that future discourses are more likely to reinscribe what is taken for granted through new and emerging technologies (Farvid & Braun, 2022).

13.2.2 Orgasmic Imperative

Modernist sex research, with plenty of help from the popular media, has created an orgasm imperative in Western culture (Tepper, 2000). Orgasm is privileged as a natural, inevitable and necessary part of sexual activity. At a single click on images of "orgasm books" on the Internet, dozens of titles appear. People can apparently eat their way to "full body orgasm" or take small steps to "make" their partner orgasm "again and again." If orgasm is so naturally inevitable, one wonders why so much help is needed to make it happen.

Persistent absence of orgasm during sexual encounters is, according to Western medical classification, *dysfunctional* – an "abnormality" that needs to be corrected. This may explain why myriad remedies exist. Orgasm has been transformed from being an incidental experience into a cultural benchmark for every sexual encounter. It is not just something that one could experience but *should* experience (Frith, 2015). As a requirement, obligation and responsibility, it is not exclusive to heterosexuals and bears the hallmark of good sex and good relationship for Anglo-Europeans.

Orgasm is a potential source of intense pleasure, yet it can be fraught with difficulty because it is, as discussed above, burdened by meanings. A study with 119 sexually experienced young people of a range of sexualities explored meanings of orgasm and pleasure during sex with a partner (Opperman et al., 2014). The participants' talk resonated strongly with widespread discourses of sexuality that prioritize coitus, orgasm and orgasm reciprocity. The experience of orgasm is so central that, in its absence, it might be faked so that relational meanings are preserved.

The subject of orgasm is an emotive one for people whose genital responsiveness has been irrevocably damaged – by genital cutting, physical health problems and/or their treatments. Feeling compelled but unable to approximate neoliberal pleasure norms can be a source of shame not just for people with variations but many other groups also.

Interests in clitoral reconstruction by women after female genital cutting in the Global North have soared, even though the safety and benefits are not clearly evidenced (Abdulcadir et al., 2015). A recent analysis observed that many help seekers, including those who already experience sexual pleasure, construct surgery as a remedy for the missing clitoris and as a way to become complete as a woman (O'Neill et al., 2021). Problematically, women from sub-Saharan origins living in the Global North are socialized into constructing female wholeness as an approximation of a white body-normality (capable of meeting white bodily pleasure norms). Similarly, prevailing norms have left people with variations and a range of physical health conditions without alternative discourses to construct pleasure on their own terms.

13.2.3   Medicalization

The co-opting of the coital and orgasmic imperatives is strategically important to enlarge the market for fixing sexual failings. Promoted as a miracle to restore relational happiness, Viagra for example trades on oppressive cultural norms (Gavey, 2011). Pharmacological and numerous other fixes, including self-help books, have their place in modern life, but they also intensify normative pressures and squeeze out any space for constructing alternative meanings.

Despite genital reconstruction (and sometimes because of it), sexual difficulties are more prevalent for people with variations compared to the general population. After surgery, the knee-jerk response to any sexual complaint is hormonal management (e.g., check hormone levels, prescribe estrogen cream). While hormones are important for urogenital and general health, research does not suggest a reliable relationship between hormonal levels and sexual experience. Hormonal treatment of sexual problems in the general population has focused almost exclusively on the use of testosterone to increase sexual desire in women. From the 2000s, a series of randomized, placebo-controlled trials of testosterone patches has been carried out with women diagnosed with premature ovarian insufficiency (POI). Women already on adequate estrogen replacement were given 300 μg testosterone patches daily for 24 weeks, in the form of a twice-weekly patch worn on the abdomen. By deploying a large number of exclusion criteria, the most intensively studied population was Caucasian (and presumably heterosexual) women without additional health complications. All of the studies involved short-term treatment and follow-up. All of them declared involvement from the pharmaceutical industry in study design, statistical analysis and in some cases assistance with the manuscript. While the studies point to a small increase in one to two satisfying sexual activities per month during treatment, the trade-off between this outcome and known and unknown adverse events renders the treatment highly dubious (see ESHRE Guideline Group on POI et al., 2016).

Disease mongering, a process that turns healthy people into patients in order to grow treatment markets, works hand in hand with disease taxonomies that classify ordinary life experiences into illnesses. Of the large number of objectors to the very idea of sexual dysfunction, the feminist sexologist Leonore Tiefer is among the most prolific and persistent. Her resistance to medical authority has taken the form of academic scholarship, media satire and street protests. Despite criticisms, many sex researchers and therapists continue to valorize pathologizing discourses, buying into the supposition that sexual deficits exist and that they can be uncovered, categorized and treated.

McCarthy and Metz (2008) suggested that since the introduction of Viagra in 1998, the focus has been on a medication approach for men to chase perfectionism, which often backfires and produces insecurities, unhappiness and perpetual dissatisfaction. To counter the pressure, the authors introduced the idea of "good enough sex" where, first of all, intimacy is the ultimate focus, secondly, pleasure is as important as function and, thirdly, mutual emotional acceptance is the environment in which sex takes place. Sex therapy is becoming more socially inclusive, but there remains a risk of universalizing sexual desire and a quickness to pathologize its absence as something to be worked on. While it is important for therapists to identify and support people whose sexual desire is compromised by psychosocial difficulties, not feeling sexual, per se, is not a problem unless the individual or couple consider it so.

13.3 Absence of Pleasure Talk

In DSD, sex is rarely discussed outside normalizing discourses. As discussed in Chapter 4, however, medical interventions can attract their own suite of abnormal life experiences. However expertly and compassionately delivered, medical fixing comes with a meta message that the body with variation is not good enough. Despite genital modification, care users' talk of sexual intimacy is characterized by fear and dread. Women with XY conditions have spoken of avoiding sex for years after vaginoplasty (Boyle et al., 2005). A woman spoke of her partner's penis feeling like "a dead weight inside" when she finally engaged in coitus (p. 582). The absence of pleasure talk in psychological research is paralleled in surgical outcome studies with women, whereby success is defined as anatomical capacity to be penetrated by an erect penis. Indeed, surgery is considered a "partial success" even if a woman experiences discomfort during coitus, provided this "did not fully impair penetration" (Azziz et al., 1990, p. 24). Although vaginal construction is fraught with difficulties (Callens et al., 2012; Liao et al., 2011), it is sought by many women who are already able to access a range of sexual experiences (Dear et al., 2019). Men with variations have likewise expressed extreme fear of sexual encounters (Chadwick et al., 2005).

13.3.1   Objectification, Aversion, Shame

Throughout this book, I discuss repeat examinations of children with genital variations as particularly toxic. Adults (with gender-normative as well as queer identities) have spoken movingly about their experiences of body shame, genital aversion and fear of intimacy (Davis & Feder, 2015). I do not suggest that medicalization causes body shame, because shame is universal and body shame extremely common. People in the general population go to inordinate lengths to conform to social norms for bodily appearance and function to avoid shame (see Dolezal, 2015). What I do suggest is that medicalization can exacerbate and prolong body shame.

Body shame refers to the experience of a bodily appearance or function as failing against an internalized norm. Some psychological researchers suggest that internalization is the mechanism that links exposure to bodily ideals to self-objectification, body shame and uptake of interventions to erase the perceived shortcoming (Fredrickson et al., 2011).

Shame of failing to meet a preconceived bodily standard is said to be associated with an array of compromised health outcomes (Goffnett et al., 2020). Sanchez and Kiefer (2007) carried out a study to examine whether body shame was related to sexual problems in a sample of 320 heterosexual men and women. Men and women's body shame was related to greater sexual self-consciousness, which in turn predicted lower sexual pleasure and sexual arousability. The study largely supported the proposition that bodily appearance concerns are associated with reduced sexual arousability and pleasure for men and women. The authors discussed their findings in terms of appearance norms in the wider culture.

In an attempt to better understand reduced sexual satisfaction among socially anxious people who are in intimate partnerships, self-report data were collected from 115 undergraduate students and their partners in monogamous, heterosexual, committed relationships (Montesi et al., 2013). Higher social anxiety predicted higher fear of intimacy, which predicted lower satisfaction with open sexual communication and which, in turn, predicted lower sexual satisfaction. The authors suggested that fear of scrutiny and negative evaluation by others is a barrier to the process of building intimacy via information sharing. These findings suggest that sex therapy for people with variations may be more effective if it could first tackle difficulties in disclosure (see Chapter 12).

Unaddressed body shame and inability to talk about variations are likely to fuel what sex therapists call *spectatoring* in sexual situations. Rather than focus on what feels good, an individual may be preoccupied with their genitals not measuring up to the imaginary penis or vagina and look for signs of aversion in the partner. Spectatoring is evident in a number of qualitative studies involving adults with variations (Boyle et al., 2005; Chadwick et al., 2005; May et al., 1996). Research participants have reported checking what surgeons have done during sex. Spectatoring pulls people out of the moment. The resultant deflating experience becomes self-fulfilling.

Although there is no research in interventions to reduce body shame and sexual anxiety for adults with variations, research in psychological interventions to tackle shame provides grounds for optimism. A recent systematic review looked at the effectiveness of psychosocial interventions to reduce shame in general (rather than body shame specifically). The review included a pooled sample of 5 128 individuals who participated across 37 intervention studies (Goffnett et al., 2020). Of these, 16 studies were randomized controlled trials (RCT) and 21 were prospective studies using pre/post measures. Shame was treated in a variety of behavioral health contexts. The most common interventions were cognitive behavioral therapy (CBT) and mindfulness. Eighty-nine percent of studies (N = 32) reported reductions in shame at post-test. Nine studies reported sustained reductions in shame over time. The authors concluded that shame experience is malleable. A Cochrane Review has found CBT to be highly effective in the treatment of body image distress (Ipser et al., 2009). Although this evidence is not specific to genital body image or sexual distress, it has implications for therapists seeking effective means to help people with variations to address body shame.

13.3.2   *Physical Health Considerations*

Factors other than genital variations can contribute to an absence of pleasure talk. Chronic conditions can have a direct impact on sexual function, or the impact could be secondary to common symptoms such as pain, fatigue and mobility restrictions. Sexual difficulties may also be secondary to anxiety and low mood as a result of living with poor physical health. Insight from research in the impact of chronic illness may be helpful for sex therapists preparing to work with people with certain sex variations. Sadly, Verschuren et al. (2010) examined the literature in diabetes, multiple sclerosis, Parkinson's disease, cardiovascular disease, spinal cord injury, traumatic brain injury and amputation and identified only a tiny percentage of publications that mentioned sexuality in the title.

Because of the long-term and sometimes irreversible nature of sexual difficulties, there is a need to examine coping and adjustment. Disappointingly, research often focuses on sexual *dysfunction* but rarely examines how couples renegotiate their sexual lives. An example that represents an exception to this trend was an interview study with 44 (mainly heterosexual) men and women impacted by different types of cancer (Ussher et al., 2013). Renegotiation of sex or intimacy was reported by 70% of participants. The interviewees talked about resisting the coital imperative to redefine "sex" and embracing intimacy. They also talked about maintaining the coital imperative by refiguring the body through techno-medicine. The authors concluded that resistance to hegemonic constructions of "sex," in particular the coital imperative, is central in negotiating sexual intimacy after cancer. In relation to adjustment, Barsky et al. (2006) put forward a model of coping that focuses on flexibility, which includes redefining sexual functioning and its centrality to an overall sense of self. Within such a model, which clearly draws on humanistic existential frameworks, sex therapy is broadly similar to generic psychological therapy.

There are many opportunities for clinicians across healthcare contexts to inquire about sexuality and adjustment. McGrath et al. (2021) carried out a systematic review of studies reporting on knowledge, attitudes and behaviors of healthcare professionals in relation to how they address sexuality concerns in the context of chronic disease and disability. Their pooled analysis showed that only 14.2% of health professionals routinely ask questions or provide information about the sexual impact of the physical health condition. In general, care providers experience significant discomfort when raising the topic of sex, especially with people living with chronic disease and disability. Surprisingly, there is no interest in inquiring into DSD clinicians' capacity to probe into care users' sexual difficulties, perhaps because, historically, there is such an overriding emphasis on mechanical approaches.

Inquiry into sexual concerns is a delicate process. Care providers need to discern whether the patient has any concern or need for support without any supposition that sex is central to the care user. A recent study provides a salutary lesson for providers keen to fix patients' sex lives. Shen and Liu (2021) examined the relationship between sexual obligation and perceived stress. Although their focus was on older adults rather than a clinical population, the findings are interesting for healthcare contexts. Using longitudinal data from three waves of the National Social Life, Health, and Aging Project, the study included 1 477 partnered, sexually active respondents aged 57–85 at the baseline survey. Sexual obligation was positively associated with perceived stress. Feeling more obligated to have sex had a significantly greater effect on older men's subjective experience of stress over time than older women's. In other words, sex therapy may involve supporting people to decentralize sexual activity rather than offering solutions to keep people sexually active.

13.4   Sex Therapy

Remedies for sexual difficulties have existed in some shape or form since antiquity but, overshadowed by pharmacological and surgical developments, research in psychosexual interventions is sparse. Sex therapy remains highly speculative, though perhaps no more so than medical interventions.

Western modernist sex therapy leans heavily on the pioneering work of Masters and Johnson (1970), who described a "normal" sexual response cycle of excitement, plateau, orgasm and resolution. Based on research with white, educated, young, nondisabled and heterosexual Americans in the 1960s, the cycle is said to dovetail between men and women. The therapy program took on what might be considered a short-term psychoeducational approach today. It combined information, communication skills training and behavioral tasks that focus upon sensuality (at first). Although the results have never been replicated, the program attracted a huge following and has given rise to a new professional identity – sex therapist.

13.4.1   Inclusivity

In an era of prohibition, inhibition and lack of information, early sex therapy programs that aimed to educate people about the sex anatomy, remove pressure from coital performance (for a time) and focus on sensual experiences and communication were a credible beginning. However, the program also subscribed to cardinal elements of the medical model: norms, expertise and classification (Tiefer, 2012). In time, some sex therapists incorporated the physical body works (e.g., directed masturbation practices) developed in the humanistic movement as optional elements of sexual exploration, but into a medical model that continues to categorize sexual experiences as "normal" or "pathological" based on the imaginary white, middle-class and (hetero)sexual dyad as the default service user.

Most structured therapy programs lend themselves to be developed into self-help formats. Before long, patients would arrive for help having already read sex manuals and tried out various techniques yet still felt dissatisfied. LoPiccolo (1994) suggested that sex therapists in the post Masters and Johnson era would need to do more than give information and teach skills. They must also explore ways in which sexual difficulties may be implicated in distance, closeness and power relationships between people. How individuals relate to culturally valorized sexualities is currently also considered to be part and parcel of sex therapy.

The greater acknowledgment of fluidity in identity, attractions and behaviors and a changing social context place new demands on sex therapists. Today's therapists must engage productively with people with diverse identities and practices including BDSM (bondage and discipline, dominance and submission, and sadism and masochism), fetishes and polyamory. The sex therapist has to be familiar with online resources in pornography/erotica and varieties of solo sex that are produced to enable people to explore new and/or alternative sexual desires and possibilities.

In a CNN article (Kinsman, 2014), intersex activist Pidgeon Pagonis quoted their therapist as saying, "Sex is 90% fiction and 10% friction!" Deconstructing oppressive norms is the most important component of contemporary sex therapy. However, whereas many people are relieved to debunk sex and body norms, many more are reluctant to relinquish the narcissistic coercive norms and scripts that proliferate in the social world. There are other limits to sex therapy. It may be appropriate to suggest sex therapy staples to some clients, such as masturbation for self-learning and self-control of sexual responses; the very idea of engaging in sex for pleasure (perhaps especially autoerotic pleasure for women) may be offensive or threatening to other clients. There is a continuing and fascinating debate on the conceptual framework of *Sensate Focus*, a key part of Masters and Johnson's program (see Section 13.4.2) on how well it serves sexual minorities (see Linschoten et al., 2016).

Berry and Lezos (2017) carried out an interview study with 34 sex therapists to identify what are considered important therapist qualities. The three clinical principles identified are therapist self-reflection, client affirmation and normalizing (of diverse experiences). To work in sex development, I would add to the list 1) connecting with advocacy groups,

2) ongoing learning with peers, 3) good self-care and 4) accessing restorative supervision with an experienced supervisor with whom to discuss personal-professional boundaries and dilemmas.

Below are some of the basic techniques that can help to reduce body shame, increase sensuality, improve communication and move away from sexual imperatives that give rise to perfectionism, self-surveillance, anxiety and avoidance. With the client's permission, the assessment could focus on developmental trajectories of the following (Liao, 2007): 1) gender positioning of self, 2) gender(s) of preferred partners, 3) body-related perceptions and emotions, 4) sexual experiences and fantasies, 5) sexual and relationship aspirations and 6) knowledge and interests relating to diverse sexual activities.

Using the techniques below, the therapist and client may move toward one or more of the following goals (Liao, 2007): 1) understanding past and present influences on the identified sexual difficulty or distress, 2) increasing awareness of variations in human sexuality, 3) decision-making about sexual activities (or not), 4) self-permission to explore a range of sexual activities – solo or partnered – with or without erotic material or mechanical aids, 5) decentralizing genital and/or penetrative sex and 6) increasing control over social and sexual situations via clear communication.

13.4.2   Sensate Focus

Sensate focus (SF) is a structured behavioral program with three phases and has remained a staple in sex therapy, if adapted creatively in response to different presentations (Weiner & Avery-Clark, 2014). In classic SF, phase 1 consists of sequential touching of the partner's body other than breasts and genitals. The toucher is guided by their own curiosity and inclination and not by trying to please the other. The touchee provides verbal feedback to the toucher about the qualities of the touch. After approximately 15 minutes, the roles are reversed. The emphasis is on sensual rather than erotic pleasure, and overt sexual activity is prohibited during this period. Phase 2 includes breast and genital touch and the goal is the same, to learn about the partner's body, rather than to create pleasure in another. Phase 3 involves mutual touching. In the original program developed by Masters and Johnson (1970), intercourse is reintroduced during this phase. The therapist seeks to monitor the couple's responses to the assignment and emphasize positive reinforcers (e.g., praise) without dwelling on negative reinforcers (e.g., criticism of self or the partner).

Table 13.1. *Prompts to encourage pleasure talk...*

"When did you first start longing to be physically close with someone?"
"What kind of scenarios played out in your mind?"
"What kind of pleasures did you lean toward?"
"For example touch, how did you like to be touched?"
"If you were to touch ___, what was that like for you?"
"What was your body doing?"
"Where in your body were the physical changes most vivid?"
"How did those touch preferences change over time, if they have?"

13.4.3   Communication

Communication is a strong predictor of relationship satisfaction. For many adults with variations, however, communication is even more difficult than sexual interaction (see Vosoughi et al., 2022; Weijenborg et al., 2019). Learning to communicate limits and construct safe words and experience bodily contact that is not penetration or genital-focused can be a useful contribution to therapy with some individuals. The idea of consensual creation of experiences of physical sensations and emotions from oft-misunderstood BDSM communities can be usefully incorporated in sexual communication and negotiation. On the note of negotiating experience, a few example questions to prompt pleasure talk are provided in Table 13.1.

13.4.4   Mind–Body Awareness

The notion of mindfulness-based sex therapy to help men to achieve erection (Bossio et al., 2018) and women to improve arousability (Stephenson & Kerth, 2017) is not a comfortable fit with the foundational value of non-striving in mindfulness. Nevertheless, mindfulness is being widely trialled with people diagnosed with *sexual dysfunction*.

   Mindfulness and SF practices can work well together. Both are aimed at helping people to focus on the moment, but the former is an especially valuable training in letting go of judging thoughts and allowing the body to have more of a say in terms of what feels good, without obstruction from the judging mind. In a cross-sectional study with a sample of college-aged women (N = 115), mindfulness practice was associated with lower body shame and higher body responsiveness as well as other health outcomes (Lamont, 2019). Although the study was carried out to examine the relationship between mindfulness and health by reducing body shame and heightening body responsiveness, the study offers additional evidence to suggest that mindfulness-based techniques are promising in sex therapy for people with body shame.

13.4.5 Cognitive and Behavioral Techniques

As discussed in Chapter 8, cognitive therapy involves guiding clients to observe how certain thoughts (e.g., "What if my sexual partner flips when I tell them?") make them feel (e.g., fear) and act (e.g., spectator-ing). The behavioral component usually involves graded exposure to what is avoided or feared, such as talking to a sexual partner about a genital variation (see practice vignette in Section 12.4 in Chapter 12). Response substitution techniques, such as paying the partner a compliment when there is an urge to self-surveillance, can pay dividends in some situations.

13.5 Practice Vignette

"Tess" is a 22-year-old woman with a childhood diagnosis of partial androgen insensitivity syndrome (PAIS). At the adult DSD service, her current care plan concerns vaginal dilation. After a year-long absence from the nurse-led dilation clinic, Tess presents herself for a review. She is accompanied by her new partner, "Milly." The couple met 15 months ago. Milly is in her mid-30s and divorced. Tess has recently moved in to live with Milly and her 6-year-old son "Franck," who gets on well with Tess because she knows how to make and repair toys with him.

Tess insists on staying on the dilation program and says she will "get back on track" when she is not so tired. The highly experienced nurse specialist "Alicia" has offered flexible and skillful support to Tess. She has checked all of Tess' medical records and sees that her hormone levels are correct and up to date. She cannot identify any medical reasons for the tiredness and wonders if Tess may be depressed. She suggests an appointment with the family physician to look into the use of antidepressants. Tess protests that she has never been happier. It is enough for her to have to use an estrogen patch – "taking more drugs is out of the question." Alicia asks the couple to meet with in-house psychological care provider "Dr. Cook."

13.5.1　Assessment

Dr. Cook refers to himself as a trans man who has grown up and lived as a woman for many years. He discloses that culturally, he is from a blue-collar background and is now aligned with a mainly white LGBT community. He asks the couple how this information might affect their work together. The couple look disinterested. He also asks to be called "Dr. C," to sound friendly yet retain a level of formality, in anticipation of the intimate conversations that are likely to ensue.

Milly begins by telling Dr. C that Tess' childhood and adolescent surgeries have not "worked" and that dilation is "not working either." While she and Tess enjoy sex, they would like to explore a fuller range of activities that include vaginal penetration. This is not possible at the moment because Tess' vagina has shrunk. Dr. C asks Tess her view of the situation. The reply is: "It's just as Milly says, the surgeries didn't work and the dilation is no good either." Dr. C is concerned that dilation is being discussed as an innocuous activity and directs the conversation to inquire about Tess' experience with it. She claims to have followed the program but does not elaborate. Dr. C can see that Tess tends to look to Milly to speak for her. He asks to spend some time with Tess alone.

With a fair amount of prompting, Tess explains to Dr. C that she is too busy to dilate. She is a full-time trainee carpenter. She often babysits Franck. She sings in the church choir. When asked exactly how many times she has dilated, the answer is: "At least twice, maybe three, four times." It takes quite a few prompts from Dr. C to realize that Tess is not talking about a few times a week but in total in the past year. This level of dilation would not have any clinical impact, but it would have given Tess enough experience to express how she feels about the program. Dr. C inquires as follows:

DR. C:　If you were to think about restarting dilation this week, what are the first words that come to mind?

TESS:　I would say, I would say, I don't have time this week. I have to . . .

DR. C:　But if you were to dilate, picture yourself dilating, what comes to mind?

TESS:　The words that come to mind are . . . boredom, effort, slow, eye rolling, looking at my watch, can't wait to stop . . .

DR. C:　I see from our records that as a teenager you found dilation difficult too after the surgery. You're in charge now, if that's how you feel, what makes you agree to dilation?

TESS:　Because I want to make the entrance bigger.

DR. C:　How would that change anything?

TESS: We can use the sex toys, Milly and me. We have a double-sided dildo. Lots of toys, stuff like that. I am the reason why we can't do new things. I have never been happier. I don't want to let Milly down.

DR. C: Suppose Milly doesn't care about penetrative sex, how would you feel about dilation then?

TESS: I mean, well, if she absolutely doesn't care, if I can be totally sure of that, I wouldn't bother with dilation.

On further questioning, Tess admits to enjoying oral-genital sex the most, but especially in the dark, when she would feel most aroused. She explains that visibility can be distracting, as she would usually "start looking around." Dr. C also asks about other bodily experiences. Tess does not like but can tolerate being touched ("It may grow me, as long as it's Milly") and says that her favorite experience is having someone brush her hair.

Tess had her first genital surgery at the age of 7 months, and then again aged 8 and 13 years old. She understands the reason as "looking too much like a boy down below." She remembers fragments of the second and third operations. The memories may have merged. She still carries an image of watching herself and everybody in a hospital ward. In that image, her father is crying and her mother comforts him with, "Don't worry, she'll be alright, the doctors know best." Tess does not know whether this image is a dream or a memory. She does not recall when it first came to mind ("it's always been there").

In between surgeries, Tess attended the hospital for follow-ups every six months. She was examined at every appointment. She was so conditioned to the routine that, as a toddler, the moment that she was in the doctor's office, she would jump onto the examining couch and lift up her skirt. Her mother still muses how cute that was. Tess does not link these early experiences to her subsequent psychological difficulties, which included the dissociation (watching herself from above) and also distressed eating from the age of 14 years. Since meeting Milly, she has been eating healthily with the rest of the household, though she still thinks a lot about becoming size zero one day. The rest of the assessment information can be seen in Table 13.2.

13.5.2   Formulation

In his systemic formulation, Dr. C understands that Tess' parents had looked to the medical profession to help them to survive their social displacement on account of their child's variation. Out of fear of exclusion, they did not talk about the variation with anyone, and their distressing thoughts and feelings remained undigested and unsaid. They became ever more dependent on medical experts. Tess is reported to be pliant with

Table 13.2. *Summary of initial assessment with Tess*

Inquiry domains	Summary of content
Goal of assessment – Information gathering for formulation and care planning as appropriate	– Tess had disengaged from the vaginal dilation program and now re-presents herself for a review. The nurse asks her to see the sex therapist to discuss her struggles with dilation that she insists on continuing.
Relationship to help – Who is referring whom for what reason – Who are in the system – Relationship with specialist services and community providers – Patterns of engagement with services	– Appointment triggered by partner Milly though Tess agrees "it's a good idea." – Tess feels cared for by the clinic with which she has an easy relationship; she does not disagree with any aspect of her management. – However, she has never been a proactive service user – her father used to arrange her travels to make sure she does not miss her appointments.
General health and psychological well-being – Current – Past	– Describes physical health as fair. – Lethargic, no zest for life, sometimes wonders if she should try antidepressant. – History of distressed eating; now eats healthily.
Personal strengths and needs – Psychosocial skills (e.g., communication, emotion regulation) – Family relationships (e.g., closeness and distances) – Peer relationships – Capacity for independence – Education, work, creativity, interests – Hopes and fears	– Quiet, does not enjoy talking in general. – Good at model making – interested and skilled. – Great singer. – Is gainfully employed. – Popular with colleagues at work. – Has good contact with both parents – warm – but not communicative. – Not sure what she wants in life, maybe have her own workshop and teach furniture making one day.
Understanding of variation and treatment past/present – Factual knowledge – Understanding of immediate and long-term MDT care plan – Knowledge of respective roles of providers involved	– Understands partial AIS but doesn't talk about it – "not worried, just just not a great talker." – Knows about past feminizing genitoplasties – has no memory of the first one, the memories of the next two are merged – may have dissociated during one of the pre-ops. – Understands the importance of taking hormones (but sometimes forgets) and regular health checks.
Emotional responses to variation and treatment past/present – Emotional reactions – Immediate and future concerns	– Cannot remember early reactions but is often portrayed by mother as a "good girl for the doctors."

Table 13.2. (*cont.*)

Inquiry domains	Summary of content
	– Has had a lot of genital examinations and thinks of them as part and parcel of her condition – looks emotionally detached and flat when asked about the experience. – Has been teased at school for being a tomboy – "I like being a tomboy but I hated being teased because it's like this, I'm at the center of attention."
Social and cultural aspects – Family relationships – Community support – Access to confiding relationships – Cultural and religious attitudes relating to diversity – Knowledge of education and support resources; and capacity to navigate	– Small family; rarely sees extended family who lives afar. – Church goer; "semi religious"; social support from church. – Was encouraged to but has so far declined peer support – reason: "I'm not a great talker."
Gender and sexuality – Sex/gender identity – Attitudes, preferences – Sexual experiences – Current relationship	– Self-identifies as female. – Only attracted to women. – Masturbated for pleasure before meeting Milly, was sometimes orgasmic. – No experience with erotica, pornography, etc. – Milly is her first stable relationship. – Feels guilty toward Milly for not including the AIS in her profile and wonders if Mily would have chosen her if she had disclosed everything. – Both enjoy oral-genital sex, but Milly wants to explore mutual penetration using sex toys. Tess is open to this but is unexcited for herself.

medical procedures. When it got too much, she blanked out certain experiences. Shortly after her third surgery she developed distressed eating.

Tess' life is coming together. She attributes this to Milly's support. They are deeply in love. Talk of marriage has been mooted. However, Tess experiences herself as a beneficiary of the relationship rather than an equal partner. She reciprocates by taking up dilation because she is aware that Milly really wants her to succeed. Deep down, Tess also feels guilty toward Milly. She met Milly through a dating app and, although she told Milly about the PAIS when they met in person, Tess feels disingenuous for not ticking the category "Intersex" in the dating app in the first place.

Penetration is integral to sex in the wider culture. Although Milly has had rather mixed experiences of penetrative sex with previous partners, it feels like a given that she would explore this with Tess. She is not aware of the fact that Tess does not feel any inclination toward it, because she has never been told.

Tess is socialized into believing in medical solutions. When dilation is again suggested, she overrides her aversion and accepts the program by minimizing her distaste for it. Although dilation can be creatively channeled as an erotic activity for some women and laudably managed by others, it can be psychologically invasive for women with genital aversion due, in Tess' case, to overexposure and not being in control in medical encounters. Milly is uninformed about the impact of medicalization on Tess' sexuality, not least because the latter has been avoiding the topic.

Dr. C establishes that dilation is not feasible for Tess without first thinking with her about certain life experiences and the ways in which different forms of power have been operating on her life. In the formulation chart in Figure 13.2, Dr. C places Tess' dilation-related experiences in a multilayered context, one of which is medicalization. Supporting Tess to dilate now would mean supporting the notion that she does not have the right equipment to enjoy sex, that her body needs to be continually medically managed and that she is not entitled to negotiate how she wants to enjoy sex with her partner. Dr. C sees the first step as support for Tess to develop a more coherent understanding of her life experiences. If she engages with therapy, there is time to help her to explore her sexual preferences later.

Dr. C intends to encourage Tess to examine the meanings of her variation and how it is managed. Her understanding of her body has so far been structured by a medical language and flavored by shaming experiences. Within a supported sense-making process, it is hoped that Tess is also guided to identify and own her power – resilience, survivorship, interests, skills, popularity at work, and so on – and then decide what the next step may be.

13.5.3   Sex Therapy

Bearing in mind what the physical clinic space may represent to Tess, Dr. C invites her to meet for three online sessions in the first instance, to try to build rapport and trust. At the end of the online appointments, he draws

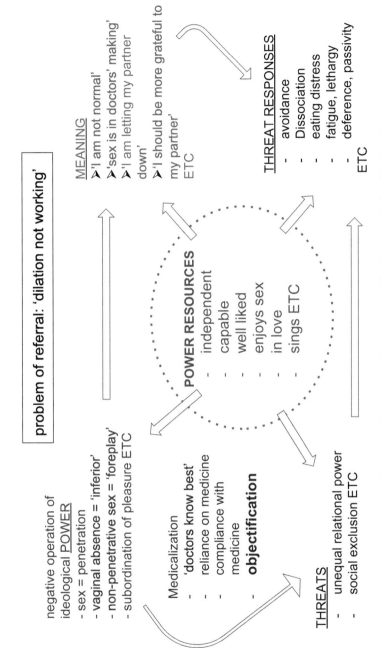

Figure 13.2 Formulation chart for Tess. A colour version of this figure can be found in the plate section.

out the following care plan for Tess but suggests that they progress flexibly at her pace:

Working individually with Tess:

1. *Story repair* (see Chapter 8) to encourage Tess to narrate her experiences, build coherence, cocreate preferred language and meanings, decolonize and reclaim her body, and take ownership of her strengths and powers
2. Explore contributions to physical well-being (e.g., tiredness) that may be mood-related and, if needs be, triage for medical input
3. Encourage Tess to take appreciative care of her body with lots of treats (e.g., reflexology, warm baths, simple stretching) and record the effects (e.g., on energy levels)
4. Explore how Tess feels about pleasuring herself and self-discover sexual responses to erotica and fantasies without external pressure

Working jointly to include Milly:

5. Invite Tess to narrate feelings about her variation and past treatments to Milly, and her feelings of guilt for not mentioning about her variation before they met
6. Sensate Focus program: mutual learning to rediscover relaxed enjoyment and communication around physical intimacy (e.g., stroking along the back, brushing each other's hair)
7. Mindfulness practices to help Tess to experience her urges to self-spectator during sex without acting on them and then substituting self-spectatoring with an alternative response, such as voicing what feels pleasurable
8. Discuss diverse ideas relating to the role of penetration in sexual intimacy and the different levels of penetration and bodily positionings
9. Discuss dilation and how to approach it (e.g., clinically or erotically) – if still relevant

Dr. C encourages Tess to create a workbook, a kind of portfolio in which to record private reflections throughout therapy, note down fantasies and dreams to mull over, rate experiences of the various home practices, collate resources that she chooses to consult and gather any new material of interest to her. As Tess becomes more proactive in learning from the experiences of other people with variations, she particularly enjoys reading the courageous story of Bria Brown-King (2019), who explained how their mixed experiences of dating, even when not all positive, had helped them to understand and accept their body:

> I've learned to ask questions of healthcare providers instead of just accepting their answers, and I've learned to be okay with the fact that my body doesn't mirror that of many women. I am okay with the fact that for my partners, this means that physical intimacy with me might require a lesson on the anatomy of a person with a nontraditional body.

13.6 Reflexivity

The inclusion of this chapter does not come with the message that sexual intimacy is a must for everyone. Rather, it reflects the struggles with sexual intimacy reported by many people with variations. Here, sex therapy, which can be with an individual or inclusive of partners, is positioned not as a path to have sex in culturally scripted ways but as an exploration of what enjoyment is possible. This usually requires interrogating oppressive sexual norms.

Far from fixing sexual problems, supporting clients to express their experiences in a preferred language and encouraging them to experience their bodies in nonsexual ways is an important part of the preparation for a more relaxed and appreciative relationship with the body. As a clinical psychologist working in sex development, I find this work – transforming aversion and judgment to self-appreciation and love – to be the most intricate and rewarding work. This work, which requires highly developed generic therapy knowledge and skills, can be integrated with a range of tools and resources associated with sex therapy to imagine a different sexual future, which may be characterized by fun and light-heartedness, excitement and intensity, or something in between.

CHAPTER 14

Childfreedom

The word family may evoke a picture of the traditional nuclear family with a father working outside the home and a mother at home with the couple's two children. This prototype began only in the 1950s in affluent communities in the West. It was not to last. Family life has been more diverse for quite some time. Today, less than a quarter of US households consist of a married couple with their own biological children. Other households include heterosexual couples with or without biological and/or adoptive children, same-gender couples with or without biological and/or adoptive children, blended families comprising parents with biological and/or adoptive children from current and/or previous relationships, one-parent households with biological and/or adoptive and/or stepchildren, multigenerational extended families living together, groups of adults and children and single adults without children. Despite substantial social changes, the heteronormative nuclear household, which is now a statistical minority, is still held to be the ideal to aspire to.

This chapter begins with a summary of the fertility potential of people with sex development variations. Spontaneous conception is technically feasible for congenital adrenal hyperplasia (CAH). People with some of the other variations can potentially access biological parenthood via assisted reproductive technology (ART), which is considerably less straightforward physically, psychologically and financially, than that which is portrayed in glossy advertisements for fertility services.

I next provide a brief overview of psychosocial research in infertility. On browsing the clinical literature on reproductive choices and outcomes in the general population, I am struck by several observations. The most obvious is that the literature is overwhelmingly dominated by reproductive biotechnology. Relative to the scale of this output is a small body of empirical research with people of childbearing age on lived experiences of current nonparenthood. This literature is characterized by 1) recruitment of research participants from fertility clinics, 2) problem-saturated accounts of nonparenthood, 3) placing the heterosexual woman at the center of analysis, 4) gender differences in experience of nonparenthood and 5) invisibility of the narratives of people not seeking parenthood. To address this imbalance, I highlight some of the more nuanced psychosocial research in childfreedom. I draw attention to studies that focus on child-freedom as an active choice and some of the difficulties in articulating this choice in a world of uncritical pronatalism.

Empowerment of and compassion for people impacted by variations in sex development is increasingly framed in terms of technocentric innovations to propel them toward the pronatalist heterosexual ideal. Such a restricted view obscures other human responses. The chapter ends with a practice vignette that explores fertility counseling with a couple, one of whom is diagnosed with Klinefelter syndrome (KS), as they navigate an ongoing dilemma.

14.1 Fertility and Variations in Sex Development

It has been said that a "dividend" of biogenetic research is improved spontaneous conception and ART outcomes in recent years for people with a uterus (Conway, 2014). Presence of a uterus is associated with 46,XX CAH, Turner syndrome (TS) and Swyer syndrome. For women with Mayer-Rokitansky-Küster-Hauser syndrome (MRKHS), who tend to have healthy ovaries and no (functional) uterus, genetic parenthood is possible via surrogacy. Ongoing animal and human experimentation in womb transplantation may have future implications for MRKHS (Brännström et al., 2019). Womb transplantation represents the most extreme technological fix yet, for human unhappiness, longing and desire in the sex development context.

Medical research has focused the most on 46,XX CAH (see Chapter 2), the majority of whom are female-assigned and identified. Fertility in women with CAH is reduced, especially in those with the salt-losing (classical) form (e.g., Hagenfeldt et al., 2008; Ogilvie et al., 2006). Reasons for reduced fertility in women with CAH are thought to be multifaceted. Ogilvie et al. (2006) critiqued fertility research that fails to make a distinction between active attempt at conception and nonattempt, which makes it difficult to estimate precise ovulation and pregnancy rates. The authors suggested that it is important to examine factors such as adrenal suppression, prevalence of polycystic ovaries leading to irregular ovulation and elevated progesterone levels during the follicular phase that result in nonimplantation.

A French study with a cohort of 190 women with nonclassical (mild, nonsalt-losing) CAH reported that pregnancy was desired by half of the sample. In the cohort, 85/190 women reported 187 pregnancies and 141 births, with 2 infants diagnosed with classical CAH (Bidet et al., 2010). The rate of miscarriage was significantly lowered by glucocorticoid treatment at 6.5%, compared to 26.3% without treatment.

It may always be difficult to separate biological from psychosocial factors in lower conception rates in CAH. The latter may include fewer heterosexual interests, sexual difficulties due to anatomical or psychological reasons, and disinterest in motherhood, which is increasingly prevalent in regions of the world where more women can access financial security and enjoy diverse social roles. There is a dearth of research on how important biological parenthood is to people with CAH. Research almost always caters to medical and technocentric possibilities.

In another substantial French study, this time in TS, Bernard et al. (2016) assessed the prevalence and outcomes of spontaneous pregnancies (SP) in 480 women in 7 endocrine services in France. TS is associated with, among other health concerns, premature ovarian insufficiency. The researchers identified 27 women (5.6%) who had a total of 52 SPs, which resulted in 30 full-term deliveries for 18 women. The strongest predictive factors for SP were spontaneous menarche (first menstrual period) and chromosomal mosaicism (combination of 45,X and 46,XX). The women took 0–84 months to conceive (median 6 months). Miscarriage was twice as prevalent as the general French population, and Caesarean sections were more than twice as prevalent. TS was diagnosed in two of the births in this cohort. The research team concluded that SP outcomes are more favorable than egg donation in TS patients and that fetal chromosomal variations were relatively high.

In terms of Swyer syndrome, which is significantly more rare than CAH and TS, a UK retrospective notes review identified a cohort of 29 women (Michala et al., 2008). Fertility was achieved with egg donation in three women, all of whom had live births and one subsequently had a second successful pregnancy. The uterine size and shape was assessed in eight women after completion of induction of puberty. The uterine cross-section was found to be significantly lower than that in non-Swyer controls. The authors concluded that early diagnosis and adequate hormone replacement might improve the uterine size and shape, which could affect pregnancy outcome.

Reports on testicular sperm extraction (TESE) combined with intra-cytoplasmic sperm injection (ICSI) to achieve conception offer the possibility of biological parenthood for people with KS. Sperm is recoverable from the testes in about half (44%–55%) of the KS population. Sperm extraction, however, does not translate directly to live births, as there are many steps between the two outcomes. Vloeberghs et al. (2018) criticized the literature for its proneness to biased reporting that can mislead people, for example by giving sperm retrieval estimates, when it is clearly live births that matter to ART consumers. The authors reported results from a lengthy follow-up of 138 KS patients having a first testicular biopsy between January 1994 and December 2013. They reported that per intention-to-treat, only 10.1% (14/138) of care users starting treatment eventually succeeded in having biological children. The report suggested that KS patients and their partners seeking treatment by TESE–ICSI should be counseled that the chance of sperm retrieval is fair but that the chance of having a genetic child is low.

Caretakers of children with certain variations can opt to have the child's gonads removed and experimentally preserved (Islam et al., 2019). Words to the effect of "reproductive potential" and "fertility preservation," even when there is no known fertility, resonate with narratives of innovation and breakthrough that characterize ART (Hodson & Bewley, 2019). These discourses justify nonconsensual gonadectomy. Postgonadectomy, the XY children will have to undergo pubertal induction. In theory, caretakers can opt for the child to have only one gonad removed. However, children who eventually have the second gonad removed will be doubling the surgical risks. The ethical implication of false hope has also been raised (Campo-Engelstein et al., 2017).

A multinational European study with a low participation rate (and therefore unknown generalizability) examined fertility outcomes in a mixed DSD cohort with a mean age of 32 years (Słowikowska-Hilczer et al., 2017). The study confirmed what is known about the variability between DSD diagnoses in terms of spontaneous conception and ART potential and that the diagnosis associated with the highest conception rates is nonclassical CAH, followed by classical CAH. Of the cohort of 1 039 people, 33% reported living with a partner; there was no report of nonlive-in partners. About 14% reported having at least one child as a result of spontaneous conception (3.5%), conception via ART (7%) or adoption (4%). The 3.5% of the sample who had reproduced without ART comprised mainly women with CAH. Among those in the overall sample who recalled receiving information about fertility and options, 53% were satisfied with the way the question of fertility was discussed. In the total cohort, 30% were neither satisfied nor dissatisfied with the information, and about 17% were not satisfied with the way fertility was discussed. These percentages offer no insight on how participants construct fertility-related concerns and the nature of their satisfaction and dissatisfaction with the information given. Attitudes to childfreedom were not assessed, even though it is blindingly obvious that this is a valid and important option for people with variations to explore with openness.

There is a dearth of research to elicit rich accounts of the diverse ways in which people with variations make sense of fertility-related concerns. Without a nuanced literature, infertility is assumed to have a blanket negative effect on service users. My actual practice experience suggests that the person with a variation is much less likely to be emotionally overwhelmed than their caretakers. The following excerpts from a qualitative study in androgen insensitivity syndrome are typical of the concerns expressed by caretakers about their child's future (Le Maréchal, 2001):

All I could think about was, you know, they can't have children. (p. 81)

So she could be a very unhappy, lonely lady in later life because . . . the one person she loves might not want her because of those reasons. (p. 102)

A study suggested that caretakers of children with KS are more likely than adult patients with KS and their partners to express a wish to use ART (Maiburg et al., 2011). My experience in counseling adolescents and adults with variations is that infertility is a concern of variable magnitude, ranging from absent distress, even relief, to high distress. Furthermore, any distress is often informed more by a fear of rejection by an actual or imaginary partner than by a strong personal desire to be a biological parent. People who are not currently in a stable relationship may imagine that they would be rejected on account of infertility. People who are in a stable relationship may imagine that the partner who has accepted their infertility would change their mind later. By far the majority of people with variations who have spoken to me about infertility and relationship concerns talk about these concerns as if they are unique to them rather than as widely shared in society.

14.2   Psychosocial Research in Infertility

Infertility, defined as an inability to conceive after 12 months of unprotected heterosexual intercourse, is surprisingly difficult to estimate. Prevalence in women aged 25–49 years ranges from 15% in high-income countries to 30% in Middle Africa between 1994 and 2000 (Petraglia et al., 2013). Lifestyle factors that affect reproductive health include delayed childbearing, obesity, nonexercise or overexercise, inappropriate diet, smoking, psychological stress, alcohol and/or caffeine consumption and exposure to environmental pollutants and chemicals. In low-income countries, genital tract infections and sexually transmitted diseases are also important factors.

Fertility problems can be temporary or permanent but, in any case, at any particular time point, it is indefinite. A primary life goal that is taken for granted is threatened with permanent loss. Psychological research is based largely on convenience samples from fertility clinics. This means that our understanding of how people experience infertility is mixed up with the psychological impact of fertility treatment. Research samples are prone to white middle-class biases, partly because of prohibiting treatment costs (in most countries) that exclude many social groups. Research is also biased toward quantifying psychological distress, which is often pathologized. Such approaches render invisible the experiences of people who do not seek treatment (Culley et al., 2013).

Experience of infertility is shaped by cultural, social and psychological factors. An individual's identities and strengths, the presence or absence of concomitant psychological difficulties, the access to a wide range of social roles and the characteristics of the partnership can determine the degree of distress and coping. Responses to infertility are also moderated by available support within the individual's social environment. Psychological distress is neither a universal nor inevitable response to infertility (e.g., Benyamini et al., 2005). A path analysis of data from a sample of 119 women in New York suggested that gender role identity, career role salience, felt societal pressure and cognitive appraisal accounted for 32% of the variance in distress (Miles et al., 2009). Boivin et al. (2007) estimated that the international prevalence of infertility (of 12 months) was about 9% and that just over half of impacted couples seek treatment. The authors suggested that the treatment rate was lower than previously cited but that they were remarkably similar between more or less developed nations.

14.2.1   Assisted Reproductive Technology

For many people whose circumstances enable them to take advantage of ART, the fertility treatment journey is one of agonizing decisions, the raising of hope and the crushing of dreams. Investigation and treatment take time; outcome is unpredictable. Major changes to lifestyle are required to accommodate multiple clinic appointments, rigid medication schedules and recovery from procedures. Career choices and other important life goals are often suspended. Given the disruptions, anxiety and mood fluctuations are hardly surprising. Women tend to undergo the bulk of the invasive procedures, are responsible for daily monitoring of their menstrual cycles and put the rest of life on hold to accommodate rigid treatment processes. For heterosexual couples, women tend to take on more of the psychological burden, even when the factor lies with the male partner. Nevertheless, interviews with heterosexual men have identified considerable distress especially in men with male-factor infertility (Throsby & Gill, 2004). Research suggested that infertile men experience low self-esteem and high levels of anxiety and that these difficulties persisted 18 months after treatment, regardless of whether a live birth was achieved (Glover et al., 1999).

ART outcome is binary – baby or no baby. For many, adjustment to childlessness is merely delayed rather than averted. Meanwhile, couples may judge themselves for being stressed, which is often believed to be causing treatment to fail. The majority of people will have tried to control their stress at some stage via a wide range of methods, some more outlandish than others. As the ART process itself is conducive to making people feel out of control, effects of these remedies, from homeopathy to acupuncture, are often transitory.

Despite the many drawbacks, business is booming. Reproductive tourism is a growing economy, due to country-specific legislation and varying access to different forms of ART. Donor egg IVF accounts for over 25 000 IVF cycles annually in Europe and 20 000 cycles in the USA (see Deveaux, 2016). Egg brokers and bankers can recruit and arrange transportation of donors and frozen eggs and embryos worldwide. The economics of course say nothing of the physical and psychological burden of and risks to both consumers and donors.

Some industrialized countries make allowance for altruistic gestational surrogacy while others ban it completely. Prohibition and/or high costs have led to individuals and couples of wealthy nations looking beyond borders for reproductive opportunities. India is well known for having turned surrogacy into a multimillion dollar market serving couples from all over the world (Arvidsson et al., 2015). It has accordingly been called "a transnational hub for surrogacy" (Kirby, 2014, p. 24). Critics highlight the stark power imbalances between commissioning parents and surrogate mothers and contend that the global fertility market is structured along class, ethnic and racial lines, with infinite potential for exploitation. The typically limited contact between commissioning parents and surrogate mothers render it impossible to obtain detailed knowledge of how surrogate mothers are treated. Research has alarmingly identified that surrogate mothers are often not properly informed about treatment and risks and therefore cannot be deemed to have given their informed consent (e.g., Tanderup et al., 2015). A study of Swedish parents' constructions of transnational surrogacy identified colliding discourses (Arvidsson et al., 2015). While the commissioning parents rejected the exploitation discourse, they also argued for regulation to protect surrogate mothers from exploitation. Reflections on the legal protection of surrogate children and the women giving birth to them were evident in the research partipants' talk.

14.2.2 Adoption

Although attitudes toward adoption have changed in a positive direction in many countries, it is still culturally constructed as second best. Adoptive parents are sometimes positioned as desperate and sometimes as heroes (Weistra & Luke, 2017). Adoption is rarely considered to have been an active choice. Innocent questions to adoptive parents include why they have not tried IVF and who are the children's "real" parents. The questions reflect the construction of adoption as a last-ditch attempt to have children when all else fails. These attitudes denigrate adoptive parents and children and are deeply disrespectful.

In such a context, a person may be revealing their biological infertility when choosing to adopt. This can be an inhibiting factor for those who might otherwise have chosen to adopt rather than have biological children. However, the biggest barrier is the level of scrutiny and testing required of adoptive parents to have the necessary skills and resources and support to meet the additional physical, emotional, developmental and educational needs of adoptees. Potential adoptive parents talk about the many hurdles in the adoption process including, for example, having to prove that they have grieved sufficiently for their losses, sometimes in writing. They have also to be open to the authorities regarding their personal financial details, their parenting role models and any experiences of trauma and difficulties in their own childhood.

14.2.3 Gender Differences

The multibillion-dollar international ART business is criticized for treating women's bodies as objects for experimentation and for both exploiting and reifying the conflation of womanhood with motherhood. The increasingly technological processes privilege medical experts and remove control from women whose body is the main object of intervention. Inhorn (2007), however, disputed earlier feminist credo that women's bodies are violated in IVF while men's bodies go untouched. Rather, new forms of ART involving testicular sperm extraction also render the recipient objectified and docile, yet male experiences of infertility and treatment are obscured. Hinton and Miller (2013) suggested that we move from a gender-difference to a gender-inclusive orientation in research and make sense of maternal and paternal identities in a context of fertility business expansion and attendant dilemmatic decision-making.

A nuanced analysis offered detailed insight into men's treatment experiences (Throsby & Gill, 2004). Compared to their partners and wives, the men were more invested in positive discourses about scientific innovation, yet they were also invested in seeing IVF as a mechanical aid to boost a natural process. An observation that resonates with my clinical experience is the way in which men frequently presented themselves as supporters and women as the decision-makers (Hinton & Miller, 2013; Throsby & Gill, 2004). Infertility in men carries the meaning of impotence. It may be face-saving for heterosexual partners to position treatment as a women's issue and men as a supportive and pragmatic bystander. But this means that many women experience their male partners as unemotional and unwilling to share their grief and many men feel that their pain is minimized.

In contrast to the aforementioned study, which observed that men tended to be scathing about low-tech approaches to enhancing their own fertility, such as dietary changes, stopping smoking and giving up alcohol (Thorsby & Gill, 2004), a recent study found that there are more male interests in lifestyle adaptations in online anonymous forums (Hanna et al., 2018). Here, male fertility is discussed as malleable; fitness to father is questioned where commitment to make lifestyle changes to boost the chance of conception is not demonstrated.

14.2.4 *Psychological Support*

Research indicates that fertility problems can precipitate a range of difficult emotions. Reports of anger, shame and guilt for failing the other partner are not uncommon. Under pressure to keep up with coital performance, many heterosexual couples report a loss of sexual spontaneity and pleasure. Research in several European countries (where treatment is free or partly free) reported that a high proportion of people had dropped out of treatment because of emotional distress (see Cousineau & Domar, 2007). In Figure 14.1, I draw on the Power Threat Meaning Framework (see Chapter 7) to make sense of individuals' and couples' fertility-related distress, responses to which are,

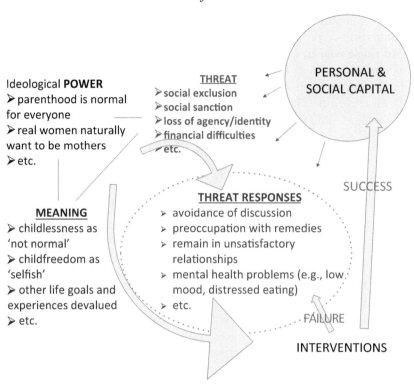

Figure 14.1   A Power Threat Meaning understanding of fertility distress. A colour version of this figure can be found in the plate section.

suffice to say, mitigated by personal factors such as the availability of social support, financial resources and alternative life goals.

Given the physical, emotional, social and financial demands, one would think that psychological preparation for treatment is the norm. Preparation might sensibly include socializing service users into an effective model of stress management prior to the start of treatment. And, given the value of social support to mitigate the ongoing effects of anxiety, stigma and powerlessness, individuals and couples could be prepared to take some risks to confide in trusted family and friends. Regular monitoring of psychological well-being might be built into fertility services. The cost of such low-tech input would be minuscule relative to the astronomical treatment fees. And yet, in my years of supporting ART consumers, the psychological presentation of women, men and couples was strongly suggestive of a culture where absence of psychological care is acceptable and where the offer of an optional rubber-stamping session with a counselor was sufficient to meet licensing requirements. Distressed ART consumers, which included many middle-aged single women and couples, were disproportionately represented in a stillbirth clinic where I provided counseling for some years. As I remember the many distraught clients, the following words of two medical experts (Bewley & Kisby Littleton, 2016) come to mind: "Assisted reproduction technology (ART) is often framed within a discourse of 'innovation,' 'break-through,' and 'success,' and less commonly in terms of 'human experimentation,' 'safety,' and 'harm' in vulnerable, infertile women" (p. 1876).

Ten sessions of group cognitive-behavioral therapy (CBT) has been shown to reduce self-reported psychological distress in infertile women, although the results require replication with tighter control (Domar et al., 2000). More recently, a randomized controlled trial compared 10 sessions of CBT with a low-dose antidepressant for women who scored themselves on a depression scale in the mild to moderate range (Faramarzi et al., 2013). These researchers conceptualized psychological outcome along five factors hypothesized to be integral to psychological distress: social concern, sexual concern, marital concern, rejection of childfree lifestyle and perceived need for parenthood. They reported that while medication resulted in a reduction of depression scores and also sexual concern scores, CBT resulted in a reduction of depression scores as well as scores on all of the five contributory concerns.

14.3   Childfree Lives

Researchers have urged for a distinction between childfreedom, which implies choice, and childlessness, which implies circumstance. However, pronatalist ideology appears to operate on childfree people in equal measure. Women especially are marked out as people who need to explain themselves for being childfree. Citing statistics in the USA, Moore (2014) reported that the rate of childfreedom is steady at just over 6% of women, who are more likely to be socially privileged and not religious (p. 162). In her research in identity construction, the author observed multiple and sometimes contradictory ways of relating to the concept of childfreedom, with some participants self-identifying as intentional nonparents and others describing themselves as being ordinary people who were uninterested in children.

A recent study of a representative sample of 981 Michigan adults aimed to estimate the prevalence of childfree individuals, to examine how childfree individuals differ from parents, not-yet-parents and childless individuals in terms of life satisfaction, political ideology and personality, and to examine whether childfree individuals are viewed as outsiders (Watling Neal & Neal, 2021). Over a quarter of the sample identified as childfree. The researchers observed no differences in life satisfaction across the groups and only limited differences in personality traits between childfree individuals and the other groups. Childfree individuals were observed to be more politically liberal than the parents in the sample. Furthermore, those who have children or those who want(ed) children expressed substantially less warmth toward the childfree individuals, suggesting that there is a level of prejudice against childfree people in the general population. These observations render it unsurprising that childfree people mobilize different discourses to justify what ought to be an equally legitimate form of existence.

As a form of ideological power, pronatalism operates selectively on lives and especially female lives (Moore, 2014). Healthy and successful white women who choose to be childfree are admonished for their selfishness. Poorer women of color are frowned upon for having too many children. Mothers with disabilities are under pressure to prove that they are deserving of motherhood.

Research with childfree women suggests that childfreedom is often constructed as a choice to have an advantageous lifestyle, such as enhancement of career and income and being carefree. Some childfree women, however, disavow the rhetoric of choice. Peterson and Engwall (2013), for example, identified essentialist explanations by Swedish childfree women as having been born without an innate urge to reproduce. It is suggested that the rhetoric of choice attracts stigma and that the positioning of childfreedom as a natural (deficit) state enables women to bypass criticism for choosing not to bear children (Morison et al., 2016). Gillespie (2003) argued that analyses of childfreedom can recast understandings of feminine identity outside the normative motherhood discourses.

Clarke et al. (2018) pointed out that the burgeoning literature in successful ART and parenthood outcomes in LGBTQ+ communities might have erased the highly meaningful experience of being childfree, in a society that continues to conflate motherhood with womanhood. They argue that in excluding the voices of women opting out of motherhood, there is a risk of excluding the experiences of those who do not fit into dominant heterosexual norms. They drew attention to the strong parenthood expectations of queer youth in a postequality era. In an attempt to redress research leaning on what motivates queer people to choose to parent rather than what motivates them to remain childfree, these authors interviewed British lesbian women about their experience. Their study suggested that even for a group for whom childlessness may be expected to be less remarkable, it is difficult to articulate a desire to remain childfree. However, the researchers noted that childfreedom was far less isolating for lesbian than for heterosexual women. In a subsequent study, the research group suggested that negotiating childfreedom was precarious and required constant maintenance (Hayfield et al., 2019). In other words, childfreedom cannot be taken for granted as a valid and ordinary form of existence.

Using a phenomenological design, Stahnke et al. (2020) interviewed 14 women over the age of 65 to gain a deeper understanding of the overall life satisfaction of older women who have not had children. They explored the following questions: 1) What is the overall sense of life satisfaction of childfree women over 65 years of age? 2) What is the lived experience of being a childfree woman in US society? 3) How does being childfree inform women's overall life satisfaction? The researchers observed that nearly all participants reported a high life satisfaction and many reported a strong sense of resilience. However, the interviewees also reported an awareness of the stigma associated with their status as nonmothers.

14.4   Practice Vignette

Below is a truncated version of a piece of work that PCP "Mike" has carried out with a couple, and his reflections on the constraints placed upon the counseling process embedded within a technocentric treatment environment.

Jas and Tim are in their mid-30s. They married three years ago and started to "try for a family" right away. After 12 months of lack of success, they were referred to a fertility clinic, where Tim was diagnosed with KS. This news came as a shock but also a relief to the couple – at least there was an explanation for their troubles, and there was still a chance for them to have biological children. They quickly decided to focus on treatment. A relaxed and experienced "Dr. Rossi," the fertility doctor at the clinic, flanked by walls of baby photos, thank-you letters and bottles of wine with gilded labels, spoke to the anxious couple as follows: "Look, there is no need to be so upset. Technology is improving all the time. You can stay hopeful. But remember, there are now a few extra steps for you to take. It's a choice, and I would be happier if you could think it over with our fertility counselor." As well as referring the couple to Mike, Dr. Rossi also refers Tim to the endocrinologist "Dr. Dowling" to assess his long-term health needs on account of the KS diagnosis.

The clinic receptionist organizes an appointment with Mike for the couple with an explanation – in a hushed tone, that "this is just routine."

At the appointment, Mike asks Jas and Tim what they would like to work on. The couple look confused. Jas says, "Oh, we thought you're here to check that we're capable of deciding because we, we're going to do the sperm suction method at this clinic."

Mike engages equally with the couple by drawing on *circular questioning* techniques, which was developed by a group of Milanese family therapists in the 1980s (see Brown, 1997). As well as eliciting thoughts and feelings informed by different ideas, circular prompts and questions offer dyads and families the opportunity to comment on the nature of their relationships with each other. The rationale of circular questioning is summarized as follows:

> The aim of circular questioning is to fix the point in the history of the system when important coalitions underwent a shift and the subsequent adaptation of that shift became problematic for the family. The information sought by circular questions is the differences in relationships the family has experienced before and after the problem began. (Penn, 1982, p. 272)

The therapist may ask questions to highlight differences between verbal and nonverbal information. For example, they may comment, "You say you're angry with your sister, but I see that you are also smiling." The therapist may also inquire into the differences between how the problem/solution is understood at different times. For example, a therapist may ask, "The meaning seems to have changed for you, I wonder what your father may have noticed." By charting differences between the views of family members and how each member may have changed their views over time, particularly around the presenting problem, relational patterns and what is up for negotiation can unfold.

In the simplified excerpt below, Mike seeks to understand how Jas and Tim relate to the KS diagnosis and its implications for their relationship:

MIKE: So which one of you knows the most about KS?

JAS: We've both read the booklet given to us by Dr. Rossi. I'm glad it's KS and nothing more. It could have been so much worse.

MIKE: [Turns to Tim] Jas thinks it could be a lot worse, what are your thoughts?

TIM: Well, it's good to know I don't have anything life threatening, but I'm still in a quandary. Put it this way, I am being told, in so many words, that I am a little bit female. That's a lot to take on. Dr. Dowling asked if I wanted to see a breast surgeon. Okay, I am not very muscular up here [puts his hand on his chest] but I thought that was me being too lazy to go to the gym. Now I, I have a gyne, I'm told I have a gynemastic condition? Wow, I didn't see that coming.

MIKE: A bit female? Gynecomastia? [Turns to Jas] What do you make of the words that Tim's just used?

JAS: He's too hung up on what he's read, what he's been told. To me he's the
        same man. Nothing's changed. I guess we'll just have to let Tim get past that.
MIKE: [Turns to Tim] You and Jas seem to have a slightly different take on KS
        at the moment, what kind of effects do these different views have?
TIM: What do you mean?
MIKE: I mean, if I knew you both before the KS diagnosis, what changes would
        I notice about you as a couple?

Throughout the conversation, Mike notices that Tim is more committed
to talking about KS than Jas. Furthermore, in terms of decision to undergo
TESE, he is much more hesitant than her:

JAS: Dr. Rossi says we can have up to a 50% chance of having a biological child
        with what they do here.
MIKE: [Turns to Tim] Do you share the same understanding as Jas?
JIM: No, no, oh no, I didn't hear 50%. I thought I heard 10%. Maybe I heard
        both 10 and 50%. That's, that's a huge difference. We can't commit to, to
        the, the TESE, without knowing more . . .
MIKE: [Turns to Jas] So Tim thinks that the chance of a biological baby between
        you two can be much less than 50%, how does that affect your view?
JAS: Oh I don't know. Let's call it 10%, it's still worth it. Someone has to be in
        the 10%, why couldn't it be us? I know it's not guaranteed, but we work
        hard, what's money for if not to invest in what we both want the most?
TIM: Well no, it's not as simple as that. I'm the one who's going to have to go
        through the extraction. First I'm told XXY, then I'm told I have a female
        body, now my, my testicles are going to be needled. I don't know if I can
        keep up with your breakneck speed, Jas.
MIKE: Jas, sounds like you're more ready for treatment to start, but Tim wants to
        think about what KS means for him first. What would you like him to do next?
JAS: You'll have to ask Tim. He's obsessed with reading about men with KS on
        the internet.
MIKE: KS men's stories, Tim?
TIM: I've actually spoken to one of the men, a dad, real nice guy, he's adopted a
        kid and very happy.
MIKE: And is adoption something to include in our conversation?
JAS: Now wait a minute, I'm confused. I have no idea that Tim has been
        talking to other people about us. [Looks surprised] [Turns to Tim] When
        did this happen? There I was, looking for a nutritionist to get you in shape
        for the TESE . . . . And there you are, getting distracted . . .

The couple acknowledge that they are "not on the same page" regarding
treatment. They agree to continue with counseling. Jas is angry with Tim
for losing his focus on the TESE–ICSI offer, which she thought they had
both signed up to. She is highly emotional when she says, "if adoption is
what you had in mind, why didn't you say so at the beginning?"

Mike experiences the medical environment as problematic for the in-depth work that he would have liked to offer Tim and Jas. In the current service context, however, the couple's entire lives are compressed into a technological frame. He shares his frustration with the couple and invites them to engage with him in a different frame, "I would have loved to know more about the non-problem part of your lives, like your strengths, interests … how did you meet, how did you fall in love, how did you decide to commit to a future together …"

Pronatalism is a pervasive ideology that "naturalizes" the desire of couples, especially heterosexuals, to have children. It does not usually require any thought. The desire not to have children, on the other hand, almost always requires continuous explanation. Most of Jas and Tim's peers have children. Jas has been reminded within her social network that her "biological clock" is ticking. She sees how the pregnant women at work are rewarded with attention and approval. She is assumed to be too "career-driven" and taking a big biological risk by waiting. This is ironic, because Jas is actually extremely jealous of colleagues going on parental leave to have children. She is too ashamed to tell friends and family about her struggles. In addition to these struggles, Tim has not wanted to have sex with her for many months. She feels rejected by the world ("I don't know who I am anymore"). Jas feels increasingly isolated and out of control.

Tim appreciates the pressure of the "biological clock" on Jas. He feels guilty for letting her down ("I can't give her a baby"). At the same time, he is somewhat taken aback at her apparent disinterest in the implications of his genetic variation. He feels that Jas is placing the potential child ahead of him. The couple are disappointed in each other's response to the challenges that they are facing. They agree to inform both sets of parents of the situation. However, they do not find either set of responses helpful.

Jas is very close to her mother "Sally," who disapproves of sperm donation as another option because that would mean that her daughter is having a child with another man. Sally advises Tim out of love – she wants him to be the "real" father: "You should have more faith in technology," she says, "doctors can make anything happen these days, just let them help you." To enthuse Tim, Sally searches the Internet for stories of success, including expectant parents into their 50s and 60s. She even drops into conversation anecdotes "incidentally" about someone who died years ago and is now "living on" in the happy child conceived posthumously with stored gametes. But, far from tempting Tim to start treatment, Sally's "medical miracles" are alienating him. His own parents' reactions are equally unhelpful, if in a different way. They worry about their son's long-term health and wonder if they may have "passed on the bad genes" to him. They resent Jas' "obsession with getting pregnant" and the attendant pressure on their son. But this is not at all how Tim experiences Jas, toward whom he feels empathy and guilt in equal measure.

Some years on, Mike still thinks about Jas and Tim and what he has learned from his work with them. The couple no longer attend clinic. Dr. Rossi remembers the couple too. She is able to recall that the TESE was successful but the ICSI was not. She does not know what happened to the couple after that.

14.5   Reflexivity

Valorization of parenthood positions childlessness as a tragedy, inconsolable distress as a natural consequence, and ART as hope and light. Psychosocial research that is complicit with the negative operation of pronatalist ideology predictably produces problem-saturated accounts, which are then framed as a medical problem that requires a medical solution. Psychosocial research that does not begin and end with pronatalist standpoints suggests that inconsolable distress is neither universal nor inevitable. This research seeks to widen the restricted view of adult possibilities and has much to offer psychological practice.

Psychological input can help individuals and couples to contemplate parenthood options but, within an intense physical treatment context involving high financial stakes, where treatment is set up as a default position, psychological exploration is compressed and distorted. It can be difficult for conversations to get beyond the pros and cons of treatment and to discuss coping strategies for surviving the highly intrusive medical process. Away from a treatment context, however, psychological input can additionally guide individuals and couples to explore personal meaning of no treatment and nonparenthood. It can facilitate service users to grieve for what is not possible, challenge feelings of deviance and shame, reengage with a range of life goals and, perhaps most important of all, recast adult identities.

References

Abdulcadir, J., Rodriguez M., & Say, L. (2015). A systematic review of the evidence on clitoral reconstruction after female genital mutilation/cutting. *International Journal of Gynaecology & Obstetrics*, *129*(2), 93–97.

Abelow Hedley, L. (2006). The seduction of the surgical fix. In E. Parens (Ed.), *Surgically shaping children: Technology, ethics, and the pursuit of normality* (pp. 43–48). Johns Hopkins University Press.

Ahmed, S. F., Achermann, J., Alderson, J., Crouch, N. S., Elford, S., Hughes, I. A., . . . Turner, H. E. (2021). Society for Endocrinology UK guidance on the initial evaluation of a suspected difference or disorder of sex development (revised 2021). *Clinical Endocrinology*, *95*(6), 818–840.

Ahmed, S. F., Gardner, M., & Sandberg, D. E. (2014). Management of children with disorders of sex development: New care standards explained. *Psychology & Sexuality*, *5*(1), 5–14.

Ahmed, S. F., Khwaja, O., & Hughes, I. A. (2000). The role of a clinical score in the assessment of ambiguous genitalia. *British Journal of Urology International*, *85*(1), 120–124.

Alderson, J., Madill, A., & Balen, A. (2004). Fear of devaluation: Understanding the experience of intersexed women with androgen insensitivity syndrome. *British Journal of Health Psychology*, *9*(1), 81–100.

Alderson, J., Skae, M., & Crowne, E. C. (2022). Parental perceptions of the necessity, benefit, and cost of early childhood clitoral surgery for congenital adrenal hyperplasia (CAH). *International Journal of Impotence Research*. https://doi.org/10.1038/s41443-022-00578-0

Alizai, N. K., Thomas, D. F. M., Lilford, R. J., Batchelor, A. G. G., & Johnson, N. (1999). Feminizing genitoplasty for congenital adrenal hyperplasia: What happens at puberty? *Journal of Urology*, *161*(5), 1588–1591.

American Academy of Pediatrics. (1995). Informed consent, parental permission, and assent in pediatric practice (RE9510). *Pediatrics*, *95*(2), 314–317.

(2000). Evaluation of the newborn with developmental anomalies of the external genitalia. *Pediatrics*, *106*(1), 138–142.

Amnesty International. (2017). *First do no harm: Ensuring the rights of children with variations of sex characteristics in Denmark and Germany*. www.amnesty.org/en/documents/euro1/6086/2017/en/

Androgen Insensitivity Syndrome Support Group Australia, Intersex Trust Aotearoa New Zealand, Organisation Intersex International Australia … Carpenter, M. (2017). *Darlington statement*. Retrieved February 22, 2022, from https://darlington.org.au/statement

Angier, A. (1996, February 4). Intersexual healing: An anomaly finds a group. *New York Times*.

Annas, G. J. (1992). The patient rights movement. In *The rights of patients* (pp. 1–16). Humana Press.

Anonymous. (1994). Once a dark secret. *British Medical Journal, 308*, 542.
  (2018, April 4). *Grieving the loss of the perfect child*. https://tripleamommy.com/2018/04/04/grieving-the-loss-of-the-perfect-child

Anonymous Parent. (2021). Parenting intersex children: Sensitive medical care and peer support that make the difference. *Journal of Pediatric Ethics, 1*(4), 169–170.

Anonymous Parents. (2021). Our beautiful child. *Journal of Pediatric Ethics, 1*(4), 165–168.

Arkowitz, H., Miller, W. R., & Rollnick, S. (Eds.). (2015). *Motivational interviewing in the treatment of psychological problems*. Guilford Publications.

Arvidsson, A., Johnsdotter, S., & Essén, B. (2015). Views of Swedish commissioning parents relating to the exploitation discourse in using transnational surrogacy. *PLoS One, 10*(5), e0126518.

Aveline, M. (2005). The person of the therapist. *Psychotherapy Research, 15*(3), 155–164.

Azziz, R., Jones, H. W., & Rock, J. A. (1990). Androgen-insensitivity syndrome: Long-term results of surgical vaginal creation. *Journal of Gynecologic Surgery, 6*(1), 23–26.

Ball, C., Kirkby, M., & Williams, S. (2003). Effect of the critical care outreach team on patient survival to discharge from hospital and readmission to critical care: Non-randomised population based study. *British Medical Journal, 327*(7422), 1014.

Bangalore Krishna, K., Kogan, B. A., Ernst, M. M., Romao, R. L. P., Mohsin, F., Serrano-Gonzalez, M., … Lee, P. A. (2020). Individualized care for patients with intersex (disorders/differences of sex development): Part 3. *Journal of Pediatric Urology, 16*(5), 598–605.

Baratz, A. B., Sharp, M. K., & Sandberg, D. E. (2014). Disorders of sex development peer support. In O. Hiort & S. F. Ahmed (Eds.), *Understanding differences and disorders of sex development (DSD)* (Endocr. Dev., Vol. 27, pp. 99–112). Karger.

Barnett, D., Clements, M., Kaplan-Estrin, M., & Fialka, J. (2003). Building new dreams: Supporting parents' adaptation to their child with special needs. *Infants & Young Children, 16*(3), 184–200.

Barsky, J. L., Friedman, M. A., & Rosen, R. C. (2006). Sexual dysfunction and chronic illness: The role of flexibility in coping. *Journal of Sex & Marital Therapy, 32*(3), 235–253.

Bellomo, R., Goldsmith, D., Uchino, S., Buckmaster, J., Hart, G., Opdam, H., . . . Gutteridge, G. (2004). Prospective controlled trial of effect of medical emergency team on postoperative morbidity and mortality rates. *Critical Care Medicine, 32*(4), 916–921.

Bennecke, E., Köhler, B., Röhle, R., Thyen, U., Gehrmann, K., Lee, P., . . . Wiesemann, C. (2021). Disorders or differences of sex development? Views of affected individuals on DSD terminology. *Journal of Sex Research, 58*(4), 522–531.

Bennecke, E., Werner-Rosen, K., Thyen, U., Kleinemeier, E., Lux, A., Jürgensen, M., . . . Köhler, B. (2015). Subjective need for psychological support (PsySupp) in parents of children and adolescents with disorders of sex development (DSD). *European Journal of Pediatrics, 174*(10), 1287–1297.

Benyamini, Y., Gozlan, M., & Kokia, E. (2005). Variability in the difficulties experienced by women undergoing infertility treatments. *Fertility and Sterility, 83*(2), 275–283.

Berenbaum, S. A., & Bailey, J. M. (2003). Effects on gender identity of prenatal androgens and genital appearance: Evidence from girls with congenital adrenal hyperplasia. *Journal of Clinical Endocrinology & Metabolism, 88*(3), 1102–1106.

Berenbaum, S. A., & Meyer-Balhburg, H. F. L. (2015). Gender development and sexuality in disorders of sex development. *Hormone Metabolism and Research, 47*(5), 361–366.

Bernard, V., Donadille, B., Zenaty, D., Courtillot, C., Salenave, S., Brac de la Perrière, A., . . . Christin-Maitre, S. (2016). Spontaneous fertility and pregnancy outcomes amongst 480 women with Turner syndrome. *Human Reproduction, 31*(4), 782–788.

Berry, M. D., & Lezos, A. M. (2017). Inclusive sex therapy practices: A qualitative study of the techniques sex therapists use when working with diverse sexual populations. *Sexual and Relationship Therapy, 32*(1), 2–21.

Bethell, G. S., Chhabra, S., Shalaby, M. S., Corbett, H., Kenny, S. E., Godse, A., . . . Kalidasan, V. (2020). Parental decisional satisfaction after hypospadias repair in the United Kingdom. *Journal of Pediatric Urology, 16*(2), 164-e1–164-e7.

Bewley, S., & Kisby Littleton, F. (2016). How should we honour and memorialise the experimental subjects who gave their hopes and lives to the development of in vitro fertilisation in Britain in the 1970s? *BJOG: An International Journal of Obstetrics & Gynaecology, 123*(11), 1876.

Bidet, M., Bellanné-Chantelot, C., Galand-Portier, M.-B., Golmard, J.-L., Tardy, V., Morel, Y., . . . Kuttenn, T. F. (2010). Fertility in women with nonclassical congenital adrenal hyperplasia due to 21-hydroxylase deficiency. *Journal of Clinical Endocrinology & Metabolism, 95*(3), 1182–1190.

Billig, M., Condor, S., Edwards, D., Gane, M., Middleton, D., & Radley, A. (1988). *Ideological dilemmas: A social psychology of everyday thinking.* Sage.

Blackless, M., Charuvastra, A., Derryck, A., Fausto-Sterling, A., Lauzanne, K., & Lee, E. (2000). How sexually dimorphic are we? Review and synthesis. *American Journal of Human Biology*, *12*(2), 151–166.

Boivin, J., Bunting, L., Collins, J. A., & Nygren, K. G. (2007). International estimates of infertility prevalence and treatment-seeking: Potential need and demand for infertility medical care. *Human Reproduction*, *22*(6), 1506–1512.

Borrill, C., West, M., Shapiro, D., & Rees, A. (2000). Team working and effectiveness in health care. *British Journal of Healthcare Management*, *6*(8), 364–371.

Bossio, J. A., Basson, R., Driscoll, M., Correia, S., & Brotto, L. A. (2018). Mindfulness-based group therapy for men with situational erectile dysfunction: A mixed-methods feasibility analysis and pilot study. *Journal of Sexual Medicine*, *15*(10), 1478–1490.

Bostock, S., & Steptoe, A. (2012). Association between low functional health literacy and mortality in older adults: Longitudinal cohort study. *BMJ*, *344*, e1602.

Boyle, M. (2020). Power in the Power Threat Meaning Framework. *Constructivist Psychology*, *35*(1), 27–40.

Boyle, M., & Johnstone, L. (2020). *A straight talking introduction to the Power Threat Meaning Framework: An alternative to psychiatric diagnosis*. PCCS Books.

Boyle, M. E., Smith, S., & Liao, L. M. (2005). Adult genital surgery for intersex: A solution to what problem? *Journal of Health Psychology*, *10*(4), 573–584.

Boyse, K. L., Gardner, M., Marvicsin, D. J., & Sandberg, D. E. (2014). "It was an overwhelming thing": Parents' needs after infant diagnosis with congenital adrenal hyperplasia. *Journal of Pediatric Nursing*, *29*(5), 436–441.

Braga, L. H., Lorenzo, A. J., Bagli, D. J., Pippi Salle, J. L., & Caldamone, A. (2016). Application of the STROBE statement to the hypospadias literature: Report of the International Pediatric Urology Task Force on Hypospadias. *Journal of Pediatric Urology*, *12*(6), 367–380.

Brännström, M., Enskog, A., Kvarnström, N., Ayoubi, J. M., & Dahm-Kähler, P. (2019). Global results of human uterus transplantation and strategies for pre-transplantation screening of donors. *Fertility & Sterility*, *112*(1), 3–10.

Brömdal, A., Rasmussen, M. L., Sanjakdar, F., Allen, L., & Quinlivan, K. (2017). Intersex bodies in sexuality education: On the edge of cultural difference. In L. Allen & M. L. Rasmussen (Eds.), *The Palgrave handbook of sexuality education* (pp. 369–390). Palgrave Macmillan.

Brown, J. (1997). Circular questioning: An introductory guide. *Australian and New Zealand Journal of Family Therapy*, *18*(2), 109–114.

Brown-King, B. (2019, October 26). What dating as an intersex person taught me about self-acceptance. *Them*. https://www.them.us/story/dating-as-an-inter sex-person

Butler, G., De Graaf, N., Wren, B., & Carmichael, P. (2018). Assessment and support of children and adolescents with gender dysphoria. *Archives of Disease in Childhood*, *103*(7), 631–636.

Cadet, P., & Feldman, M. D. (2012). Pretense of a paradox: Factitious intersex conditions on the internet. *International Journal of Sexual Health, 24*(2), 91–96.

Callens, N., De Cuypere, G., Wolffenbuttel, K. P., Beerendonk, C. C., van der Zwan, Y. G., Van den Berg, M., ... Cools, M. (2012). Long-term psychosexual and anatomical outcome after vaginal dilation or vaginoplasty: A comparative study. *Journal of Sexual Medicine, 9*(7), 1842–1851.

Campo-Engelstein, L., Chen, D., Baratz, A. B., Johnson, E. K., & Finlayson, C. (2017). The ethics of fertility preservation for pediatric patients with differences (disorders) of sex development. *Journal of the Endocrine Society, 1*(6), 638–645.

Canning, D. A. (2015). Can we correct hypospadias with a staged operation? If not, are we bold enough to report it? *Journal of Urology, 194*(2), 284–285.

Carpenter, M. (2018a). What do intersex people need from doctors? *O&G Magazine, 20*(4), 32–33. https://www.ogmagazine.org.au/20/4-20/what-do-intersex-people-need-from-doctors/

(2018b). The "normalisation" of intersex bodies and "othering" of intersex identities. In J. Scherpe, A. Dutta, & T. Helms (Eds.), *The legal status of intersex persons* (pp. 445–514). Intersentia.

Carroll, L., Graff, C., Wicks, M., & Diaz Thomas, A. (2020). Living with an invisible illness: A qualitative study exploring the lived experiences of female children with congenital adrenal hyperplasia. *Quality of Life Research, 29*(3), 673–681.

Cecchin, G., Lane, G., & Ray, W. A. (1993). From strategizing to nonintervention: Toward irreverence in systemic practice. *Journal of Marital and Family Therapy, 19*(2), 125–136.

Chadwick, P. M., Liao, L. M., & Boyle, M. (2005). Size matters: Experiences of atypical genital and sexual development in males. *Journal of Health Psychology, 10*(4), 529–543.

Chadwick, P. M., Smyth, A., & Liao, L. M. (2014). Improving self-esteem in women diagnosed with Turner syndrome: Results of a pilot intervention. *Journal of Pediatric and Adolescent Gynecology, 27*(3), 129–132.

Chambers, C. (2008). *Sex, culture, and justice: The limits of choice.* Penn State University Press.

Chase, C. (1998). Hermaphrodites with attitude: Mapping the emergence of intersex political activism. *GLQ, 4*(2), 189–211.

(2003). What is the agenda of the intersex patient advocacy movement? *The Endocrinologist, 13*(3), 240–242.

Chivers, C., Burns, J., & Deiros Collado, M. (2017). Disorders of sex development: Mothers' experiences of support. *Clinical Child Psychology and Psychiatry, 22*(4), 675–690.

Clarke, V., Hayfield, N., Ellis, S. J., & Terry, G. (2018). Lived experiences of childfree lesbians in the United Kingdom: A qualitative exploration. *Journal of Family Issues, 39*(18), 4133–4155.

Coldicott, Y., Nesheim, B. I., MacDougall, J., Pope, C., & Roberts, C. (2003). The ethics of intimate examinations – teaching tomorrow's doctors.

Commentary: Respecting the patient's integrity is the key. Commentary: Teaching pelvic examination – putting the patient first. *BMJ, 326*(7380), 97–101.

Consortium on the Management of Disorders of Sex Development. (2006a). *Clinical guidelines for the management of disorders of sex development in childhood.* https://dsdguidelines.org/htdocs/clinical/

(2006b). *Handbook for parents.* https://dsdguidelines.org/files/parents.pdf

Conway, G. S. (2014). Disorders of sex development (DSD): An overview of recent scientific advances. *Psychology & Sexuality, 5*(1), 28–33.

(2022). Differences in sex development (DSD) and related conditions: Mechanisms, prevalences and changing practice. *International Journal of Impotence Research,* forthcoming.

Cools, M., Nordenström, A., Robeva, R., Hall, J., Westerveld, P., Flück, C., . . . Pasterski, V. (2018). Caring for individuals with a difference of sex development (DSD): A consensus statement. *Nature Reviews Endocrinology, 14*(7), 415–429.

Coughlin, M. B., & Sethares, K. A. (2017). Chronic sorrow in parents of children with a chronic illness or disability: An integrative literature review. *Journal of Pediatric Nursing, 37,* 108–116.

Cousineau, T. M., & Domar, A. D. (2007). Psychological impact of infertility. *Best Practice & Research Clinical Obstetrics and Gynaecology, 21*(2), 293e308.

Creighton, S., Alderson, J., Brown, S., & Minto, C. L. (2002). Medical photography: Ethics, consent and the intersex patient. *BJU International, 89*(1), 67–72.

Creighton, S., Chernausek, S. D., Romao, R., Ransley, P., & Salle, J. P. (2012). Timing and nature of reconstructive surgery for disorders of sex development – introduction. *Journal of Pediatric Urology, 8*(6), 602–610.

Creighton, S. M., Minto, C. L., Liao, L. M., Alderson, J., & Simmonds, M. (2004). Meeting between experts: Evaluation of the first UK forum for lay and professional experts in intersex. *Patient Education and Counseling, 54*(2), 153–157.

Creighton, S. M., Minto, C. L., & Steele, S. J. (2001). Objective cosmetic and anatomical outcomes at adolescence of feminising surgery for ambiguous genitalia done in childhood. *The Lancet, 358*(9276), 124–125.

Crissman, H. P., Warner, L., Gardner, M., Carr, M., Schast, A., Quittner, A. L., . . . Sandberg, D. E. (2011). Children with disorders of sex development: A qualitative study of early parental experience. *International Journal of Pediatric Endocrinology, 2011*(1), 1–11.

Crocetti, D., Monro, S., Vecchietti, V., & Yeadon-Lee, T. (2020). Towards an agency-based model of intersex, variations of sex characteristics (VSC) and DSD/dsd health. *Culture, Health & Sexuality, 23*(4), 500–515.

Crossley, M. L. (2000). *Introducing narrative psychology.* McGraw-Hill Education.

Crouch, N. S., Liao, L. M., Woodhouse, C. R., Conway, G. S., & Creighton, S. M. (2008). Sexual function and genital sensitivity following feminizing genitoplasty for congenital adrenal hyperplasia. *Journal of Urology, 179*(2), 634–638.

Cull, M. L., & Simmonds, M. (2010). Importance of support groups for intersex (disorders of sex development) patients, families and the medical profession. *Sexual Development, 4*(4–5), 310–312.

Culley, L., Hudson, N., & Lohan, M. (2013). Where are all the men? The marginalization of men in social scientific research on infertility. *Reproductive BioMedicine Online, 27*(3), 225–235.

D'Alberton, F. (2010). Disclosing disorders of sex development and opening the doors. *Sexual Development, 4*, 304–309.

Davies, J. H., Knight, E. J., Savage, A., Brown, J., & Malone, P. S. (2011). Evaluation of terminology used to describe disorders of sex development. *Journal of Pediatric Urology, 7*(4), 412–415.

Davis, G. (2015). *Contesting intersex: The dubious diagnosis*. New York University Press.

Davis, G., & Feder, E. (Eds.). (2015). Narrative symposium: Intersex. *Narrative Inquiry in Bioethics, 5*(2), 87–150.

Dear, J., Creighton, S. M., Conway, G. S., Williams, L., & Liao, L. M. (2019). Sexual experience before treatment for vaginal agenesis: A retrospective review of 137 women. *Journal of Pediatric & Adolescent Gynecology, 32*(3), 300–304.

De Clercq, E. (2022). Intersex in fictional films throughout history: Towards a cinema of inclusion?. In M. Walker (Ed.), *Interdisciplinary and global perspectives on intersex* (pp. 17–38). Palgrave Macmillan.

Delimata, N., Simmonds, M., O'Brien, M., Davis, G., Auchus, R., & Lin-Su, K. (2018). Evaluating the term 'disorders of sex development': A multidisciplinary debate. *Social Medicine, 12*(1), 98–107.

de Neve-Enthoven, N. G., Callens, N., Van Kuyk, M., Van Kuppenveld, J. H., Drop, S. L., Cohen–Kettenis, P. T., & Dessens, A. B. (2016). Psychosocial well-being in Dutch adults with disorders of sex development. *Journal of Psychosomatic Research, 83*, 57–64.

Deveaux, M. (2016). Exploitation, structural injustice, and the cross-border trade in human ova. *Journal of Global Ethics, 12*(1), 48–68.

Devore, H. (1999). Growing up in the surgical maelstrom. In A. D. Dreger (Ed.), *Intersex in the age of ethics* (pp. 79–89). University Publishing Group.

DiSandro, M., Merke, P., & Rink, R. C. (2015). Review of current surgical techniques and medical management considerations in the treatment of pediatric patients with disorders of sex development. *Hormone & Metabolism Research, 47*(5), 321–328.

Dittmann, R. W., Kappes, M. E., & Kappes, M. H. (1992). Sexual behavior in adolescent and adult females with congenital adrenal hyperplasia. *Psychoneuroendocrinology, 17*(2–3), 153–170.

Dodds, P. R., Batter, S. J., Shield, D. E., Serels, S. R., Gavafalo, F. A., & Maloney, P. K. (2008). Adaptation of adults to uncorrected hypospadias. *Urology, 71*(4), 682–685.

Dolezal, L. (2015). *The body and shame: Phenomenology, feminism, and the socially shaped body*. Lexington Books.

Domar, A. D. (1986). Psychological aspects of the pelvic exam. *Women & Health*, *10*(4), 75–90.

Domar, A. D., Clapp, D., Slawsby, E., Kessel, B., Orav, J., & Freizinger, M. (2000). The impact of group psychological interventions on distress in infertile women. *Health Psychology*, *19*(6), 568–575.

Donahoe, P. K. (1987). The diagnosis and treatment of infants with intersex abnormalities. *Pediatric Clinics of North America*, *34*(5), 1333–1348.

  (1991). Clinical management of intersex abnormalities. *Current Problems in Surgery*, *28*(8), 519–579.

Donahoe, P. K., Powell, D. M., & Lee, M. M. (1991). Clinical management of intersex abnormalities. *Current Problems in Surgery*, *28*(8), 519–579.

Donahoe, P. K., & Gustafson, M. L. (1994). Early one-stage surgical reconstruction of the extremely high vagina in patients with congenital adrenal hyperplasia. *Journal of Pediatric Surgery*, *29*(2), 352–358.

Doka, K. (2017). *Grief is a journey*. Atria Books.

Downing, L., Morland, I., & Sullivan, N. (2014). *Fuckology: Critical essays on John Money's diagnostic concepts*. University of Chicago Press.

Dreger, A. D. (1998). *Hermaphrodites and the medical invention of sex*. Harvard University Press.

  (Ed.). (1999). *Intersex in the age of ethics*. University Publishing Group.

Dreger, A. D., & Chase, C. (1999). A mother's care: An interview with 'Sue' and 'Margaret.' In A. D. Dreger (Ed.), *Intersex in the age of ethics* (pp. 83–89). University Publishing Group.

dsdfamilies. (n.d.). *Top tips for dilation*. Retrieved on February 22, 2022, from https://dsdfamilies.org/application/files/4515/3632/8183/Dilation-booklet-Feb-16-ecopy.pdf

  (2018a). *First days – when your baby is born with genitals that look different*. Retrieved on February 22, 2022, from https://dsdfamilies.org/application/files/1615/4236/8548/firstdays-dsdfamilies.pdf

  (2018b). *Top tips for talking about differences of sex development*. Retrieved on February 22, 2022, from https://www.dsdfamilies.org/application/files/4115/3780/1476/Top_Tips_for_Talking.pdf

  (2019). *The story of sex development*. Retrieved on February 22, 2022, from https://dsdfamilies.org/application/files/4915/7386/0021/ECOPY_Story_of_Sex_Dev_Nov_2019.pdf

Egan, S. K., & Perry, D. G. (2001). Gender identity: A multidimensional analysis with implications for psychosocial adjustment. *Developmental Psychology*, *37*(4), 451–463.

Ellens, R. E. H., Bakula, D. M., Mullins, A. J., Reyes, K. J. S., Austin, P., & Baskin, L. (2017). Psychological adjustment of parents of children born with atypical genitalia 1 year after genitoplasty. *Journal of Urology*, *198*(4), 914–920.

Ellerkamp, V., Rall, K. K., Schaefer, J., Stefanescu, D., Schoeller, D., Brucker, S., & Fuchs, J. (2021). Surgical therapy after failed feminizing genitoplasty in young adults with disorders of sex development: Retrospective analysis and review of the literature. *Journal of Sexual Medicine*, *18*(10), 1797–1806.

Engberg, H., Butwicka, A., Nordenström, A., Hirschberg, A. L., Falhammar, H., Lichtenstein, P., . . . Landén, M. (2015). Congenital adrenal hyperplasia and risk for psychiatric disorders in girls and women born between 1915 and 2010: A total population study. *Psychoneuroendocrinology*, *60*, 195–205.

Engberg, H., Möller, A., Hagenfeldt, K., Nordenskjöld, A., & Frisén, L. (2016). The experience of women living with congenital adrenal hyperplasia: Impact of the condition and the care given. *Clinical Endocrinology*, *85*(1), 21–28.

Engel, G. L. (1977). The need for a new medical model: A challenge for biomedicine. *Science*, *196*(4296), 129–136.

Enzendorfer, M., & Haller, P. (2020). Intersex and education: What can schools and queer school projects learn from current discourses on intersex in Austria?. In D. A. Francis, J. I. Kjaran, & J. Lehtonen (Eds.), *Queer social movements and outreach work in schools* (pp. 261–284). Palgrave Macmillan.

Ernst, M. E., Sandberg, D. E., Keegan, C., Quint, E. H., Lossie, A. C., & Yashar, B. M. (2016). The lived experience of MRKH: Sharing health information with peers. *Journal of Pediatric and Adolescent Gynecology*, *29*(2), 154–158.

Ernst, M. M., Chen, D., Kennedy, K., Jewell, T., Sajwani, A., Foley, C., & Sandberg, D. E. (2019). Disorders of sex development (DSD) web-based information: Quality survey of DSD team websites. *International Journal of Pediatric Endocrinology*, *2019*(1), 1–11.

Ernst, M. M., Gardner, M., Mara, C. A., Délot, E. C., Fechner, P. Y., Fox, M., . . . Sandberg, D. E. (2018). The DSD-translational research network leadership group and psychosocial workgroup. Psychosocial screening in disorders/differences of sex development: Psychometric evaluation of the psychosocial assessment tool. *Hormone Research in Paediatrics*, *90*(6), 368–380.

Ernst, M. M., Kogan, B. A., & Lee, P. A. (2020). Gender identity: A psychosocial primer for providing care to patients with a disorder/difference of sex development and their families [individualized care for patients with intersex (Disorders/differences of sex development): Part 2]. *Journal of Pediatric Urology*, *16*(5), 606–611.

Ernst, M. M., Liao, L.-M, Baratz, A. B., & Sandberg, D. S. (2018). Disorders of sex development/intersex: Gaps in psychosocial care for children. *Pediatrics*, *142*(2), e20174045.

ESHRE Guideline Group on POI, Webber, L., Davies, M., Anderson, R., Bartlett, J., Braat, D., . . . Vermeulen, N. (2016). ESHRE guideline: Management of women with premature ovarian insufficiency. *Human Reproduction*, *31*(5), 926–937.

Fairbank, C. (2011). Men's health: It is imperative to teach scrotal and rectal examination. *Clinical Teaching*, *8*(2), 101–104.

Faramarzi, M., Pasha, H., Esmailzadeh, S., Kheirkhah, F., Heidary, S., & Afshar, Z. (2013). The effect of the cognitive behavioral therapy and pharmacotherapy on infertility stress: A randomized controlled trial. *International Journal of Fertility & Sterility*, *7*(3), 199–206.

Farvid, P., & Braun, V. (2022). A critical encyclopedia of heterosex. In K. Hall & R. Barrett (Eds.), *The Oxford handbook of language and sexuality* (pp. 1–21). Oxford University Press.

Faustino, M. J. (2018). Rebooting an old script by new means: Teledildonics – the technological return to the 'coital imperative.' *Sexuality & Culture, 22*(1), 243–257.

Fausto-Sterling, A. (2000). *Sexing the body: Gender politics and the construction of sexuality.* Basic Books.

Feder, E. K. (2002). Doctor's orders: Parents and intersexed children. In E. F. Kittay & E. K. Feder (Eds.), *The subject of care: Feminist perspectives on dependency* (pp. 294–320). Rowman & Littlefield.

 (2006). "In their best interests": Parents' experience of atypical genitalia. In E. Parens (Ed.), *Surgically shaping children, technology, ethics, and the pursuit of normality* (pp. 189–210). Johns Hopkins University Press.

 (2014). *Making sense of intersex: Changing ethical perspectives in biomedicine.* Indiana University Press.

Fernández-Ávalos, M. I., Pérez-Marfil, M. N., Ferrer-Cascales, R., Cruz-Quintana, F., & Fernández-Alcántara, M. (2021). Feeling of grief and loss in parental caregivers of adults diagnosed with intellectual disability. *Journal of Applied Research in Intellectual Disabilities, 34*(3), 712–723.

Fichtner, J., Filipas, D., Mottrie, A. M., Voges, G. E., & Hohenfellner, R. (1995). Analysis of meatal location in 500 men: Wide variation questions need for meatal advancement in all pediatric anterior hypospadias cases. *Journal of Urology, 154*(2), 833–834.

Fiddes, P., Scott, A., Fletcher, J., & Glasier, A. (2003). Attitudes towards pelvic examination and chaperones: A questionnaire survey of patients and providers. *Contraception, 67*(4), 313–317.

Freda, M. F., Dicé, F., Auricchio, M., Salerno, M., & Valerio, P. (2015). Suspended sorrow: The crisis in understanding the diagnosis for the mothers of children with a disorder of sex development. *International Journal of Sexual Health, 27*(2), 186–198.

Fredrickson, B. L., Hendler, L. M., Nilsen, S., O'Barr, J. F., & Roberts, T. A. (2011). Bringing back the body: A retrospective on the development of objectification theory. *Psychology of Women Quarterly, 35*(4), 689–696.

Frith, H. (2015). The orgasmic imperative. In *Orgasmic bodies* (pp. 22–42). Palgrave Macmillan.

Garland, F., Thomson, M., Travis, M., & Warburton, J. (2021). Management of 'disorders of sex development'/intersex variations in children: Results from a freedom of information exercise. *Medical Law International, 21*(2), 116–146.

Gastaud, F., Bouvattier, C., Duranteau, L., Brauner, R., Thibaud, E., Kutten, F., & Bougneres, P. (2007). Impaired sexual and reproductive outcomes in women with classical forms of congenital adrenal hyperplasia. *Journal of Clinical Endocrinology & Metabolism, 92*(4), 1391–1396.

Gavey, N. (2011). Viagra and the coital imperative. In S. Seidman, N. L. Fischer, C. Meeks (Eds.), *Introducing the new sexuality studies* (2nd ed.; pp. 135–141). Routledge.

Ghidini, F., Sekulovic, S., & Castagnetti, M. (2016). Parental decisional regret after primary distal hypospadias repair: Family and surgery variables, and repair outcomes. *Journal of Urology, 195*(3), 720–724.

Gillespie, R. (2003). Childfree and feminine: Understanding the gender identity of voluntarily childless women. *Gender & Society, 17*(1), 122–136.

Glover, L., Gannon, K., & Abel, P. D. (1999). Eighteen-month follow-up of male subfertility clinic attenders: A comparison between men whose partner subsequently became pregnant and those with continuing subfertility. *Journal of Reproductive and Infant Psychology, 17*(1), 83–87.

Goffman, E. (1974). *Frame analysis: An essay on the organization of experience.* Harper & Row.

Goffnett, J., Liechty, J. M., & Kidder, E. (2020). Interventions to reduce shame: A systematic review. *Journal of Behavioral and Cognitive Therapy, 30*(2), 141–160.

Goldschmidt, R. (1917). Intersexuality and the endocrine aspect of sex. *Endocrinology, 1*(4), 433–456.

Goldstein, E., Murray-García, J., Sciolla, A. F., & Topitzes, J. (2018). Medical students' perspectives on trauma-informed care training. *The Permanente Journal, 22*, 17–126.

Gong, E. M., & Cheng, E. Y. (2017). Current challenges with proximal hypospadias: We have a long way to go. *Journal of Pediatric Urology, 13*(5), 457–467.

González, R., & Ludwikowski, B. M. (2018). Is it beneficial to patients to include congenital adrenal hyperplasia (CAH) among the disorders of sex development (DSD)?. *Frontiers in Pediatrics, 6*, 344.

Gough, B., Weyman, N., Alderson, J., Butler, G., & Stoner, M. (2008). 'They did not have a word': The parental quest to locate a 'true sex' for their intersex children. *Psychology & Health, 23*(4), 493–507.

Goulet, C., Bell, L., St-Cyr Tribble, D., Paul, D., & Lang, A. (1998). A concept analysis of parent-infant attachment. *Journal of Advanced Nursing, 28*(5), 1071–1081.

Gramc, M., Streuli, J., & De Clercq, E. (2021). Multidisciplinary teams caring for people with variations of sex characteristics: A scoping review. *BMJ Paediatrics Open, 5*(1).

Guntram, L. (2013). "Differently normal" and "normally different": Negotiation of female embodiment in women's account of "atypical" sex development. *Social Science & Medicine, 98*, 232–238.

Guntram, L., & Zeiler, K. (2016). "You have all those emotions inside that you cannot show because of what they will cause": Disclosing the absence of one's uterus and vagina. *Social Science & Medicine, 167*, 63–70.

Hagenfeldt, K., Janson, P. O., Holmdahl, B., Falhammar, H., Filipsson, H., Frisén, L., Thorén, M., & Nordenskjöld, A. (2008). Fertility and pregnancy outcome in women with congenital adrenal hyperplasia due to 21-hydroxylase deficiency. *Human Reproduction, 23*(7), 1607–1613.

Hallam, R. (2015). *The therapy relationship: A special kind of friendship.* Karnac.

Hampson, J. G. (1955). Hermaphrotic genital appearance, rearing and eroticism in hyperadrenocorticism. *Bulletin of the Johns Hopkins Hospital, 96*(6), 265–273.

Hanna, E., Gough, B., & Hudson, N. (2018). Fit to father? Online accounts of lifestyle changes and help-seeking on a male infertility board. *Sociology of Health & Illness, 40*(6), 937–953.

Hayfield, N., & Clarke, V. (2012). "I'd be just as happy with a cup of tea": Women's accounts of sex and affection in long-term hetero-sexual relationships. *Women's Studies International Forum, 35*(2), 67–74.

Hayfield, N., Terry, G., Clarke, V., & Ellis, S. (2019). "Never say never?" Heterosexual, bisexual, and lesbian women's accounts of being childfree. *Psychology of Women Quarterly, 43*(4), 526–538.

Hays, P. A., & Iwamasa, G. Y. (2006). *Culturally responsive cognitive-behavioral therapy: Assessment, practice, and supervision.* American Psychological Association.

Hegarty, P., Prandelli, M., Lundberg, T., Liao, L. M., Creighton, S., & Roen, K. (2021). Drawing the line between essential and nonessential interventions on intersex characteristics with European health care professionals. *Review of General Psychology, 25*(1), 101–114.

Hendricks, M. (1993, November). Is it a boy or a girl? *Johns Hopkins Magazine,* 10–16.

Henretty, J. R., & Levitt, H. M. (2010). The role of therapist self-disclosure in psychotherapy: A qualitative review. *Clinical Psychology Review, 30*(1), 63–77.

Hensle, T. W., Shabsigh, A., Shabsigh, R., Reiley, E. A., & Meyer-Bahlburg, H. F. (2006). Sexual function following bowel vaginoplasty. *Journal of Urology, 175*(6), 2283–2286.

Hines, M. (2004). *Brain gender.* Oxford University Press.
    (2020). Neuroscience and sex/gender: Looking back and forward. *Journal of Neuroscience, 40*(1), 37–43.

Hinton, L., & Miller, T. (2013). Mapping men's anticipations and experiences in the reproductive realm: (In)fertility journeys. *Reproductive BioMedicine Online, 27*(3), 244–252.

Hiort, O., Birnbaum, W., Marshall, L., Wünsch, L., Werner, R., Schröder, T., ... Holterhus, P. M. (2014). Management of disorders of sex development. *Nature Reviews Endocrinology, 10*(9), 520–529.

Hodson, N., & Bewley, S. (2019). Abuse in assisted reproductive technology: A systematic qualitative review and typology. *European Journal of Obstetrics & Gynecology and Reproductive Biology, 238,* 170–177.

Hoffman, L. (1990). Constructing realities: An art of lenses. *Family Process, 29*(1), 1–12.

Holmes, M. M. (2009). Straddling past, present and future. In *Critical intersex* (pp. 1–12). Ashgate.

Holmes, T. H., & Rahe, R. H. (1967). The social readjustment rating scale. *Journal of Psychosomatic Research, 11*(2), 213–218.

Hughes, I. A. (2002). Intersex. *BJU International, 90*(8), 769–776.
    (2010). The quiet revolution. *Best Practice & Research Clinical Endocrinology & Metabolism, 24*(2), 159–162.

Hughes, I. A., Nihoul-Fékété, C., Thomas, B., & Cohen-Kettenis, P. T. (2007). Consequences of the ESPE/LWPES guidelines for diagnosis and treatment of disorders of sex development. *Best Practice & Research Clinical Endocrinology & Metabolism, 21*(3), 351–365.

Human Rights Watch. (2017). *"I want to be like nature made me": Medically unnecessary surgeries on intersex children in the U.S.* https://www.hrw.org/sites/default/files/report_pdf/lgbtintersex0717_web_0.pdf

Inhorn, M. C. (2007). Masturbation, semen collection and men's IVF experiences: Anxieties in the Muslim world. *Body & Society, 13*(3), 37–53.

Ipser, J. C., Sander, C., & Stein, D. J. (2009). Pharmacotherapy and psychotherapy for body dysmorphic disorder. *Cochrane Database of Systematic Reviews, 1*, CD005332.

Islam, R., Lane, S., Williams, S. A., Becker, C. M., Conway, G. S., & Creighton, S. M. (2019). Establishing reproductive potential and advances in fertility preservation techniques for XY individuals with differences in sex development. *Clinical Endocrinology, 91*(2), 237–244.

Jääskeläinen, J., Tiitinen, A., & Voutilainen, R. (2001). Sexual function and fertility in adult females and males with congenital adrenal hyperplasia. *Hormone Research in Paediatrics, 56*(3–4), 73–80.

Jennings, L., & Skovholt, T. M. (1999). The cognitive, emotional, and relational characteristics of master therapists. *Journal of Counseling Psychology, 46*(1), 3–11.

Jericho, B., Luo, A., & Berle, D. (2021). Trauma-focused psychotherapies for post-traumatic stress disorder: A systematic review and network meta-analysis. *Acta Psychiatrica Scandinavica, 145*(2), 132–155.

Johnson, E. K., Rosoklija, I., Finlayson, C., Chen, D., Yerkes, E. B., Madonna, M. B., ... Cheng, E. Y. (2017). Attitudes towards "disorders of sex development" nomenclature among affected individuals. *Journal of Pediatric Urology, 13*(6), 608-e1–608.e8.

Johnstone, L., & Boyle, M. (2018). *The Power Threat Meaning Framework: Overview*. British Psychological Society.

Jordal, M., Sigurjonsson, H., Griffin, G., & Wahlberg, A. (2021). The benefits and disappointments following clitoral reconstruction after female genital cutting: A qualitative interview study from Sweden. *PLoS One, 16*(7), e0254855.

Jordan-Young, R. M. (2011). *Brain storm: The flaws in the science of sex differences*. Harvard University Press.

Kabat-Zinn, J. (2013). *Full catastrophe living, revised edition: How to cope with stress, pain and illness using mindfulness meditation*. Hachette UK.

Kaltiala, R., Bergman, H., Carmichael, P., de Graaf, N. M., Egebjerg Rischel, K., Frisen, L., ... Waehre, A. (2020). Time trends in referrals to child and adolescent gender identity services: A study in four Nordic countries and in the UK. *Nordic Journal of Psychiatry, 74*(1), 40–44.

Karkazis, K. A. (2008). *Fixing sex: Intersex, medical authority, and lived experience*. Duke University Press.

Karkazis, K., Tamar-Mattis, A., & Kon, A. A. (2010). Genital surgery for disorders of sex development: Implementing a shared decision-making approach. *Journal of Pediatric Endocrinology & Metabolism, 23*(8), 789–805.

Kazak, A. E., Simms, S., & Rourke, M. T. (2002). Family systems practice in pediatric psychology. *Journal of Pediatric Psychology, 27*(2), 133–143.

Kessler, S. (1998). *Lessons from the intersexed.* Rutgers University Press.

Kinsey, C. B., & Hupcey, J. E. (2013). State of the science of maternal–infant bonding: A principle-based concept analysis. *Midwifery, 29*(12), 1314–1320.

Kinsman, K. (2014, April 15). *Intersex dating: Finding love across the intersection.* CNN. http://edition.cnn.com/2014/04/15/living/intersex-dating-relate/index.html

Kirby, J. (2014). Transnational gestational surrogacy: Does it have to be exploitative?. *American Journal of Bioethics, 14*(5), 24–32.

Knox, S., & Hill, C. E. (2003). Therapist self-disclosure: Research-based suggestions for practitioners. *Journal of Clinical Psychology, 59*(5), 529–539.

Koyama, E. (2003). *Teaching intersex issues: A guide for teachers in women's gender and queer studies* (2nd ed.). Intersex Initiative Portland. www.ipdx.org

Krege, S., Walz, K. H., Hauffa, B. P., Körner, I., & Rübben, H. (2000). Long-term follow-up of female patients with congenital adrenal hyperplasia from 21-hydroxylase deficiency, with special emphasis on the results of vaginoplasty. *BJU International, 86*(3), 253–258.

Kreukels, B. P., Cohen-Kettenis, P. T., Roehle, R., van de Grift, T. C., Slowikowska-Hilczer, J., Claahsen-van der Grinten, H., ... dsd-LIFE Group. (2019). Sexuality in adults with differences/disorders of sex development (DSD): Findings from the dsd-LIFE study. *Journal of Sex & Marital Therapy, 45*(8), 688–705.

Kreukels, B. P., Köhler, B., Nordenström, A., Roehle, R., Thyen, U., Bouvattier, C., ... Szarras-Czapnik, M. (2018). Gender dysphoria and gender change in disorders of sex development/intersex conditions: Results from the dsd-LIFE study. *Journal of Sexual Medicine, 15*(5), 777–785.

Kyriakou, A., Dessens, A., Bryce, J., Iotova, V., Juul, A., Krawczynski, M., ... Ahmed, S. F. (2016). Current models of care for disorders of sex development: Results from an international survey of specialist centres. *Orphanet Journal of Rare Diseases, 11*(1), 1–10.

Lamont, J. M. (2019). The relationship of mindfulness to body shame, body responsiveness, and health outcomes. *Mindfulness, 10*(4), 639–649.

Lazarus, R. S. (1996). The role of coping in the emotions and how coping changes over the life course. In C. Magai & S. H. McFadden (Eds.), *Handbook of emotion, adult development, and aging* (pp. 289–306). Academic Press.

Lee, P. A., Houk, C. P., Ahmed, S. F., & Hughes, I. A. (2006). Consensus statement on management of intersex disorders. In collaboration with the participants in the international consensus conference on intersex organized by the Lawson Wilkins Pediatric Endocrine Society the European Society for Paediatric Endocrinology. *Pediatrics, 118*(2), e488–e500.

Lee, P. A., Nordenstrom, A., Houk, C. P., Ahmed, S. F., Auchus, R., Baratz, A., ... The Global DSD Update Consortium. (2016). Global disorders of sex development update since 2006: Perceptions, approach and care. *Hormones Research in Paediatrics, 85*(3), 158–180.

Le Maréchal, K. (2001). *Bringing up an XY girl: Parents' experience of having a child with androgen insensitivity syndrome.* Unpublished DClinPsy Thesis, University College London, UK.

Lesnik-Oberstein, M., Cohen, L., & Koers, A. J. (1982). Research in the Netherlands on a theory of child abuse: A preliminary report. *Child Abuse & Neglect, 6*(2), 199–206.

Leuzinger-Bohleber, M. (2001). The "Medea fantasy": An unconscious determinant of psychogenic sterility. *International Journal of Psychoanalysis, 82*(2), 323–345.

Lewis, C., Roberts, N. P., Andrew, M., Starling, E., & Bisson, J. I. (2020). Psychological therapies for post-traumatic stress disorder in adults: Systematic review and meta-analysis. *European Journal of Psychotraumatology, 11*(1), 1729633.

Liao, L. M. (2003). Learning to assist women born with atypical genitalia: Journey through ignorance, taboo and dilemma. *Journal of Reproductive and Infant Psychology, 21*(3), 229–238.

   (2007). Towards a clinical-psychological approach for addressing the heterosexual concerns of intersexed women. In V. Clarke & E. Peel (Eds.), *Out in psychology: Lesbian gay bisexual transgender and queer perspectives* (pp. 391–408). Wiley.

Liao, L. M., Baker, E., Boyle, M. E., Woodhouse, C. R. J., & Creighton, S. M. (2014). Experiences of surgical continence management approaches for cloacal anomalies: A qualitative analysis based on 6 women. *Journal of Pediatric and Adolescent Gynecology, 27*(5), 266–270.

Liao, L. M., Chadwick, P. M., & Tamar-Mattis, A. (2018). Informed consent in pediatric and adolescent gynecology: From ethical principles to ethical behavior. In S. Creighton, A. Balen, L. Breech, & L. M. Liao (Eds.), *Pediatric and adolescent gynaecology: A problem-based approach* (pp. 45–52). Cambridge University Press.

Liao, L. M., Conway, G. S., Ismail-Pratt, I., Bikoo, M., & Creighton, S. M. (2011). Emotional and sexual wellness and quality of life in women with Rokitansky syndrome. *American Journal of Obstetrics and Gynecology, 205*(2), 117-e1–117-e6.

Liao, L. M., Doyle, J., Crouch, N. S., & Creighton, S. M. (2006). Dilation as treatment for vaginal agenesis and hypoplasia: A pilot exploration of benefits and barriers as perceived by patients. *Journal of Obstetrics and Gynaecology, 26*(2), 144–148.

Liao, L. M., Green, H., Creighton, S. M., Crouch, N. S., & Conway, G. S. (2010). Service users' experiences of obtaining and giving information about disorders of sex development. *BJOG: An International Journal of Obstetrics & Gynaecology, 117*(2), 193–199.

Liao, L. M., Hegarty, P., Creighton, S., Lundberg, T., & Roen, K. (2019). Clitoral surgery on minors: An interview study with clinical experts of differences of sex development. *BMJ Open, 9*(6), e025821.

Liao, L. M., & Roen, K. (2014). Intersex/DSD post-Chicago: New developments and challenges for psychologists. *Psychology & Sexuality, 5*(1), 1–4.

(2021). The role of psychologists in multi-disciplinary teams for intersex/diverse sex development: Interviews with British and Swedish clinical specialists. *Psychology & Sexuality, 12*(3), 202–216.

Liao, L. M., & Simmonds, M. (2013). Communicating about diverse sex development. In J. Wiggens & A. Middleton (Eds.), *Getting the message across: Practical advice for genetics health care professionals* (pp. 42–60). Oxford University Press.

(2014). A values-driven and evidence-based health care psychology for diverse sex development. *Psychology & Sexuality, 5*(1), 83–101.

Liao, L.-M., Wood, D., & Creighton, S. M. (2015). Parental choice on normalising cosmetic genital surgery. *BMJ, 351*, h5124.

Lima, M., Ruggeri, G., Randi, B., Dòmini, M., Gargano, T., La Pergola, E., & Gregori, G. (2010). Vaginal replacement in the pediatric age group: A 34-year experience of intestinal vaginoplasty in children and young girls. *Journal of Pediatric Surgery, 45*(10), 2087–2091.

Linschoten, M., Weiner, L., & Avery-Clark, C. (2016). Sensate focus: A critical literature review. *Sexual & Relationship Therapy, 31*(2), 230–247.

Lin-Su, K., Lekarev, O., Poppas, D. P., & Vogiatzi, M. G. (2015). Congenital adrenal hyperplasia patient perception of "disorders of sex development" nomenclature. *International Journal of Pediatric Endocrinology, 2015*(1), 1–7.

Lloyd, J., Crouch, N. S., Minto, C. L., Liao, L. M., & Creighton, S. M. (2005). Female genital appearance: "Normality" unfolds. *BJOG: An International Journal of Obstetrics & Gynaecology, 112*(5), 643–646.

LoPiccolo, J. (1994). The evolution of sex therapy. *Sexual and Marital Therapy, 9* (1), 5–7.

Lorenzo, A. J., Pippi Salle, J. L., Zlateska, B., Koyle, M. A., Bägli, D. J., & Braga, L. H. (2014). Decisional regret after distal hypospadias repair: Single institution prospective analysis of factors associated with subsequent parental remorse or distress. *Journal of Urology, 191*(5S), 1558–1563.

Lucas, J., Hightower, T., Weiss, D. A., Van Batavia, J., Coelho, S., Srinivasan, A. K., . . . Long, C. J. (2020). Time to complication detection after primary pediatric hypospadias repair: A large, single center, retrospective cohort analysis. *Journal of Urology, 204*(2), 338–344.

Lundberg, T., Hegarty, P., & Roen, K. (2018). Making sense of "intersex" and "DSD": How laypeople understand and use terminology. *Psychology & Sexuality, 9*(2), 161–173.

Lundberg, T., Lindström, A., Roen, K., & Hegarty, P. (2017). From knowing nothing to knowing what, how and now: Parents' experiences of caring for their children with congenital adrenal hyperplasia. *Journal of Pediatric Psychology, 42*(5), 520–529.

Lundberg, T., Roen, K., Kraft, C., & Hegarty, P. (2021). How young people talk about their variations in sex characteristics: Making the topic of intersex talkable via sex education. *Sex Education, 21*(5), 552–567.

Magritte, E. (2012). Working together in placing the long term interests of the child at the heart of the DSD evaluation. *Journal of Pediatric Urology, 8*(6), 571–575.

Maiburg, M. C., Hoppenbrouwers, A. C., van Stel, H. F., & Giltay, J. C. (2011). Attitudes of Klinefelter men and their relatives towards TESE-ICSI. *Journal of Assisted Reproduction and Genetics, 28*(9), 809–814.

Malouf, M. A., Inman, A. G., Carr, A. G., Franco, J., & Brooks, L. M. (2010). Health-related quality of life, mental health and psychotherapeutic considerations for women diagnosed with a disorder of sexual development: Congenital adrenal hyperplasia. *International Journal of Pediatric Endocrinology, 2010*, 253465.

Malta. (2015). *Gender Identity, Gender Expression and Sex Characteristics Act.* https://legislation.mt/eli/act/2015/11.

Marmot, M. (2015). *The health gap: The challenge of an unequal world.* Bloomsbury.

Marsac, M. L., Kassam-Adams, N., Hildenbrand, A. K., Nicholls, E., Winston, F. K., Leff, S. S., & Fein, J. (2016). Implementing a trauma-informed approach in pediatric health care networks. *JAMA Pediatrics, 170*(1), 70–77.

Marsh, J. L. (2006). To cut or not to cut? A surgeon's perspective on surgically shaping children. In E. Parens (Ed.), *Surgically shaping children, technology, ethics, and the pursuit of normality* (pp. 113–134). Johns Hopkins University Press.

Masters, W., & Johnson, V. E. (1970). *Human sexual inadequacy.* Little, Brown and Company.

May, B., Boyle, M., & Grant, D. (1996). A comparative study of sexual experiences: Women with diabetes and women with congenital adrenal hyperplasia due to 21-hydroxylase deficiency. *Journal of Health Psychology, 1*(4), 479–492.

McCarthy, B. W., & Metz, M. E. (2008). The "Good-Enough Sex" model: A case illustration. *Sexual and Relationship Therapy, 23*(3), 227–234.

McCarthy, V. (1997). The first pelvic examination. *Journal of Pediatric Health Care, 11*(5), 247–249.

McGrath, M., Low, M. A., Power, E., McCluskey, A., & Lever, S. (2021). Addressing sexuality among people living with chronic disease and disability: A systematic mixed methods review of knowledge, attitudes and practices of health care professionals. *Archives of Physical Medicine and Rehabilitation, 102* (5), 999–1010.

McPhillips, K., Braun, V., & Gavey, N. (2001). Defining (hetero) sex: How imperative is the "coital imperative"? *Women's Studies International Forum, 24*(2), 229–240.

Meldrum, K. K., Mathew, R., & Gearhart, J. P. (2001). Hugh Hampton Young: A pioneer in pediatric urology. *Journal of Urology, 166*(4), 1415–1417.

Mendez, J. E. (2014, February 1). *Report of the Special Rapporteur on torture, and other cruel, inhuman and degrading punishment.* 22nd Session of the UN Human Rights Council. A/ HRC/22/53. http://www.ohchr.org/Documents/HRBodies/HRCouncil/RegularSession/Session22/A.HRC.22.53_English.pdf

Menon, M., Menon, M., Cooper, P. J., Pauletti, R. E., Tobin, D. D., Spatta, B. C., ... Perry, D. G. (2017). Do securely and insecurely attached children derive well-being from different forms of gender identity? *Social Development, 26*(1), 91–108.

Meoded Danon, L. (2022). The geneticisation of intersex bodies in Israel. In M. Walker (Ed.), *Interdisciplinary and global perspectives on intersex* (pp. 219–240). Palgrave Macmillan.

Meyer-Bahlburg, H. N. L. (1999). Gender assignment and reassignment in 46, XY pseudohermaphroditism and related conditions. *Journal of Clinical Endocrinology & Metabolism, 84*(10), 3455–3458.

Meyer-Bahlburg, H. F. L. (2022). The timing of genital surgery in somatic intersexuality: Surveys of patients' preferences. *Hormone Research in Pediatrics, 95,* 12–20.

Meyer-Bahlburg, H. F., Khuri, J., Reyes-Portillo, J., Ehrhardt, A. A., & New, M. I. (2018). Stigma associated with classical congenital adrenal hyperplasia in women's sexual lives. *Archives of Sexual Behavior, 47*(4), 943–951.

Meyer-Bahlburg, H. F., Khuri, J., Reyes-Portillo, J., & New, M. I. (2017). Stigma in medical settings as reported retrospectively by women with congenital adrenal hyperplasia (CAH) for their childhood and adolescence. *Journal of Pediatric Psychology, 42*(5), 496–503.

Michala, L., Goswami, D., Creighton, S. M., & Conway, G. S. (2008). Swyer syndrome: Presentation and outcomes. *British Journal of Obstetrics & Gynaecology, 115*(6), 737–741.

Michala, L., Liao, L. M., Wood, D., Conway, G. S., & Creighton, S. M. (2014). Practice changes in childhood surgery for ambiguous genitalia? *Journal of Pediatric Urology, 10*(5), 934–939.

Miles, L. M., Keitel, M., Jackson, M., Harris, A., & Licciardi, F. (2009). Predictors of distress in women being treated for infertility. *Journal of Reproductive and Infant Psychology, 27*(3), 238–257.

Mills, L., & Thompson, S. (2020). Parental responsibilities and rights during the "gender reassignment" decision-making process of intersex infants: Guidance in Terms of Article 5 of the Convention on the Rights of the Child. *International Journal of Children's Rights, 28*(3), 547–570.

Minto, C. L., Liao, L. M., Woodhouse, C. R., Ransley, P. G., & Creighton, S. M. (2003a). The effect of clitoral surgery on sexual outcome in individuals who have intersex conditions with ambiguous genitalia: A cross-sectional study. *The Lancet, 361*(9365), 1252–1257.

Minto, C. L., Liao, K. L. M., Conway, G. S., & Creighton, S. M. (2003b). Sexual function in women with complete androgen insensitivity syndrome. *Fertility and Sterility, 80*(1), 157–164.

Money, J., Hampson, J. G., & Hampson, J. L. (1955a). An examination of some basic sexual concepts: The evidence of human hermophroditism. *Bulletin of the Johns Hopkins Hospital, 97*(4), 301–319.

(1955b). Hermaphroditism: Recommendations concerning assignment of sex, change of sex and psychologic management. *Bulletin of the Johns Hopkins Hospital, 97*(4), 284–300.

Money, J., & Lamacz, M. (1987). Genital examination and exposure experienced as nosocomial sexual abuse in childhood. *Journal of Nervous & Mental Disease, 175*(12), 713–721.

Montesi, J. L., Conner, B. T., Gordon, E. A., Fauber, R. L., Kim, K. H., & Heimberg, R. G. (2013). On the relationship among social anxiety, intimacy, sexual communication, and sexual satisfaction in young couples. *Archives of Sexual Behavior, 42*(1), 81–91.

Moore, J. (2014). Reconsidering childfreedom: A feminist exploration of discursive identity construction in childfree LiveJournal communities. *Women's Studies in Communication, 37*(2), 159–180.

Moreno, A. (1999). In Amerika they call us hermaphrodites. In A. D. Dreger (Ed.), *Intersex in the age of ethics* (pp. 137–139). University Publishing Group.

Morison, T., Macleod, C., Lynch, I., Mijas, M., & Shivakumar, S. T. (2016). Stigma resistance in online childfree communities: The limitations of choice rhetoric. *Psychology of Women Quarterly, 40*(2), 184–198.

Morland, I. (2009). Between critique and reform: Ways of reading the intersex controversy. In M. Holmes (Ed.), *Critical intersex* (pp. 191–213). Ashgate.

Mouriquand, P., Caldamone, A., Malone, P., Frank, J. D., & Hoebeke, P. (2014). The ESPU/SPU standpoint on the surgical management of disorders of sex development (DSD). *Journal of Pediatric Urology, 10*(1), 8–10.

Murray, M. (2017). The pre-history of health psychology in the United Kingdom: From natural science and psychoanalysis to social science, social cognition and beyond. *Journal of Health Psychology, 23*(2), 1–21.

Newman, K., Randolph, J., & Anderson, K. (1992). The surgical management of infants and children with ambiguous genitalia: Lessons learned from 25 years. *Annals of Surgery, 215*(6), 644–653.

NHS England. (2014). *Multi-disciplinary team handbook*. Retrieved on July 7, 2022, from https://www.england.nhs.uk/wp-content/uploads/2015/01/mdt-dev-guid-flat-fin.pdf.

Nicolson, P. (2011). *Postnatal depression: Facing the paradox of loss, happiness and motherhood*. John Wiley & Sons.

Nordenskjöld, A., Holmdahl, G., Frisén, L., Falhammar, H., Filipsson, H., Thorén, M., Olof Janson, P., & Hagenfeldt, K. (2008). Type of mutation and surgical procedure affect long-term quality of life for women with congenital adrenal hyperplasia. *Journal of Clinical Endocrinology & Metabolism, 93*(2), 380–386.

Ogilvie, C. M., Crouch, N. S., Rumsby, G., Creighton, S. M., Liao, L. M., & Conway, G. S. (2006). Congenital adrenal hyperplasia in adults: A review of medical, surgical and psychological issues. *Clinical Endocrinology, 64*(1), 2–11.

Ogilvy-Stuart, A. L., & Brain, C. E. (2004). Early assessment of ambiguous genitalia. *Archives of Disease in Childhood, 89*(5), 401–407.

O'Neill, S., Richard, F., Vanderhoven, C., & Caillet, M. (2021). Pleasure, womanhood and the desire for reconstructive surgery after female genital cutting in Belgium. *Anthropology & Medicine.* https://doi.org/10.1080/13648470.2021.1994332

Opperman, E., Braun, V., Clarke, V., & Rogers, C. (2014). "It feels so good it almost hurts": Young adults' experiences of orgasm and sexual pleasure. *Journal of Sex Research, 51*(5), 503–515.

Orlinsky, D. E. (2009). The "generic model of psychotherapy" after 25 years: Evolution of a research-based metatheory. *Journal of Psychotherapy Integration, 19*(4), 319–339.

Panagopoulou, E., Mintziori, G., Montgomery, A., Kapoukranidou, D., & Benos, A. (2008). Concealment of information in clinical practice: Is lying less stressful than telling the truth?. *Journal of Clinical Oncology, 26*(7), 1175–1177.

Parikh, N., Saruchera, Y., & Liao, L. M. (2020). It is a problem and it is not a problem: Dilemmatic talk of the psychological effects of female genital cutting. *Journal of Health Psychology, 25*(12), 1917–1929.

Parry, V. (2006, August 22). *What does it mean to be normal?* BBC News. http://news.bbc.co.uk/1/hi/health/5273936.stm

Pasterski, V., Prentice, P., & Hughes, I. A. (2010). Consequences of the Chicago Consensus on disorders of sex development (DSD): Current practices in Europe. *Archives of Disease in Childhood, 95*(8), 618–623.

Penn, P. (1982). Circular questioning. *Family Process, 21*(3), 267–280.

Pennebaker, J. W., & Smyth, J. M. (2016). *Opening up by writing it down: How expressive writing improves health and eases emotional pain* (3rd ed.). Guildford Press.

Perez-Palacios, G., & Jaffe, R. B. (1972). The syndrome of testicular feminization. *Pediatric Clinics of North America, 19*(3), 653–668.

Perry-Parrish, C., Copeland-Linder, N., Webb, L., & Sibinga, E. M. (2016). Mindfulness-based approaches for children and youth. *Current Problems in Pediatric and Adolescent Health Care, 46*(6), 172–178.

Peterson, H., & Engwall, K. (2013). Silent bodies: Childfree women's gendered and embodied experiences. *European Journal of Women's Studies, 20*(4), 376–389.

Petraglia, F., Serour, G. I., & Chapron, C. (2013). The changing prevalence of infertility. *International Journal of Gynecology & Obstetrics, 123*(Suppl. 2), S4–S8.

Pianta, R. C., Marvin, R. S., Britner, P. A., & Borowitz, K. C. (1996). Mothers' resolution of their children's diagnosis: Organized patterns of caregiving representations. *Infant Mental Health Journal, 17*(3), 239–256.

Pitts, M., & Rahman, Q. (2001). Which behaviors constitute "having sex" among university students in the UK? *Archives of Sexual Behavior, 30*(2), 169–176.

Platt, F. W., & Keating, K. N. (2017). Differences in physician and patient perceptions of uncomplicated UTI symptom severity: Understanding the communication gap. *International Journal of Clinical Practice, 61*(2), 303–308.

Prandelli, M., & Testoni, I. (2021). Inside the doctor's office: Talking about intersex with Italian health professionals. *Culture, Health & Sexuality, 23*(4), 484–499.

Preves, S. E. (2003). *Intersex and identity: The contested self.* Rutgers University Press.

   (2005). Out of the O.R. and into the streets: Exploring the impact of the intersex media activism. *Cardozo Journal of Law & Gender, 12*(1), 247–288.

Prigerson, H. G., Vaughan, S. C., & Lichtenthal, W. G. (2016). The hidden dangers of a cancer diagnosis. *BMJ, 354*, i4446.

Purkey, E., Patel, R., & Phillips, S. P. (2018). Trauma-informed care: Better care for everyone. *Canadian Family Physician, 64*(3), 170–172.

Raja, S., Hasnain, M., Hoersch, M, Gove-Yin, S., & Rajagopalan, C. (2015). Trauma informed care in medicine: Current knowledge and future research directions. *Family Community Health, 38*(3), 216–226.

Randolf, J., & Hung, W. (1970). Reduction clitoroplasty in females with hyper-trophied clitoris. *Journal of Pediatric Surgery, 5*(2), 224–231.

Reder, P., & Fredman, G. (1996). The relationship to help: Interacting beliefs about the treatment process. *Clinical Child Psychology and Psychiatry, 1*(3), 457–467.

Reilly, J. M., & Woodhouse, C. R. J. (1989). Small penis and the male sexual role. *Journal of Urology, 142*(2), 569–571.

Reis, E. (2009). *Bodies in doubt: An American history of intersex.* Johns Hopkins University Press.

Rink, R. C., & Adams, M. C. (1998). Feminizing genitoplasty: State of the art. *World Journal of Urology, 16*(3), 212–218.

Roen, K., Creighton, S. M., Hegarty, P., & Liao, L. M. (2018). Vaginal construction and treatment providers' experiences: A qualitative analysis. *Journal of Pediatric and Adolescent Gynecology, 31*(3), 247–251.

Roen, K., & Hegarty, P. (2018). Shaping parents, shaping penises: How medical teams frame parents' decisions in response to hypospadias. *British Journal of Health Psychology, 23*(4), 967–981.

Roen, K., & Lundberg, T. (2020). Intersex mental health. In E. Rothblum (Ed.), *The Oxford handbook of sexual and gender minority mental health* (pp. 305–317). Oxford University Press.

Rolston, A. M., Gardner, M., van Leeuwen, K., Mohnach, L., Keegan, C., Délot, E., ... Advisory Network Accord Alliance. (2017, June). Disorders of sex development (DSD): Clinical service delivery in the United States. *American Journal of Medical Genetics Part C: Seminars in Medical Genetics, 175*(2), 268–278.

Rosen, M. A., DiazGranados, D., Dietz, A. S., Benishek, L. E., Thompson, D., Pronovost, P. J., & Weaver, S. J. (2018). Teamwork in healthcare: Key discoveries enabling safer, high-quality care. *American Psychologist, 73*(4), 433–450.

Royal College of Physicians. (2017). *Improving teams in health care – Resource 1: Building effective teams.* Retrieved February 22, 2022, from https://www.rcplondon.ac.uk/file/8202/download?token=AFPPJhkl:

Sanchez, D. T., & Kiefer, A. K. (2007). Body concerns in and out of the bedroom: Implications for sexual pleasure and problems. *Archives of Sexual Behavior, 36*(6), 808–820.

Sandberg, D. E., Gardner, M., Callens, N., Mazur, T., & DSD-TRN Psychosocial Workgroup, the DSD-TRN Advocacy Advisory Network, and Accord Alliance. (2017, June). Interdisciplinary care in disorders/differences of sex development (DSD): The psychosocial component of the DSD–translational research network. *American Journal of Medical Genetics Part C: Seminars in Medical Genetics, 175*(2), 279–292.

Sandberg, D. E., Gardner, M., Kopec, K., Urbanski, M., Callens, N., Keegan, C. E., ... Siminoff, L. A. (2019). Development of a decision support tool in pediatric differences/disorders of sex development. *Seminars in Pediatric Surgery, 28*(5), 1508–1538.

Sandberg, D. E., & Voss, L. D. (2002). The psychosocial consequences of short stature: A review of the evidence. *Best Practice & Research Clinical Endocrinology and Metabolism, 16*(3), 449–463.

Sanders, C., & Carter, B. (2015). A qualitative study of communication between young women with disorders of sex development and health professionals. *Advances in Nursing, 2015*, 653624.

Sanders, C., Carter, B., & Goodacre, L. (2008). Parents' narratives about their experiences of their child's reconstructive genital surgeries for ambiguous genitalia. *Journal of Clinical Nursing, 17*(23), 3187–3195.

(2011). Searching for harmony: Parents' narratives about their child's genital ambiguity and reconstructive genital surgeries in childhood. *Journal of Advanced Nursing, 67*(10), 2220–2230.

(2012). Parents need to protect: Influences, risks and tensions for parents of prepubertal children born with ambiguous genitalia. *Journal of Clinical Nursing, 21*(21–22), 3315–238.

Sanders, C., Carter, B., & Lwin, R. (2015). Young women with a disorder of sex development: Learning to share information with health professionals, friends and intimate partners about bodily differences and infertility. *Journal of Advanced Nursing, 71*(8), 1904–1913.

Sanders, C., Edwards, Z., & Keegan, K. (2017). Exploring stakeholder experiences of interprofessional teamwork in sex development outpatient clinics. *Journal of Interprofessional Care, 31*(3), 376–385.

Sanders, S. A., & Reinisch, J. M. (1999). Would you say you had sex if...?. *Journal of the American Medical Association, 281*(3), 275–277.

Sax, L. (2002). How common is intersex? A response to Anne Fausto-Sterling. *Journal of Sex Research, 39*(3), 174–178.

Schilte, A. F., Portegijs, P. J., Blankenstein, A. H., van der Horst, H. E., Latour, M. B., van Eijk, J. T. M., & Knottnerus, J. A. (2001). Randomised controlled trial of disclosure of emotionally important events in somatisation in primary care. *BMJ, 323*(7304), 86.

Schneuer, F. J., Holland, A. J. A., Pereira, G., Bower, C., & Nassar, N. (2015). Prevalence, repairs and complications of hypospadias: An Australian population-based study. *Archives of Disease in Childhood, 100*(11), 1038–43.

Schönbucher, V., Schweizer, K., & Richter-Appelt, H. (2010). Sexual quality of life of individuals with disorders of sex development and a 46, XY karyotype: A review of international research. *Journal of Sex & Marital Therapy, 36*(3), 193–215.

Schützmann, K., Brinkmann, L., Schacht, M., & Richter-Appelt, H. (2009). Psychological distress, self-harming behavior, and suicidal tendencies in adults with disorders of sex development. *Archives of Sexual Behavior, 38* (1), 16–33.

Schweizer, K., Brunner, F., Handford, C., & Richter-Appelt, H. (2014). Gender experience and satisfaction with gender allocation in adults with diverse intersex conditions (divergences of sex development, DSD). *Psychology & Sexuality, 5*(1), 56–82.

Selye, H. (1956). *The stress of life*. McGraw-Hill.

Shao, S., Wang, X., Lei, X., Hua, K., & Zhang, Y. (2022). Psychological intervention in women with Mayer-Rokitansky-Küster-Hauser syndrome after artificial vaginoplasty: A prospective study. *International Urogynecology Journal, 33*, 723–729.

Sharpe, D., & Rossiter, L. (2002). Siblings of children with a chronic illness: A meta-analysis. *Journal of Pediatric Psychology, 27*(8), 699–710.

Sheehan, P., & Guerin, S. (2018). Exploring the range of emotional response experienced when parenting a child with an intellectual disability: The role of dual process. *British Journal of Learning Disabilities, 46*(2), 109–117.

Shen, S., & Liu, H. (2021). Sexual obligation and perceived stress: A national longitudinal study of older adults. *Clinical Gerontologist, 44*(3), 259–272.

Simmonds, M. (2004). Patients and parents in decision making and management. In A. H. Balen, S. M. Creighton, M. C. Davies, J. MacDougall, & R. Stanhope (Eds.), *Paediatric and adolescent gynaecology: A multidisciplinary approach* (pp. 205–228). Cambridge University Press.

(2007). Was "variations of reproductive development" considered? *Archives of Diseases in Childhood, 92*(1), 89.

Slepian, M. L., & Moulton-Tetlock, E. (2019). Confiding secrets and well-being. *Social Psychological and Personality Science, 10*(4), 472–484.

Slijper, F. M., Frets, P. G., Boehmer, A. L., Drop, S. L., & Niermeijer, M. F. (2000). Androgen insensitivity syndrome (AIS): Emotional reactions of parents and adult patients to the clinical diagnosis of AIS and its confirmation by androgen receptor gene mutation analysis. *Hormone Research, 53*(1), 9–15.

Słowikowska-Hilczer, J., Hirschberg, A. L., Claahsen-van der Grinten, H., Reisch, N., Bouvattier, C., Thyen, U., ... Nordenstrom, A. (2017). Fertility outcome and information on fertility issues in individuals with different forms of disorders of sex development: Findings from the dsd-LIFE study. *Fertility & Sterility, 108*(5), 822–831.

Solnit, A. J., & Stark, M. J. (1961, 2017). Mourning and the birth of a defective child. *Psychoanalytic Study of the Child, 16*(1), 523–537. https://doi.org/10.1080/00797308.1961.11823222

Sparks, J. A., Duncan, B. L., & Miller, S. D. (2008). Common factors in psychotherapy. In J. L. Lebow (Ed.), *Twenty-first century psychotherapies: Contemporary approaches to theory and practice* (pp. 453–498). Wiley.

Speiser, P. W., Azziz, R., Baskin, L. S., Ghizzoni, L., Hensle, T. W., Merke, D. P., ... White, P. C. (2010). Congenital adrenal hyperplasia due to steroid 21-hydroxylase deficiency: An endocrine society clinical practice guideline. *Journal of Clinical Endocrinology and Metabolism, 95*(9), 4133–4160. https://doi.org/10.1210/jc.2009-2631

Stahnke, B., Blackstone, A., & Howard, H. (2020). Lived experiences and life satisfaction of childfree women in late life. *The Family Journal, 28*(2), 159–167.

Stam, H. J. (2015). A critical history of health psychology and its relationship to biomedicine. In M. Murray (Ed.), *Critical health psychology* (2nd ed., pp. 19–35). Palgrave Macmillan.

Stam, H. J., Murray, M., & Lubek, I. (2018). Health psychology in autobiography: Three Canadian critical narratives. *Journal of Health Psychology, 23*(3), 506–523.

Steers, D. M., Andrews, G. L., Wiltshire, E. J., Ballantyne, A. J., Collings, S. C., & Stubbe, M. H. (2020). Young people with a variation in sex characteristics in Aotearoa/New Zealand: Identity, activism and healthcare decision-making. *Culture, Health & Sexuality, 23*(4), 457–471.

Stephenson, K. R., & Kerth, J. (2017). Effects of mindfulness-based therapies for female sexual dysfunction: A meta-analytic review. *Journal of Sex Research, 54*(7), 832–849.

Stewart, J. L., Spivey, L. A., Widman, L., Choukas-Bradley, S., & Prinstein, M. J. (2019). Developmental patterns of sexual identity, romantic attraction, and sexual behavior among adolescents over three years. *Journal of Adolescence, 77*, 90–97.

Stewart, M. (2001). Towards a global definition of patient centred care. *BMJ, 322*(7284), 444–445.

Stout, S. A., Litvak, M., Robbins, N. M., & Sandberg, D. E. (2010). Congenital adrenal hyperplasia: Classification of studies employing psychological endpoints. *International Journal of Pediatric Endocrinology, 2010*, 1–11.

Streuli, J. C., Vayena, E., Cavicchia-Balmer, Y., & Huber, J. (2013). Shaping parents: Impact of contrasting professional counseling on parents' decision making for children with disorders of sex development. *Journal of Sexual Medicine, 10*(8), 1953–1960.

Stroebe, M., & Schut, H. (1999). The dual process model of coping with bereavement: Rationale and description. *Death Studies, 23*(3), 197–224.

Suorsa-Johnson, K. I., Gardner, M. D., Baskin, A., Gruppen, L. D., Rose, A., Rutter, M. M., . . . Sandberg, D. E. (2021). Defining successful outcomes and preferences for clinical management in differences/disorders of sex development: Protocol overview and a qualitative phenomenological study of stakeholders' perspectives. *Journal of Pediatric Urology, 18*(1), 36.e1–36.e17.

Suris, J. C., Michaud, P. A., & Viner, R. (2004). The adolescent with a chronic condition. Part I: Developmental issues. *Archives of Disease in Childhood, 89* (10), 938–942.

Tamar-Mattis, A., Baratz, A., Baratz Dalke, K., & Karkazis, K. (2014). Emotionally and cognitively informed consent for clinical care for differences of sex development. *Psychology & Sexuality, 5*(1), 44–55.

Tanderup, M., Reddy, S., Patel, T., & Nielsen, B. B. (2015). Informed consent in medical decision-making in commercial gestational surrogacy: A mixed methods study in New Delhi, India. *Acta Obstetricia et Gynecologica Scandinavica, 94*(5), 465–472.

Tepper, M. S. (2000). Sexuality and disability: The missing discourse of pleasure. *Sexuality & Disability, 18*(4), 283–290.

Thornton, M., Harcourt, D., Deave, T., Kiff, J., & Williamson, H. (2021). "Have we done enough?" A cross-condition exploration of the experiences of parents caring for a child with an appearance-affecting condition or injury. *Developmental Neurorehabilitation, 24*(6), 418–428.

Throsby, K., & Gill, R. (2004). "It's different for men": Masculinity and IVF. *Men and Masculinities, 6*(1), 330–348.

Tiefer, L. (1995). *Sex is not a natural act & other essays.* Westview Press.

(2012). Medicalizations and demedicalizations of sexuality therapies. *Journal of Sex Research, 49*(4), 311–318.

Timmermans, S., Yang, A., Gardner, M., Keegan, C. E., Yashar, B. M., Fechner, P. Y., . . . Sandberg, D. E. (2018). Does patient-centered care change genital surgery decisions? The strategic use of clinical uncertainty in disorders of sex development clinics. *Journal of Health & Social Behavior, 59*(4), 520–535.

(2019). Gender destinies: Assigning gender in disorders of sex development-intersex clinics. *Sociology of Health & Illness, 41*(8), 1520–1534.

Tishelman, A. C., Shumer, D. E., & Nahata, L. (2017). Disorders of sex development: Pediatric psychology and the genital exam. *Journal of Pediatric Psychology, 42*(5), 530–543.

Tuck, E. (2009). Suspending damage: A letter to communities. *Harvard Educational Review, 79*(3), 409–428.

United Nations. (2015). *Ending violence and discrimination against lesbian, gay, bisexual, transgender and intersex people.* http://www.ohchr.org/Documents/Issues/Discrimination/Joint_LGBTI_Statement_ENG.PDF

Ussher, J., Perz, J., Gilbert, E., Wong, W. K. T., & Hobbs, K. (2013). Renegotiating sex and intimacy after cancer, resisting the coital imperative. *Cancer Nursing, 36*(6), 454–462.

van Anders, S. M. (2013). Beyond masculinity: Testosterone, gender/sex, and human social behavior in a comparative context. *Frontiers in Neuroendocrinology*, *34*(3), 198–210.

van Anders, S. M., Steiger, J., & Goldey, K. L. (2015). Effects of gendered behavior on testosterone in women and men. *PNAS*, *112*(45), 13805–13810.

van de Grift, T. C. (2021). Condition openness is associated with better mental health in individuals with an intersex/differences of sex development condition: Structural equation modeling of European multicenter data. *Psychological Medicine*, 1–12.

van der Straaten, S., Springer, A., Zecic, A., Hebenstreit, D., Tonnhofer, U., Gawlik, A., ... Cools, M. (2020). The External Genitalia Score (EGS): A European multicenter validation study. *Journal of Clinical Endocrinology & Metabolism*, *105*(3), e222–e230.

van der Zwan, Y. G., Callens, N., van Kuppenveld, J., Kwak, K., Drop, S. L., Kortmann, B., ... Dutch Study Group on DSD. (2013). Long-term outcomes in males with disorders of sex development. *Journal of Urology*, *190*(3), 1038–1042.

Van Seters, A. P., & Slob, A. K. (1988). Mutually gratifying heterosexual relationship with micropenis of husband. *Journal of Sex & Marital Therapy*, *14*(2), 98–107.

Vavilov, S., Smith, G., Starkey, M., Pockney, P., & Deshpande, A. V. (2020). Parental decision regret in childhood hypospadias surgery: A systematic review. *Journal of Paediatrics and Child Health*, *56*(10), 1514–1520.

Verschuren, J. E. A., Enzlin, P., Dijkstra, P. U., Geertzen, J. H. B., & Dekker, R. (2010). Chronic disease and sexuality: A generic conceptual framework. *Journal of Sex Research*, *47*(2–3), 153–170.

Verveen, A., Kreukels, B. P. C., de Graaf, N. M., & Steensma, T. D. (2021). Body image in children with gender incongruence. *Clinical Child Psychology & Psychiatry*, *26*(3), 839–854.

Vloeberghs, V., Verheyen, G., Santos-Ribeiro, S., Staessen, C., Verpoest, W., Gies, I., & Tournaye, H. (2018). Is genetic fatherhood within reach for all azoospermic Klinefelter men?. *PLoS One*, *13*(7), e0200300.

Vosoughi, N., Maasoumi, R., Mehrizi, A. A. H., & Ghanbari, Z. (2022). The effect of psychosexual education on promoting sexual function, genital self-image and sexual distress among women with Rokitansky syndrome: A randomized controlled clinical trial. *Journal of Pediatric and Adolescent Gynecology*, *35*(1), 73–81.

Vreeman, R., Gramelspacher, A. M., Gisore, P. O., Scanlon, M. L., & Winstone, M. N. (2013). Disclosure of HIV status to children in resource-limited settings: A systematic review. *Journal of International AIDS Society*, *16*(1), 18466.

Warne, G. (2003). Support groups for CAH and AIS. *Endocrinologist*, *13*, 175–178.

Warne, G. L. (2004). Management of ambiguous genitalia at birth. In A. Balen, S. Creighton, M. Davies, J. MacDougall, & R. Stanhope (Eds.), *Paediatric & adolescent gynaecology: A multi-disciplinary approach* (pp. 97–103). Cambridge University Press.

Watling Neal, J., & Neal, Z. P. (2021). Prevalence and characteristics of childfree adults in Michigan (USA). *PLoS One, 16*(6), e0252528.

Weijenborg, P. T. M., Kluivers, K. B., Dessens, A. B., Kate-Booij, M. J., & Both, S. (2019). Sexual functioning, sexual esteem, genital self-image and psychological and relational functioning in women with Mayer–Rokitansky–Küster–Hauser syndrome: A case-control study. *Human Reproduction, 34* (9), 1661–1673.

Weijenborg, P. T., & ter Kuile, M. M. (2000). The effect of a group programme on women with the Mayer-Rokitansky-Küster-Hauser syndrome. *BJOG: An International Journal of Obstetrics & Gynaecology, 107*(3), 365–368.

Weiner, L., & Avery-Clark, C. (2014). Sensate focus: Clarifying the Masters and Johnson's model. *Sexual & Relationship Therapy, 29*(3), 307–319.

Weistra, S., & Luke, N. (2017). Adoptive parents' experiences of social support and attitudes towards adoption. *Adoption & Fostering, 41*(3), 228–241.

West, M. A., & Lyubovnikova, J. (2013). Illusions of team working in health care. *Journal of Health Organization and Management, 27*(1), 134–142.

Wilkins, L. (1960). Abnormalities of sex differentiation: Classification, diagnosis, selection of gender of rearing and treatment. *Pediatrics, 26*(5), 846–857.

Williams, J. (2020). Tale of a good GP. *British Journal of General Practice, 70* (701), 598–599.

Williams, N. (2002). The imposition of gender: Psychoanalytic encounters with genital atypicality. *Psychoanalytic Psychology, 19*(3), 455–474.

Wilson, C., Christie, D., & Woodhouse, C. R. (2004). The ambitions of adolescents born with exstrophy: A structured survey. *BJU International, 94*(4), 607–612.

Wischmann, T. H. (2003). Psychogenic infertility – myths and facts. *Journal of Assisted Reproduction and Genetics, 20*(12), 485–494.

Wood, D., Baird, A., Luca Carmignani, L., De Win, G., Hoebeke, P., Holmdahl, G., ... Tekgul, S. (2019). Lifelong congenital urology: The challenges for patients and surgeons. *European Urology, 75*(6), 1001–1007.

Wood, D., & Wilcox, D. (2022). Hypospadias – Lessons learned: An overview of incidence, epidemiology, surgery, research, complications and outcomes. *International Journal of Impotence Research,* https://doi.org/10.1038/s41443-022-00563-7.

World Health Organization. (2021). *Gender definitions.* https://www.euro.who.int/en/health-topics/health-determinants/gender/gender-definitions

Zeeck, A., Orlinsky, D. E., Hermann, S., Joos, A., Wirsching, M., Weidmann, W., & Hartmann, A. (2012). Stressful involvement in psychotherapeutic work: Therapist, client and process correlates. *Psychotherapy Research, 22*(5), 543–555.

Index